INTRODUCTION TO HEALTH CARE ECONOMICS & FINANCIAL MANAGEMENT

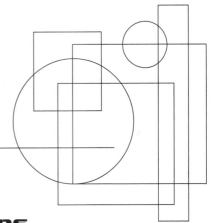

Fundamental Concepts With Practical Applications

Susan J. Penner, RN, MN, MPA, DrPH

PT Faculty
California State University, Hayward
Hayward, CA

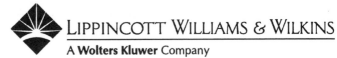

LIPPINCOTT WILLIAMS & WILKINS
A **Wolters Kluwer** Company
Philadelphia • Baltimore • New York • London
Buenos Aires • Hong Kong • Sydney • Tokyo

Acquisitions Editor: Margaret Zuccarini
Managing Editor: Joseph Morita
Editorial Assistant: Carol DeVault
Production Editor: Diane Griffith
Senior Production Manager: Helen Ewan
Managing Editor/Production: Erika Kors
Art Director: Carolyn O'Brien
Design: B.J. Crim
Manufacturing Manager: William Alberti
Indexer: Greystone Indexing
Compositor: TechBooks
Printer: R.R. Donnelly/Crawfordsville

9 8 7 6 5 4 3 2 1

Library of Congress Cataloging-in-Publication Data

Penner, Susan J.
    Introduction to health care economics and financial management : fundamental concepts
with practical applications / Susan J. Penner.
        p. cm.
    Includes bibliographical references and index.
    ISBN 0-7817-4019-3 (alk. paper)
    1. Nursing—Economic aspects.   2. Medical economics.   I. Title.

RT86.7.P46 2003
338.4′33621′088613—dc21

                                                                        2003055247

LWW.com

Reviewers

Marsha L. Conroy, RN, MSN
Faculty, Practical Nursing & Associate Nursing
  Programs
Cuyahoga Community College
Highland Hills, OH

Mary S. Tilbury, EdD, RN
Assistant Professor
University of Maryland School of
  Nursing
Baltimore, MD

Suzette Cardin, RN, DNSc, FAAN
Adjunct Assistant Professor
UCLA School of Nursing
Los Angeles, CA

Thomas R. Clancy, BSN, MA, MBA
Vice President, Nursing
Mercy Hospital
Iowa City, IA

Nashat Zuraikat, PhD, RN
Professor and Graduate Coordinator
Indiana University of Pennsylvania
Indiana, PA

Diane L. Huber, PhD, RN, FAAN, CNAA
Associate Professor
University of Iowa, College of Nursing
Iowa City, IA

Jean Ann Seago, PhD, RN
Assistant Professor
University of California San Francisco
San Francisco, CA

Mary S. Tilbury, EdD, RN, CNAA, BC
Assistant Professor
University of Maryland
Baltimore, MD

Judith Lloyd Storfjell, PhD, RN
Associate Professor
University of Illinois at Chicago
Chicago, IL

Arlene Lowenstein, PhD, RN
Professor and Director, Graduate Program in
  Nursing
MGH Institute of Health Professions
Boston, MA

Debra C. Hampton, RN, MSN, PhD
Director of Nursing, Part-Time Faculty
University of Kentucky, College of Nursing
Lexington, KY

Claudette Spalding, MSN, ARNP, CNAA
Assistant Professor, Director, Nursing
  Administration Specialty
Barry University
Miami Shores, FL

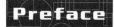

Preface

Health professionals face the effects of economics, finance, and budgeting every day, whether as budget cutbacks, cost control efforts, or complicated insurance guidelines. In any type of health care setting—inpatient or outpatient, private practice or nationwide health care system—monetary concerns influence day-to-day performance and long-term survival. It is more important than ever for health professionals to obtain at least an introductory understanding of the fundamentals of health care economics, finance, and budgeting in order to obtain, justify, and manage resources needed to provide health care.

Unfortunately, many health professionals lack any formal preparation in the basics of economics and financial management. For example, in a study of 86 American staff nurses, Caroselli (1996) found that only 26 of these nurses had obtained any general knowledge of budgeting or finance. Of the 26 nurses, only 4 reported they obtained this knowledge from a nursing instructor, and the largest number, 11, reported they were self-taught. Further, the economic awareness of these 86 staff nurses was not shown to increase based on factors such as age, work experience, education, or even management experience.

Although there is little study of the knowledge of health professionals regarding economics and financial management, informal observations indicate that this paucity of information is similar across health care disciplines. As a result, few health professionals know how to review, monitor, and control a budget, or to develop a business plan or program grant proposal that would fund important health care services, nor are they capable of conducting financial analyses to effectively evaluate programs and services.

When teaching courses in health care economics, finance, and budgeting for undergraduate (RN to BSN) and master's level nurses, I am frustrated by problems with textbooks and course materials. Although texts are available in both the field of health care economics and the field of finance, I cannot find a current text that combines introductory concepts from both fields, and includes basic information on reviewing, monitoring, and preparing budgets. Moreover, I wanted a textbook that helps students develop practical applications of the skills they learn in the course by writing a business plan or program grant proposal. *Health Care Economics, Financial Management and Budgeting: Fundamental Concepts With Practical Applications* is intended to meet these needs.

Contents

This text is designed to first give an overview of health economics, then build and develop budgeting and financial analysis skills, culminating in the ability to combine budgeting and financial analysis in writing a business plan or grant proposal. Part One of the text therefore introduces health economics and managed care systems. Chapter 1 discusses fundamental principles of health care economics including relationships between supply, demand, and price. Fundamental concepts relevant to health insurance and managed care are presented in Chapter 2, with instruction in Chapter 3 on financial reporting in managed care settings.

Part Two of this text focuses on budgets, budget monitoring, and budget preparation, with additional information on cost allocation and cost-finding. Chapter 4 presents an introductory overview of the types of budgets reviewed in health care settings. Budget monitoring and control is the focus of Chapter 5, emphasizing concepts of budget variance. Chapter 6 discusses budget preparation, including methods to forecast or otherwise estimate budgets for future time periods. Chapter 7 provides an overview of cost allocation and cost-finding.

Part Three presents break-even analysis, cost-benefit analysis, and cost-effectiveness analysis as tools used in basic financial analysis. Chapter 8 presents break-even analysis, including concepts of cost. Cost-benefit analysis and cost-effectiveness analysis are presented in Chapter 9, with concepts about valuing human life and program evaluation.

Part Four presents the review and use of financial reports. Chapter 10 presents a basic introduction to financial reporting, including the review of an income statement, balance sheet, and statement of cash flows. Additional techniques for financial analysis, such as ratio analysis, are provided in Chapter 11.

Part Five shows how to apply skills in budgeting and financial analysis to the preparation of business plans and grant proposals. Chapter 12 covers information needed in writing a business plan. Guidelines for writing a grant proposal are in Chapter 13.

Part Six is the last part of the text, covering international perspectives and future trends. Chapter 14 discusses issues of health care economics and financing among other countries in the world, and compares their health care systems to those of the United States. Future trends in health care economics, financial analysis, and budgeting are discussed in Chapter 15 with suggestions on how to keep up-to-date.

Textbook Features

The textbook uses practical case examples drawn from actual health care settings throughout each chapter to illustrate the application of content. This technique assists students in developing "hands-on" approaches to working with financial data and financial concerns. Health care professionals will learn theory and develop fundamental skills in using tools to help them understand the economic and financial forces driving today's health care system, and to prepare budgets, business plans, and health program grant proposals with practical application in their work settings.

Each chapter begins with a set of key learning objectives and a summary of terms introduced in the chapter and defined in the glossary at the end of the book. Tables, figures, and text boxes help illustrate and summarize the concepts covered throughout the chapter. Exercises at the end of each chapter help students apply and review skills they have learned, and may be adapted or tailored by faculty to meet their unique needs and the learning objectives for their courses. For example, all exercise sets could be adapted for nurses and nursing courses in economics, finance, and budgeting. Chapter appendices include sample reports or financial data to provide actual examples to use as guides for application. Most of the chapters include a text box featuring current Internet resources for further review and exploration of concepts, and all chapters include references.

An important feature of this book is its focus on experiential learning. Rather than emphasizing memorization and completion of multiple choice questions with answer sets, students are encouraged to examine or develop real-life examples and apply skills discussed in each chapter. The use of exercises and the development of a business plan or health program grant proposal are not so much focused on "the right answer" as on critical thinking and building skills in budgeting and financial analysis. Suggestions for enhancing experiential learning are provided in the following sections directed to faculty and students using this book.

This text lends itself to distance learning or to courses enhanced by the use of on-line software. The CD-ROM contains sample financial reports and data tables available to each student for practice and for source material in completing exercises. The emphasis on interdisciplinary skill building, the adaptability of exercises and projects (such as a business plan or program grant proposal) to either group or individual work, and the focus on experiential learning enhance the independent learning context in which distance education takes place.

Suggestions for Faculty

One suggestion for faculty using this textbook is to adapt the book and its features to meet the needs of their programs, courses, and levels of students. This text is designed for master's level students in clinical programs, although it also could be assigned to students in undergraduate clinical programs, or in an introductory course for health administration students.

Although the number of chapters approximate the number of weeks in an academic semester, it may be more meaningful to selectively emphasize some chapters more than others rather than assigning one chapter each week, particularly for undergraduate courses. Topics such as cost allocation, financial reports, financial ratios, and discounting may be considered too advanced, depending on course objectives and the student's academic level. Some faculty may want to selectively expand on topics, such as a more extensive discussion of discounting.

Because the target audience is considered to have no prior instruction in economics, finance, or budgeting, discussions of some topics, such as capital budgeting and discounting, are limited. It is expected that health professionals making decisions for high budget long-term expenditures, such as construction, major renovation, or major purchases, would obtain further education or experience (or both) beyond the scope of this text and the courses using this text. As a result, most examples used in this text are at the level of an annual operating budget for a program or department. Students are expected to build on skills developed from reading this text to eventually work with financial officers on more complex and long-term analyses, should their job so require.

This text takes a multidisciplinary perspective. It is assumed that regardless of discipline, health professionals responsible for financial management must work with other health professionals from a variety of departments and disciplines, including financial officers. In many cases, it is assumed that finance departments produce the budgets, financial reports, and financial analyses for review and monitoring by the health professionals involved (such as department directors). As a result, the text describes the components of documents, such as a step-down distribution cost allocation report or an income statement, assuming that students will be reviewing, interpreting, and monitoring such reports over the course of their careers, but not preparing these reports.

Again and again, students (and faculty) are also reminded that terminology, approaches, and reporting differ from one health care setting to another and may differ from the examples discussed in this text. The text provides a foundation, not an absolute set of rules.

The exercises at the end of each chapter may be adapted as in-class (or on-line) group work or as take-home work to be turned in to the instructor for evaluation. Most of the exercises allow students from various health care disciplines to develop examples relevant to their disciplines and work settings. Generic students who do not yet have a work setting to draw from may develop examples that are of interest or use budget and other financial information available in the text to work their exercises. Exercises may also be used to develop critical-thinking and examination questions for student evaluation.

Another suggestion for faculty is to collect health care budgets, financial reports, and financial analyses for students to review and use in working on group exercises and developing critical thinking skills. The institutional sources of these documents can be concealed for confidentiality. Students, working in settings where they have permission to do so, should be encouraged to obtain, review, and, if possible, exchange copies of financial documents, concealing the source as appropriate. Students will learn that approaches to financial reporting vary and will gain practice interpreting these approaches and reviewing concepts presented in the text.

A final suggestion is for faculty to use Chapter 12 or Chapter 13 as the basis for a "capstone" project for students taking the course for which this text is assigned. These chapters show how the student's skills in budgeting and financial analysis may be applied in work settings by developing a business plan or health program grant proposal. In programs and courses that focus on student writing, the business plan or grant proposal serves a dual purpose of written work that demonstrates acquisition of financial skills. The business plan or grant proposal also may be adapted for group work as well as distance learning.

Suggestions for Students and Practitioners

One suggestion is for students and practitioners to look over the basic math review on our Connection site at connection.lww.com/go/penner if there are any concerns about the math skills needed to understand the tables or calculations used in this text. If students are concerned about obtaining resources for projects, such as a business plan or grant proposal, the site also includes suggestions for obtaining financial data.

Another suggestion for students is to use examples within the chapters and end-of-chapter exercises to review the concepts presented. It is assumed that health care economics, finance, and budgeting are new to the reader, even if they have years of health care experience. Just as it takes practice to build clinical skills, it takes practice to develop skills in financial review, analysis, and reporting.

As opportunity allows, students are encouraged to review budgets and other financial reports for health care settings whenever possible. Of course, it is essential to remember that these documents are frequently considered confidential and proprietary. They should only be obtained with permission, and the source identity concealed if policy so requires. However, if available, these documents provide valuable hands-on learning experience.

A final word to the student is to remember that you are the future of health care and health care economics, finance, and budgeting. There are tremendous challenges facing health professionals and the institutions in which they work to provide access to high quality care at a reasonable cost. The skills you learn from this textbook and related assignments will provide capabilities and insights throughout your career to help meet these challenges.

References

Caroselli, Cynthia. (Sept–Oct 1996). Economic awareness of nurses: relationship to budgetary control. *Nursing Economics* 14(5):292–297.

Acknowledgments

I would like to thank the people who contributed to this book by reviewing and providing input to the content of chapters, by sharing budget and financial reports, and by helping in many other ways. Their assistance was invaluable and greatly appreciated. Thanks to Rebecca Allen-Bouska, Ellyn V. Bloomfield, Annie Buerhaus, Lori Cooper, Steven Crane, E. Sue Denger, Glenn W. Fisher, Mary Frazier, Shyrl Hayman, Ellen Hayward, Nanette Kamran, Joe Kinsella, Patricia G. Komlenic, Evelyn Lopez, Peter Nanopolous, Glen Price, Judy Quittman, Andrea Rataczak, Margaret Schultz, Marty Shawver, Cliff Skinner, and Silas Ting.

I want to thank Joe Morita and Margaret Zuccarini at Lippincott Williams & Wilkins for their encouragement and advice as I embarked on the adventure of developing a new textbook. I would also like to thank Karen Holroyd for getting all this started.

This book would not have been possible without the help of Maury Penner, who supported my efforts throughout.

Contents

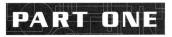

PART ONE

Introduction to Health Economics and Managed Care

CHAPTER 1

Fundamental Principles of Health Care Economics

Learning Objectives

1. Explain why health care is an important segment of the U.S. economy.
2. Define demand and identify two examples of demand shifters.
3. Differentiate between the disequilibrium states of surplus and shortage.
4. Identify two factors influencing the health care labor market for your profession.

Key Terms

Allocative efficiency
Average cost
Capital
Ceteris paribus
Complement
Costs
Demand
Demand curve
Derived demand
Disequilibrium
Dynamic labor shortage
Economy of scale
Economy of scope
Efficiency
Elasticity
Equilibrium

Externality
Factor substitute
Free rider problem
Gross domestic product (GDP)
Gross national product (GNP)
Inferior good
Information problem
Input
Law of diminishing marginal utility
Marginal cost
Marginal product
Marginal utility
Market
Market failure
Monopoly
Monopoly rent

...continued

Key Terms (continued)

Monopsony	Productivity
Natural monopoly	Profit
Normal good	Public good
Opportunity cost	Shifter
Output	Shortage
Pareto efficiency	Supply
Pareto improvement	Supply curve
Perfect competition	Surplus
Perfect information	Technical efficiency
Political monopoly	Total cost
Private good	Trade-off
Production efficiency	Utility
Production function	Wage stickiness
Production possibilities curve	Welfare loss

"If we raised RNs' salaries, we'd be able to solve the nursing shortage." "We can't do anything about rising health care costs—health care isn't like other businesses." "To save money, we should replace most of our physical therapists with physical therapy aides." "If we reduce costs for hospital services, we'll lower the quality of care."

One overhears these and many other statements about issues and solutions related to health care economics. This chapter focuses on providing a better awareness of the dynamics of the economics of health care—how factors such as supply, demand, and price not only affect health care goods and services (products) but how these factors interact with each other. In many cases, the answers to health care dilemmas such as lack of access to health care, labor shortages or surpluses, and rising costs are far from simple. An introduction to the fundamentals of health economics helps one to understand why health care issues and solutions are complex and often difficult to address. The final section discusses the extent to which health care does or does not differ from other industries.

The extent to which health care differs from other industries may be debated. However, there are some differences in the expectations of consumers and producers between health care services and many other industries that do not provide health care. When consumers purchase a non-health good or service, the typical expectation is that quality, cost, and availability (or speedy delivery) are exchangeable. In other words, if a product is of high quality and promptly delivered (or readily available), it is likely to cost more than a product of lower quality that is delivered less quickly. The same expectations and relationships apply to the typical supplier or producer. Units of goods or services may be produced quickly and at lower cost, but are not expected to be of as high quality as products produced that require more time and higher cost. The consumer or producer of many non-health care products thus focuses preferences on any two of the three expectations of cost, quality, and availability. The third expectation is given up at the expense of the other two, because all three expectations cannot be satisfied simultaneously.

Figure 1-1 illustrates fundamental expectations and relationships applicable to health care production and consumption. The health care expectation of "access" corresponds to the business expectation of "speed." The difference, according to this text's author, between health care expectations and business expectations is that clients, providers, and payers of health care goods and services are typically unwilling or far less willing to accept the sacrifice of cost, quality, or access accepted in many other business transactions. In other words, whether patients, health care professionals providing care, health care organizations, or makers of health care policy, we "want it all." People expect to receive and provide ready access to high-quality health care while controlling costs.

U.S. Health Care Economy

Health care is an important part of the overall economy in the United States and is increasing in importance. Table 1-1 shows total and per capita U.S. national health expenditures, population, and health expenditures as a percent of **gross domestic product (GDP)**. GDP (the value of all the goods and services a nation produces within its borders within a year) is used to measure change in a given country's economy over time, as well as to compare one country's economic status to another. Box 1-1 explains the difference between GDP and a previous measure of a nation's economy, **gross national product (GNP)**.

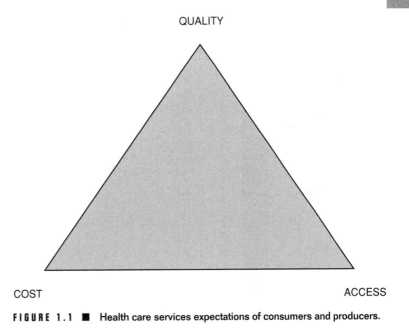

QUALITY

COST   ACCESS

FIGURE 1.1 ■ Health care services expectations of consumers and producers.

Table 1-1 shows the steady increases in health care costs (and projected costs) since 1980. National health expenditures increased from $245.8 billion in 1980 to $1,299.5 billion in 2000 (4.3 times) and are projected to increase to $2,815.8 billion by 2011 (10.5 times). National health expenditures as a percent of GDP increased from 8.8% in 1980 to 13.2% in 2000 (50%) and are projected to increase to 17% by 2011 (93.2%). Health care expenditures per capita increased from $1,067 in 1980 to $4,637 in 2000 (3.3 times) and are projected to increase to $9,216 by 2011 (7.6 times). Over the same time period, the U.S. population increased from 230.4 million in 1980 to 280.2 million in 2000 (21.6%) and is projected to increase to 305.5 million by 2011 (32.6%).

☐ B O X   1 · 1

GDP or GNP?

For many years, economists reported the **gross national product (GNP)** as the total value of all goods and services produced by a country over a year. This estimate enabled economists to compare a given country's economic performance over time, or to compare one country's economic performance to that of another.

In the 1990s, the measure changed from the GNP to the **gross domestic product (GDP).** The GNP counts the earnings in the home country of the owner of an asset, while the GDP counts the earnings in the country in which the assets are located. The actual amount of difference between the GNP and the GDP is negligible in the U.S. economy.

○ TABLE 1-1

National Health Expenditures and Selected Economic Indicators for Selected Calendar Years, 1980–2011[1]

Item	1980	1990	1999	2000	2001	2002	2003	2004	2005	2010	2011
National health expenditures (billions)	$245.8	$696.0	$1,215.6	$1,299.5	$1,423.8	$1,545.9	$1,653.4	$1,773.4	$1,902.2	$2,639.2	$2,815.8
National health expenditures as a percent of gross domestic product	8.8%	12.0%	13.1%	13.2%	14.0%	14.7%	15.0%	15.3%	15.6%	16.8%	17.0%
National health expenditures per capita	$1,067	$2,738	$4,377	$4,637	$5,039	$5,427	$5,757	$6,126	$6,519	$8,704	$9,216
U.S. population[2] (millions)	230.4	254.2	277.7	280.2	282.5	284.9	287.2	289.5	291.8	303.2	305.5

SOURCE: Centers for Medicare & Medicaid Services, Office of the Actuary. Retrieved June 15, 2002. http://www.hcfa.gov/stats/nhe%2Dproj/proj2001/tables/t1.htm

[1] The health spending projections were based on the 2000 version of the National Health Expenditures released in January 2002.

[2] July 1 Census resident based population estimates.

NOTE: Numbers and percents may not add to totals because of rounding.

Table 1-2 presents a more detailed report of the types of national health expenditures estimated or projected from 1980 to 2011. For example, expenditures for hospital care increased from $101.5 billion in 1980 to $412.1 billion in 2000 (3.1 times) and are projected to increase to $774.5 billion by 2011 (6.6 times). Prescription medications increased from $12 billion in 1980 to $121.8 billion in 2000 (9.2 times) and are projected to increase even more rapidly, to $413.9 billion by 2011 (33.5 times).

Table 1-3 shows total and per capita health care expenditures by the source of payment. For example, total out-of-pocket payments increased from $58.2 billion in 1980 to $194.5 billion in 2000 (2.3 times) and are projected to increase to $395.6 billion by 2011 (5.8 times). Per capita out-of-pocket payments increased from $253 in 1980 to $694 in 2000 (1.7 times) and are projected to increase to $1,295 by 2011 (4.1 times). Per capita expenditures for third-party payments for private health insurance increased from $263 in 1980 to $1,394 in 2000 (4.3 times) and are projected to increase to $2,763 by 2011 (9.5 times). Medicare expenditures increased from $36.3 billion in 1980 to $217 billion in 2000 (5 times) and are projected to increase to $437.3 billion by 2011 (11 times).

In summary, U.S. health costs are substantial and rising. Chapter 14 presents and compares health costs and trends in other countries, and Chapter 15 offers further discussion about future trends in health care costs in the United States. The following sections discuss some principles that affect health care expenditures and changes in health care expenditures.

Markets

Economists define a **market** as a mechanism that facilitates the efficient allocation of resources. One assumption about markets is that resources are limited at best and often are relatively scarce. The assumption of resource scarcity further implies that the various parties involved in the market (suppliers, sellers, consumers, payers) must make choices, such as what products to produce, how these products are best produced and supplied, and who receives these products. Recall that the expectations of consumers, providers, and payers in health care are to achieve high quality and ready access while controlling costs. However, choices about resource allocation in health care often make it difficult to reach these expectations.

An important concept throughout this chapter is *ceteris paribus,* a Latin term frequently used in presenting economic examples that means "all else remaining constant." For example, if a table or graph illustrates the effects of a change in price, the assumption is that none of the other variables in the example undergo changes except as influenced by the change in price. Of course, in actual health care settings several variables, such as the quantity supplied, the quantity demanded, and price, may be changing simultaneously. However, for simplicity and understanding, the assumption of *ceteris paribus* holds unless otherwise specified.

Efficiencies

Efficiency (maximizing the production of goods or services while minimizing the resources required for production) is an important concept in examining the health care market. Four types of efficiency may be attained. **Technical efficiency** represents the production of the maximum amount of **outputs** (goods or services that are produced) given the minimum amount of **inputs** (resources used to produce goods or services), or maximizing outputs for a given set of inputs.

For example, inpatient hospital care to receive intravenous cancer medications requires a fairly intensive combination of inputs such as nursing services, dietary and housekeeping services, medical supplies such as bed linens and medications, equipment, and a patient room. If patients can instead receive the same intravenous medications in an outpatient clinic, the intensity of inputs is reduced and of a shorter duration. Many of the inputs, such as 24-hour nursing supervision, dietary services, some medical supplies, and a patient room, are not required or are needed at a substantially reduced level. Technical efficiency is achieved

TABLE 1-2

National Health Expenditure Amounts for Selected Calendar Years, 1980–2011[1] (amounts in billions)

Type of expenditure	1980	1990	1999	2000	2001	2002	2003	2004	2005	2010	2011
National health expenditures	$245.8	$696.0	$1,215.6	$1,299.5	$1,423.8	$1,545.9	$1,653.4	$1,773.4	$1,902.2	$2,639.2	$2,815.8
Health services and supplies	233.5	669.6	1,175.0	1,255.5	1,377.3	1,497.0	1,601.3	1,717.8	1,842.9	2,556.9	2,727.8
Personal health care	214.6	609.4	1,062.6	1,130.4	1,235.2	1,332.4	1,425.0	1,530.8	1,642.3	2,267.2	2,416.7
Hospital care	101.5	253.9	392.2	412.1	446.3	476.1	501.6	532.4	565.2	737.3	774.5
Professional services	67.3	216.9	397.0	422.1	459.2	495.8	533.3	573.7	615.8	848.7	906.2
Physician and clinical services	47.1	157.5	270.2	286.4	310.6	336.0	361.2	387.8	415.4	559.4	593.3
Other professional services	3.6	18.2	36.7	39.0	42.7	46.6	50.4	54.4	58.5	78.2	82.6
Dental services	13.3	31.5	56.4	60.0	64.4	68.1	71.8	76.0	79.9	99.9	104.6
Other personal health care	3.3	9.6	33.7	36.7	41.5	45.0	49.9	55.5	62	111.2	125.8
Nursing home and home health	20.1	65.3	121.6	124.7	135.1	143.7	149.9	158.8	168.4	224.0	237.2
Home health care	2.4	12.6	32.3	32.4	35.9	39.9	42.8	45.9	48.9	66.6	70.8
Nursing home care	17.7	52.7	89.3	92.2	99.2	103.8	107.1	112.9	119.5	157.4	166.4
Retail outlet sales of medical products	25.7	73.3	151.8	171.5	194.5	216.8	240.2	265.9	292.9	457.2	498.7
Prescription drugs	12.0	40.3	103.9	121.8	141.8	160.9	181.5	203.8	227.8	376.0	413.9
Other medical products	13.7	33.1	48.0	49.7	52.7	55.9	58.7	62.1	65.2	81.2	84.9
Durable medical equipment	3.9	10.6	17.6	18.5	19.9	21.1	22.2	23.5	24.8	32.1	33.9

Other non-durable medical products	9.8	22.5	30.4	31.2	32.8	34.8	36.5	38.5	40.4	49.1	51.0
Government administration and net cost of private health insurance	12.1	40.0	71.5	80.9	92.7	107.2	112.2	116.4	123.2	170.8	182.2
Government public health activities	6.7	20.2	40.9	44.2	49.5	57.4	64.1	70.6	77.4	118.9	128.9
Investment	12.3	26.4	40.5	43.9	46.4	48.9	52.1	55.6	59.3	82.4	88.0
Research[2]	5.5	12.7	23.1	25.3	26.6	27.9	29.8	31.9	34.1	47.8	51.2
Construction	6.8	13.7	17.5	18.6	19.8	21.0	22.3	23.7	25.1	34.6	36.8

SOURCE: Centers for Medicare & Medicaid Services, Office of the Actuary. Retrieved June 15, 2002. http://www.hcfa.gov/stats/nhe%2Dproj/proj2001/tables/t2.htm

[1] The health spending projections were based on the 2000 version of the National Health Expenditure (NHE) released in January 2002.

[2] Research and development expenditures of drug companies and other manufacturers and providers of medical equipment and supplies are excluded from research expenditures. These research expenditures are implicitly included in the expenditure class in which the product falls, in that they are covered by the payment received for that product.

NOTE: Numbers may not add to totals because of rounding.

◯ TABLE 1-3

Personal Health Care Expenditures Aggregate and Per Capita Amounts for Selected Calender Years, 1980-2011[1]

Year	Total	Out-of-Pocket Payments	Third-Party-Payments							
			Total	Private Health Insurance	Other Private Funds	Public			Medicare[3]	Medicaid[4]
						Total	Federal[2]	State and Local[2]		
Historical Estimates	Amount in Billions									
1980	$214.6	$58.2	$156.4	$60.6	$9.2	$86.6	$62.8	$23.8	$36.3	$24.7
1990	609.4	137.3	472.1	203.6	30.6	237.9	174.2	63.7	107.3	69.7
1995	865.7	146.5	719.2	289.1	44.3	385.8	295.0	90.8	178.2	135.3
1998	1,009.9	174.5	835.4	342.7	54.7	438.0	334.2	103.8	203.4	160.1
1999	1,062.6	184.4	878.2	363.9	56.3	458.0	346.8	111.3	205.3	174.1
2000	1,130.4	194.5	935.9	390.7	56.1	489.0	370.4	118.6	217.0	188.5
Projected										
2001	1,235.2	210.4	1,024.7	423.9	59.7	541.1	409.0	132.1	238.2	210.3
2002	1,332.4	226.9	1,105.5	462.4	64.5	578.6	436.1	142.5	251.4	229.5
2003	1,425.0	242.7	1,182.3	502.2	68.8	611.3	459.1	152.2	261.4	247.5
2004	1,530.8	259.2	1,271.6	544.6	73.4	653.7	490.1	163.5	277.7	269.0
2005	1,642.3	276.2	1,366.1	587.5	77.9	700.7	524.8	175.8	296.0	292.7
2010	2,267.2	372.4	1,894.8	797.4	99.8	997.6	741.9	255.7	407.8	446.2
2011	2,416.7	395.6	2,021.1	844.1	103.6	1,073.4	797.6	275.8	437.3	485.3

Historical Estimates	Per Capita Amount									
1980	$931	$253	$679	$263	$40	$376	$272	$103	n/a	n/a
1990	2,398	540	615	801	120	936	685	251	n/a	n/a
1999	3,826	664	3,162	1,310	203	1,649	1,249	401	n/a	n/a
2000	4,034	694	3,340	1,394	200	1,745	1,322	423	n/a	n/a
Projected										
2001	4,372	745	3,627	1,500	211	1,915	1,448	467	n/a	n/a
2002	4,677	797	3,881	1,623	226	2,031	1,531	500	n/a	n/a
2003	4,962	845	4,117	1,749	240	2,129	1,599	530	n/a	n/a
2004	5,288	895	4,393	1,881	254	2,258	1,693	565	n/a	n/a
2005	5,628	947	4,682	2,013	267	2,401	1,799	603	n/a	n/a
2010	7,477	1,228	6,249	2,630	329	3,290	2,447	843	n/a	n/a
2011	7,910	1,295	6,615	2,763	339	3,513	2,611	903	n/a	n/a

SOURCE: Centers for Medicare & Medicaid Services, Office of the Actuary. Retrieved June 15, 2002. http://www.hcfa.gov/stats/nhe%2Dproj/proj2001/tables/t5.htm

[1] The health spending projections were based on the 2000 version of the National Health Expenditures (NHE) released in January 2002.

[2] Includes Medicaid SCHIP Expansion and SCHIP.

[3] Subset of federal funds.

[4] Subset of federal and state and local funds. Includes Medicaid SCHIP expansion.

NOTES: Per capita amounts based on July 1 Census resident based population estimates. Numbers and percents may not add to totals because of rounding.

because the same or greater level of outputs is possible with fewer inputs—the same number of patients can be served with fewer inputs, or more patients are served with the same amount of inputs.

Production efficiency represents minimizing the costs of producing outputs, or maximizing the production of outputs at a given cost. Instead of focusing on the inputs, or the actual resources required to produce outputs, the focus is on the costs of those inputs. For example, if the outpatient clinic manager can negotiate a substantial discount on the cost of intravenous medication needles, tubing, and related supplies, the clinic can manage the same number of patients receiving intravenous cancer medications at less cost, or more patients at the same cost, thus achieving production efficiency.

Allocative efficiency represents minimizing the amount or cost of inputs while maximizing the value or benefit of outputs, or producing outputs of maximum value or benefit for a given amount or cost of inputs. For example, the outpatient clinic might offer videotapes educating the patient about the cancer medications and other health topics while in the waiting room or while receiving the intravenous medications. Follow-up assessments might be scheduled in coordination with medication administration. These inputs might be small or relatively low cost but add substantially to the value of the outpatient visit, thus achieving allocative efficiency.

Pareto efficiency (named after an early Italian economist) represents a condition in which the amount or value of outputs cannot be increased for one party without increasing inputs or costs (or decreasing the amount or value of outputs) for another party. In other words, unlike technical, production, and allocative efficiency, it is not possible to make one or more parties better off without making another party (or parties) worse off. Pareto efficiency is a type of **trade-off,** or situation in which to increase or acquire a benefit or value, one must give up all or part of another benefit or value. By contrast, a **Pareto improvement** is a condition in which a more efficient use of inputs improves the amount or value of outputs for one or more parties without making another party (or parties) worse off.

For example, the outpatient clinic has a finite capacity for patient services, whether for cancer patients or other patients. Once technical, production, and allocative efficiencies are realized, services for outpatients receiving intravenous cancer medications cannot be increased without reducing resources or benefits for other outpatients. If the outpatient clinic manager decides to increase services for the cancer medication outpatients, services for the clinic's other outpatients must be reduced as a trade-off once the clinic has achieved full efficiency. Problems involving trade-offs are often seen at the state or federal level when funding decisions are made focusing on age groups in need (such as the Medicare program); programs for the poor (such as the Medicaid program); or serious, costly, and growing disorders, such as HIV infection.

A concept related to trade-offs is **opportunity cost,** or the economic value of an alternative benefit that could result during the same time period or with the same amount of resources as invested in the current activity. For example, the outpatient clinic manager estimates that the inputs (staff time, equipment, supplies, and other resources) required for a cancer outpatient's services are approximately twice that of other outpatients. Assuming that the clinic is fully efficient, the clinic therefore serves one cancer patient at the opportunity cost of two other outpatients who cannot be served. Conversely, the opportunity cost of serving two other outpatients is one cancer outpatient who cannot be served, assuming the clinic operates at full efficiency.

Table 1-4 illustrates the relationships between the production of other outpatient clinic services, services for cancer patients, and the corresponding opportunity costs. The numbers represent the number of patients served. For example, at maximum production entirely focused on services other than cancer treatment, the outpatient clinic can manage 75,000 patients a year. However, when inputs are allocated so that 5,000 cancer patients are served, only 65,000 other clinic patients may be served, assuming that the overall amount of inputs remains the same, as the care for one cancer patient requires the same inputs as for two other outpatients. As the number of cancer patients increases, the capacity to serve other outpatients decreases accordingly. By estimating the relative requirements for inputs for various types of production and tabulating their relationships, it is possible to identify a mix of goods or services that is optimal.

Production Possibilities Curve

The **production possibilities curve (PPC)** is a graphic illustration of the trade-offs between two categories of goods or services, within a specified set of constraints. Figure 1-2 shows the outpatient clinic example graphed as a PPC. The points OC_1, OC_2, and OC_3 represent various possible levels of inputs for other clinic services, with OC_1 the lowest and OC_3 the highest of the three points. The points CA_1, CA_2, and CA_3 represent various levels of inputs for cancer outpatient services, with CA_3 the lowest and CA_1 the highest of the three points. The points along the PPC at which the lines for other clinic services and cancer outpatient services intersect indicate two of many possible combinations of services. Note that the mix of other clinic and cancer outpatient services is efficient (making full use of the resources available) at any point along the PPC.

TABLE 1-4

Relationship of Production (Volume) of Other Clinic Services, Cancer Services and Opportunity Costs (amounts represent patients)[1]

Other Clinic Services	Cancer Services	Opportunity Cost[2]
75,000	0	—
65,000	5,000	10,000
55,000	10,000	20,000
45,000	15,000	30,000
35,000	20,000	40,000
25,000	25,000	50,000
15,000	30,000	60,000
5,000	35,000	70,000
0	37,500	75,000

[1] Figures represent volume (number of patients).
[2] One cancer patient requires same inputs as two other clinic patients.

The location of the points on the curve shown in Figure 1-2 are examples of the mix of inputs made by the other clinic and cancer services. For example, the intersection of OC_1 and CA_1 shows efficient production, with a higher production (volume of patients) and use of inputs by cancer outpatients compared to other outpatient services. The intersection of OC_3 and CA_3 also shows efficient production, but with a higher production and use of inputs by other outpatient clinic services compared to cancer outpatient services.

The intersection of OC_2 and CA_2 shows an example of inefficient production, or production below the clinic's actual capacity given the amount of inputs available (see Fig. 1-2). Points of inefficient production fall inside the PPC—the further the point from the PPC, the less efficient the mix of services. The arrow connecting the intersection of OC_2 and CA_2 with the PPC represents a Pareto improvement, as both other and cancer outpatient services could be increased to extend the intersection to

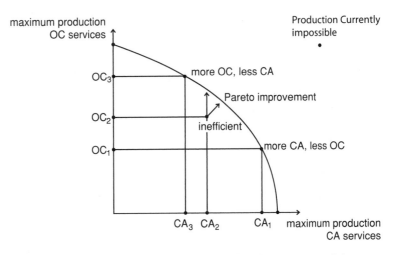

FIGURE 1.2 ■ Production possibilities curve for other outpatient clinic services (OC) vs. cancer outpatient services (CA).

the curve without requiring trade-offs of either service. The other arrow moving from the point of intersection of OC_2 and CA_2 also represents a Pareto improvement. Even though the point indicated by this arrow does not touch the PPC (and thus is not fully efficient), it is closer to the PPC, and thus more efficient than the intersection of OC_2 and CA_2.

The point outside and beyond the PPC shown in Figure 1-3 represents a mix of services that is currently impossible for the outpatient clinic. If inputs are sufficiently increased and allocated, or if productivity increases, this higher level of production that is currently beyond the level of maximum efficiency may be realized. Any point located beyond the PPC is currently impossible because of resource constraints.

Demand

In economic markets, persons or parties (consumers) are willing and able to purchase goods or services. **Demand** refers to the quantity (Q) of a good or service for which a consumer is able and willing to pay, typically over a specific time period. In most markets, if the price (P) of a good or service increases, the quantity demanded will fall. Conversely, if the price of a good or service decreases, the quantity demanded will rise. This principle is illustrated by the graphic illustration of the **demand curve** as shown in Figure 1-3, which shows the quantities demanded in a specific market over a specific time period for each possible price.

Movement along the demand curve is illustrated by the points P_1Q_1, in which the quantity demanded is comparatively low given the comparatively high price, and P_2Q_2, in which the quantity demanded increases as the price decreases. For example, many consumers purchase eyeglasses. Figure 1-3 shows that at the higher price, P_1, consumers demand fewer pairs of glasses than at a lower price, P_2 (as shown by Q_1, which is lower than Q_2).

Demand Shifters

The two lines on either side of the original demand curve in Figure 1-3 show changes in the quantity demanded brought about by **shifters,** or factors other than price that influence the quantity demanded for a good or service. Many factors influence or shift the quantity demanded, causing it to increase or decrease over time for various goods and services. One powerful influence on the quantity of a product demanded by consumers is income—an increase in income increases the quantity demanded, and a decrease in income decreases the quantity demanded for most products. If a consumer's income increases, he or she is more likely to purchase new glasses than during a time of income reduction.

Chapter 2 points out that the effect of insurance is similar to the income effect, increasing the quantity of the product

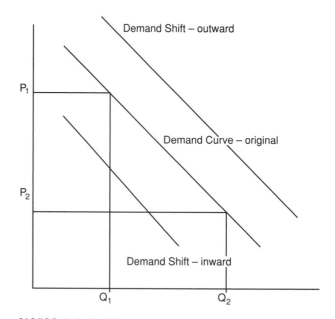

FIGURE 1.3 ■ Movement along the demand curve and shifts in demand.

covered by insurance that consumers demand, because the goods or services are largely paid for by the insurer. For example, consumers with vision insurance covering new glasses are likely to purchase new glasses more frequently than consumers with similar incomes who must pay out-of-pocket. On the other hand, an increase in opportunity costs, such as waiting time, decreases the quantity demanded, and vice versa. For example, assuming the price of new glasses remains the same, a consumer is more likely to purchase glasses if the time waiting to receive the vision examination and to receive the glasses is shorter rather than longer. If improvements in diagnostic equipment enabled optometrists to reduce appointment time substantially (thus reducing opportunity costs), the quantity of prescription eyeglasses demanded would be expected to increase.

The price of substitutes is another demand shifter. If a substitute product is available at a lower price, the quantity demanded for the substitute will increase relative to the original good or service. For example, as the price of contact lenses falls over time, consumers substitute contact lenses for prescription eyeglasses, and the quantity demanded for contact lens increases relative to prescription eyeglasses.

The price of **complements** (products associated with a specific good or service) has an opposite influence in shifting the quantity demanded than the price of substitutes—an increase in the price of complements decreases the quantity demanded, and vice versa. For example, if the price of contact lens cleansing solution and equipment increased substantially, the quantity of contact lens demanded relative to prescription glasses would be expected to decrease.

Events of various types may shift the quantity demanded up or down. For example, a disaster such as an earthquake may increase the quantity demanded for intravenous fluids, blood products, and intravenous tubing. The poisoning of a few bottles of Tylenol some years ago caused a substantial drop in the quantity demanded of that product, until consumer safety caps replaced the regular caps. Regulations to improve the quality of care in skilled nursing facilities increase the quantity of certified nursing assistants demanded.

As shown in Figure 1-3, the line indicating a demand shift outward from the original demand curve reflects an overall increase in the quantity demanded given each possible price. Factors shifting the demand curve outward include increased consumer income or insurance coverage, reduced opportunity costs, increases in the price of substitutes, decreases in the price of complements, or events that increase the quantity demanded. The line indicating a demand shift inward from the original demand curve reflects an overall decrease in the quantity demanded given each possible price. Factors shifting the demand curve inward include decreased consumer income or insurance coverage, increased opportunity costs, decreases in the price of substitutes, increases in the price of complements, or events that reduce the quantity demanded.

Utility

Utility represents the amount of satisfaction that results from consumption of a product sold in the economic market. Personal preferences and tastes, beliefs, cultural values, and styles influence an individual's perception of utility. For many health care products, a consumer's perception of positive utility is based on improved health, recovery from disability, and comfort. Negative utility is associated with the risk of harmful complications or discomfort.

For example, laser eye surgery to correct vision problems has substantial utility because the personal preferences, cultural values, and style of many consumers is to avoid wearing glasses. The surgery itself is brief and not particularly uncomfortable, with little risk of complications. Some consumers with vision problems are at higher risk for complications or cannot be successfully treated with laser surgery. For those consumers, the procedure has no or negative utility.

Consumers seek to maximize utility—in other words, to obtain the maximum value for the money spent on goods and services. However, beyond the financial and opportunity costs of consumption, there is an inherent limit to how much utility may be maximized for most products beyond a given level. The more a product is consumed by an individual, the greater total utility, until the individual is saturated. **Marginal utility** represents the rate of change in total utility given a one-unit change in consumption. Once the individual is saturated, additional consumption results in no additional utility, or in negative utility (dissatisfaction or harm). In other words, as consumption increases, marginal utility decreases; the **law of diminishing marginal utility.**

There are many examples in health care of the law of diminishing marginal utility. For example, most medications must be taken as prescribed. If the patient takes too little of the medication, it typically is not effective (so little or no utility results from consumption). If the patient takes too much of most medications, there is a risk of serious side effects, physical harm, and in some cases death. Regardless of income, few people own more than one or two pairs of prescription glasses because the utility of each additional pair of glasses becomes smaller with each pair purchased.

Elasticities

Earlier in this section the influence of price and income on the quantity demanded was discussed. **Elasticity** is a measure of responsiveness in the quantity demanded by consumers given the amount of change in price or income. Elasticities are calculated by determining the percent change in the quantity demanded (D) that results from a 1% change in price (P) or income (I). Demand is considered elastic if the amount of elasticity is greater than 1 or less than −1.

Before calculating an elasticity, it is necessary to calculate the percent change. The percent change is calculated by dividing the amount of change in the quantity demanded, the price, or the income at a specified time by the original (old or baseline) amount of demand, price, or income. For example, the old price for a product is $10,000 and the new price for that same product is now $12,000. The percent change in price is calculated as follows:

$$\text{Percent Change} = (\text{New Value} - \text{Old Value}) \div \text{Old Value}$$

$$20\% \text{ Increase} = (\$12,000 - \$10,000) \div \$10,000$$

If instead the old price for a product is $10,000 and the new price is $8,000, the amount of change is a $2,000 decrease, and the percent of change is a 20% decrease (or −20%).

The elasticity of demand with respect to price measures the effect of a 1% change in the price of a given product on the percent change in the quantity demanded for that product. Table 1-5 shows examples based on Sunshine Optical, with the baseline (old or original) price at $350 per pair and baseline demand at 12,000 pairs over the course of a year. A decline in price of $50 to $300 is a 14.3% decrease in price. Assuming that the demand for glasses, given the reduction in price, is 15,500 for the year, there is a 29.2% increase in the quantity demanded. The price elasticity of demand with respect to price is calculated as follows:

$$\text{Elasticity} = \text{Percent Change in Demand} \div \text{Percent Change in Price}$$

$$-2.0 = 29.2\% \div -14.3\%$$

In this example, it is also assumed that a 14.3% increase in price (to $400) results in a 29.2% decrease in demand (to 8,500 pairs over the year), so that the elasticity of demand with respect to price remains at −2. It appears that the demand for eyeglasses is price elastic and negative—as price increases by 1%, demand decreases by 2%, and vice versa.

The elasticity of demand with respect to income measures the effect of a 1% change in the income of a given product on the percent change in the quantity demanded for that product. Recall that as income increases, the quantity of a product demanded increases (at least to the point of saturation of utility). The amount of the consumer's budget required to purchase a product increases elasticity of demand with respect to income—the higher the proportion of income required, the more sensitive the consumer is to price. Therefore, as the income of consumers rises, they become less sensitive to the price of eyeglasses, and the quantity demanded may continue to increase.

The quality or utility of substitutes is another factor in the elasticity of demand with respect to income, because if cheaper alternatives are readily available that are acceptable, the consumer is more sensitive to price and income. Elasticity of demand with respect to income is positive for a **normal good** but negative for an **inferior good.** For example, as income rises, consumers might demand more prescription eyeglasses (in this case a normal good) and fewer over-the-counter eyeglasses purchased at a pharmacy (in this case an inferior good). Note that in this context the term "inferior" does not mean that the product is necessarily of poorer quality, but rather that it has less utility for consumers compared to the normal good.

Table 1-6 shows examples based on Sunshine Optical prescription glasses (in this example assumed to be a normal good) and over-the-counter glasses (in this example assumed to be an inferior good), with the baseline income at $35,000 per year and baseline demand at 12,000 pairs over the course of a year. A decline in income of $5,000 to $30,000 is a 14.3% decrease in income. Assuming that the quantity demanded for Sunshine Optical glasses, given the reduction in income, is 8,500 for the year, there is a 29.2% decrease in the quantity demanded. The elasticity of demand with respect to income is calculated in the same way as price elasticity, as follows:

$$\text{Elasticity} = \text{Percent Change in Demand} \div \text{Percent Change in Price}$$

$$-2.0 = 29.2\% \div -14.3\%$$

◯ T A B L E 1 - 5

Elasticity of Demand with Respect to the Price of Sunshine Optical Glasses

P	% Change P	D	% Change D	Price Elasticity
$300	−14.3%	15,500	29.2%	−2.0
$350	—	**12,000**	—	—
$400	14.3%	8,500	−29.2%	−2.0

◯ T A B L E 1 - 6

Elasticity of Demand with Respect to Income for Sunshine Optical vs. Over-the-Counter Glasses

Income (I)	% Change I	D Sunshine (normal good)	% Change D	Income Elasticity (normal good)	D OTC (inferior good)	% Change D	Income Elasticity (inferior good)
$30,000	−14.3%	8,500	−29.2%	2.0	15,500	29.2%	−2.0
$35,000	—	**12,000**	—	—	**12,000**	—	—
$40,000	14.3%	15,500	29.2%	2.0	8,500	−29.2%	−2.0

In other words, as income decreases by 1%, the quantity of a normal good demanded (Sunshine Optical glasses) decreases by 2%, and vice versa. The elasticity of demand with respect to income of an inferior good, in this case over-the-counter glasses, is also 2 as calculated in this example, but is negative; as the income increases by 1%, the quantity of the inferior good demanded decreases by 2%, and vice versa.

Demand is inelastic if the quantity of a product demanded is insensitive to price or income, in which case the amount of elasticity is less than one. Two factors help determine the inelasticity of the demand for many health care products. In the first place, products essential to a consumer's well-being are inelastic. Second, products are inelastic when the consumer lacks the time, ability, or knowledge to review choices and make informed decisions about price and substitutes. For these reasons, products such as medications and emergency services are relatively inelastic with respect to price or income, as are health care goods and services covered by insurance. As a result, many health care goods and services are relatively inelastic with respect to price or income.

Supply

Supply represents the quantity of a product that producers are able and willing to sell at a given price over a specific time period. The effect of price on the quantity supplied is opposite to the effect of price on the quantity demanded. As the price of a product increases, the quantity supplied increases, and vice versa. Figure 1-4 shows a **supply curve** depicting the quantities supplied in a specific market over a specific time period for each possible price. As in the case of demand curves, movement along the supply curve is illustrated by the points P_2Q_2, in which the quantity supplied is comparatively low given the comparatively low price, and P_1Q_1, in which the quantity supplied increases as the price increases. One example is the production of eyeglasses. Figure 1-5 shows that at the higher price, P_1, producers supply more pairs of glasses than at a lower price, P_2 (as shown by Q_2, which is lower than Q_1).

Supply Shifters

As in the case of the quantity demanded, there are many influences affecting the quantity supplied. The two lines on either side of the supply curve in Figure 1-5 show shifts in the quantity supplied, or increased and decreased levels of the quantity supplied caused by factors other than price. The following sections discuss supply shifters in more detail.

Costs

Costs represent the resources (inputs) required to produce goods or services. Cost is a very important supply shifter because the more costly it becomes to produce a good or service, the more the price for that product must increase, or production (the quantity supplied) falls. As production (the quantity supplied) increases, the cost of production increases.

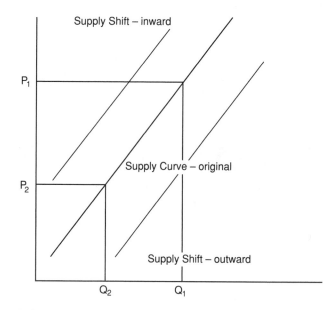

FIGURE 1.4 ■ Movement along the supply curve and shifts in supply.

For example, pharmaceutical companies must recover the costs of research and development when setting the price for new medications, or they cannot continue to produce new medications. Changes in the costs of production-related inputs also shift the quantity supplied. For example, if the cost of medical supplies rises sharply, the costs of operating a hospital (supplying hospital services) increases.

Total costs (TC) are the cost of all inputs needed to produce a given level of output. Total costs are expected to increase as output increases. For example, a certain amount of labor, equipment, supplies, and space in a building is required to produce eyeglasses. If the volume (amount) of eyeglasses produced increases, the total costs are expected to increase.

Average cost (AC) represents the total cost of producing a product over a specified time period divided by the quantity produced over the same time period. For example, Sunshine Optical has total costs of $5 million over a given year and produces 15,000 pairs of eyeglasses that same year. The average cost per pair of eyeglasses is calculated as follows:

$$AC = TC \div Q$$

$$\$333 = \$5,000,000 \div 15,000$$

Sunshine Optical's average cost to produce a pair of glasses over a given year is $333.

The **marginal cost** (MC) represents the amount of increase in total costs given one unit of additional output. For example, the additional costs in terms of labor and supplies to produce one more pair of glasses at Sunshine Optical is the marginal cost of production. The law of increasing costs is that marginal costs increase with increased output, so total costs increase at an increasing rate as production increases. For example, the marginal cost associated with increasing Sunshine Optical's annual production from 15,000 pairs of eyeglasses (at an MC of $340 per pair) to 17,000 pairs of eyeglasses is more per pair ($400) than increasing output from 15,000 pairs to only 15,500 pairs ($345). Many chapters in this text, including Chapters 4 through 8, discuss cost in more detail.

Economies of Scale and Scope

The size and capacity of the business also affects the quantity supplied. **Economy of scale** is a situation in which the long-run average costs decline as output increases, thus enabling the producer to maximize profits. Although reduction in cost may also benefit the consumer by reducing the price, the producer's incentive in economy of scale is profit maximization (profit maximization is further discussed in a following section). For example, economy of scale may be achieved with the purchase of diagnostic radiology equipment. This equipment represents a high total cost, but the long-term average cost of each additional diagnostic procedure decreases as output increases. Once the equipment is purchased, a minimum of labor and supplies are required for each additional procedure, so that a high output of procedures is possible with a relatively small amount of additional inputs.

Economy of scope is a situation in which a producer can jointly produce two or more products at a lower cost than producing each of these goods or services separately. The producer thus maximizes profits by minimizing total costs. For example, a hospital might organize services to provide skilled nursing care and home health care in addition to acute inpatient care. These three products could all be located within the same physical plant, share housekeeping, dietary, laundry, and other services, and reduce marketing costs, as patients could be referred from one service to another within the same organization. The total costs would be less than if a separate business were created independently for each product.

Other Supply Shifters

Changes in technology may shift the quantity supplied. A new technology for grinding lenses may enable Sunshine Optical to produce more eyeglasses at a lower total cost than before. Cataract surgery, which 30 years ago was difficult and expensive, is now a routine outpatient procedure with largely successful outcomes and minimal complications.

Events may shift the quantity supplied as well as the quantity demanded. New regulations or disasters may reduce the quantity supplied or increase the costs of inputs. For example, the HIV epidemic and more stringent infection-control requirements led to a global shortage of the supply of latex and a shortage of latex gloves several years ago.

As shown in Figure 1-4, the line indicating a supply shift outward from the original supply curve reflects an overall increase in the quantity supplied given each possible price. Factors shifting the supply curve outward include reduced costs of production, changes in technology or events that increase production or decrease production costs, increased economies of scale and scope, or events that increase the quantity supplied. The line indicating a supply shift inward from the original supply curve reflects an overall decrease in the quantity supplied given each possible price. Factors shifting the supply curve inward include increased costs of production, changes in technology or events that decrease production or increase production costs, decreased economies of scale and scope, or events that reduce the quantity supplied. Box 1-2 summarizes the shifters of demand and supply, as well as their effects.

Profit Maximization

Consumers seek to maximize utility, while producers seek to maximize **profit,** or the price per unit of a product sold less the production cost per unit (also discussed in Chap. 8). The profit maximization incentive encourages current producers to increase production as the price increases because they will increase their profits. Prospective producers are encouraged to enter the market and further increase the quantity supplied when prices increase. For example, when Medicare reimbursement for home health services was fairly generous, many producers entered the home health market, from individual health professionals starting their own business to hospital corporations adding home health services as another product.

☐ B O X 1 · 2

Demand and Supply Shifters in Competitive Markets

Demand Shifters
- As income increases, the quantity demanded (Q) increases.
- As insurance coverage increases, the quantity demanded (Q) increases.
- As opportunity costs increase, the quantity demanded (Q) decreases.
- As the price of substitutes increases, the quantity demanded (Q) increases.
- As the price of complements increases, the quantity demanded (Q) decreases.
- Events may increase or decrease the quantity demanded (Q).

Supply Shifters
- As production costs increase, the quantity supplied (Q) decreases.
- As economies of scale or scope increase, the quantity supplied (Q) increases.
- As new technology increases in adoption (assuming the technology reduces production costs or increases production), the quantity supplied (Q) increases.
- Events may increase or decrease the quantity supplied (Q).

Note: Decreases in the above economic factors operate in the reverse direction as increases.

Producers maximize profit when they can produce at the level of output in which the marginal cost equals the price. If the marginal costs are lower than the price, the producer must increase output to maximize profits. If marginal costs are higher than the price, the producer must reduce output to maximize profit.

For example, the marginal cost of an additional laboratory test at Accurate Labs is $175 and the price is $200, so a profit of $25 is generated by performing the additional test. Accurate Labs continues to make a profit up to the point of profit maximization, when the marginal cost and the price both equal $200. Should Accurate Labs continue to perform tests so that the marginal cost becomes $225 with the price remaining at $200, there is a loss of $25 for the additional test, and the number of tests should be reduced to maximize profits. Unless the price is increased, profit maximization requires the marginal cost not exceed $200 per test.

However, if consumers (or insurance plans paying the charges) can obtain the laboratory test at $200 per test from a competing laboratory with no additional opportunity costs, the amount of demand for the test at Accurate Labs is likely to fall if the price per test is increased beyond $200. Consumers (or payers) will attempt to maximize profits by purchasing a competing or substitute product at the lowest possible price. Thus, the "pull" from producers to increase the quantity supplied when prices increase is countered by a "pull" from consumers paying for the product to increase the quantity demanded when prices decrease.

Equilibrium and Disequilibrium

Equilibrium represents the situation in which the quantities supplied and demanded are balanced, so that the quantity of products producers want to sell and consumers want to buy are equal at a price that equals the marginal cost of production. Figure 1-5 shows equilibrium of the quantity supplied and demanded at the equilibrium price (p*), which is also the marginal cost, and equilibrium quantity (q*). For example, equilibrium is achieved if Sunshine Optical produces (indicating the quantity supplied) and sells (indicating the quantity demanded) 15,000 pairs of eyeglasses in a year at a price equaling the marginal cost of $340 per pair.

Disequilibrium occurs when the quantities supplied and demanded are not in balance. A **surplus** represents market disequilibrium in which there is an excess in the quantity supplied or a sudden drop in the quantity demanded. Surpluses occur when the market price is higher than the equilibrium price (MC) so that producers generate a quantity supplied that exceeds the quantity demanded (see the lines for P_1 and Q_1 in Figure 1-5). As a result, producers reduce the product's price, which increases the quantity demanded and brings the market to competitive equilibrium. For example, Sunshine Optical produced 17,000 pairs of glasses at a marginal cost (price) of $400 per pair ($P_1$), but the market price remained at the p* amount of $340 per pair. Sunshine Optical reduced its price from $400 to $340 to sell the excess.

A **shortage** represents market disequilibrium in which there is an excess in the quantity demanded or a sudden drop in the quantity supplied. Shortages occur when the market price is lower

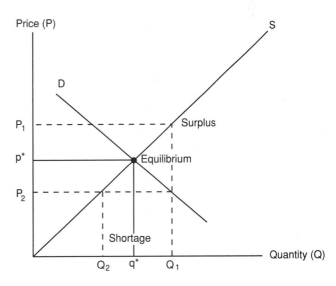

FIGURE 1.5 ■ Effects on a competitive market of changes in price.

than the equilibrium price (MC) so that the quantity demanded exceeds the quantity supplied. As a result, consumers are willing to pay a higher price for the product, and as the price increases, the quantity supplied increases, which brings the market to competitive equilibrium. In Figure 1-5, P_2 indicates that the price for eyeglasses at Sunshine Optical dropped below p* to $275 per pair, and production dropped below q* to 12,000 pairs. However, although the quantity of glasses demanded increased to Q_1, or 18,000 pairs, the quantity supplied dropped to Q_2, or 12,000 pairs, because the price is not sufficient for production. As the price of glasses increased to the p* of $340 per pair, the quantity supplied increased (and demand decreased) to address the shortage and achieve equilibrium at 15,000 pairs.

Market Failures

Markets operate under **perfect competition** given that certain conditions are fulfilled. In perfectly competitive markets, there is no market power over price or barriers to entry by either producers or consumers. Producers and consumers have perfect information and can make rational decisions to maximize their profits or utility. Producers bear all the costs of production, and consumers bear all the costs of consumption. As a result, the market price in a perfectly competitive market is established at the point in which marginal cost and the quantities supplied and demanded reach competitive equilibrium, as shown in Figure 1-5.

Market failure represents a situation in which a market cannot reach a reasonably competitive (efficient) equilibrium. Equilibrium may be reached under conditions of market failure; however, the equilibrium does not reflect the most efficient use of resources. As a result, the distribution of income or production is not socially optimal. Causes of market failure most relevant to health care settings include market power concentration among a limited number of producers or consumers, information or rational decision-making problems, and unequal distribution of the costs or benefits of production or consumption. It is frequently the responsibility of government to address market failures.

In practice, economic theory does not operate in its "pure," most extreme form. There are no purely competitive markets, for as in most health care settings and industries, some form of regulation and standards are typically required to ensure public safety, and these create barriers to entry. Likewise, there are no complete market failures, because despite considerable problems regarding information and rational decision making, many health care consumers experience highly beneficial outcomes at a reasonable price. Box 1-3 summarizes the characteristics of competitive markets and market failures.

☐ B O X　1 - 3

Features of Competitive Markets vs. Market Failures in Health Care

Competitive Markets
- No market power over price or barriers to entry by either producers or consumers
- Producers and consumers have perfect information and can make rational decisions
- Producers bear all the costs of production; consumers bear all the costs of consumption

Market Failures
- Concentrated market power so the producer or consumer controls prices or wages
- Information or rational decision-making problems
- Production of public goods and externalities

Market Power

According to economic theory, one condition for perfect competition requires that neither consumers nor producers are able to control the market price. The market price is established when the quantities supplied and demanded reach competitive equilibrium at the marginal cost of production. If either the producer (seller) or the consumer (purchaser) can control the market price, then market power leads to market failure.

Monopoly

A **monopoly** occurs under conditions in which there are only a few competitors, so market power is concentrated among only a few producers who are therefore able to control both production and price. No close substitutes exist for the product, so consumers must purchase the product at the price set by the producer, or do without. Barriers to entry (such as regulations or high production costs) may also exist for producers wanting to enter the market and increase competition. Many situations in health care markets represent monopolies—for example, the rural hospital that is the only provider of acute inpatient care in the community.

One type of monopoly is the **natural monopoly,** in which the average cost per unit of production falls as output increases because the marginal cost of production is relatively low. For example, a pharmaceutical company might have a monopoly on a medication that has no close substitutes that it is able to produce because of substantial economies of scale. Once the equipment is obtained at a relatively high production cost, the output of the medication may be increased with a relatively low marginal cost of inputs required to manufacture the medication. As a result, the average cost per unit of medication produced falls as the company increases its output.

Political monopolies are created by regulatory requirements that create barriers to entry, thus reducing competition. For example, hospitals are closely regulated, so a group of health professionals who might want to create their own hospital may be unable to meet the regulatory guidelines to do so. Most health care professions have established standards and regulations for licensure, so that unlicensed persons are barred from practice unless they meet the educational, training, and licensure requirements.

Monopoly rent represents excess profit from charging a price to the consumer that exceeds the marginal cost per unit. One reason many persons demonstrate an immediately negative reaction to the concept of monopoly is because of the commonly shared feeling that monopoly rents are unfair to the consumer. Although economists agree with this perception of unfairness, the primary economic problem with monopolies is that they are inefficient compared to competitive markets. In a competitive (efficient) market, a producer's increased price would be accompanied by an increase in the quantity supplied; in a monopoly, resources are misallocated so that society bears a loss in welfare or benefits. Economic benefits that in a competitive market would favor the consumer (society) are instead allocated to the producers, even though production is inefficient.

Figure 1-6 shows an example that may be applied to a pharmaceutical company producing a medication needed for the welfare of its consumers, with no close substitutes or competitors. The company charges a price (P_m) exceeding marginal costs or equilibrium price (P_c). However, instead of increasing the supply of the medication beyond the equilibrium quantity (q^*), which would occur if the price increased in a competitive market, the company holds production to Q_m even though it is charging a higher price.

In a competitive market, the equilibrium price at Q_m would be P_c, the competitive price for the quantity supplied. The monopoly rent is the amount between P_c and P_m or the price charged in excess of marginal cost (which also equals the competitive equilibrium price, P_c). The inefficiency of the monopoly market is measured by the triangle bounded by the lines for P_c, Q_m, and the demand curve. This triangle represents the **welfare loss,** or amount of loss to society from the misallocation of resources caused by the monopoly market.

As mentioned earlier, one role of government is to intervene in cases of market failure. The pharmaceutical company mentioned in the discussion of natural monopolies may have few if any competitors, with no

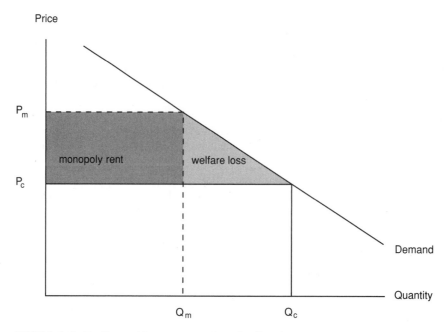

FIGURE 1.6 ■ Competition vs. monopoly and welfare loss.

substitutes among which consumers may choose. In cases in which the welfare loss brought about by the company's market power raises societal concerns, the government may intervene on behalf of the consumers. One intervention is for the government to take over as the producer of the medication. This intervention is often unpopular in the United States, where consumers believe that private markets are more competitive and efficient. Another intervention is price regulation, so that the pharmaceutical company may continue as the only producer but is not permitted to charge a price for the medication in excess of that set by regulators. Yet another choice of government is to allow the monopoly on the medication to operate with little regulation, as over time competitors may enter the market with their own products that provide the same benefits, and reduce inefficiency and welfare loss.

Monopsony

A frequently observed market failure in the health care labor market is **monopsony.** Recall that a monopoly is a form of market failure in which one supplier controls the price paid by consumers. By contrast, a monopsony is a situation in which a limited number of purchasers (consumers) control the price paid to many suppliers. In the health care labor market, a limited number of hospitals are likely to hire most of the health care workers in the community, thus controlling the price (wages) paid. As a result, local hospitals typically establish the wage levels of workers such as RNs, physical and occupational therapists, and laboratory technicians. Market failures in the health care labor market are discussed in more detail later in this chapter.

Information and Rational Decision-Making Problems

Optimum rational decision making occurs under conditions of **perfect information,** when an individual can compare prices among various goods or services and select the optimal quantity and quality to meet preferences (or needs) within budget constraints. Under conditions of perfect information, consumers are as knowledgeable as sellers. However, as Chapter 2 discusses in more detail, there are many examples in health care settings of **information problems,** or the inability of patients, providers, or payers to possess all of the information needed for completely rational decision making. In many cases otherwise rational consumers must rely on physicians and other health care professionals who possess knowledge and information the consumer lacks for advice and decisions regarding their treatment interventions.

In other situations, consumers, even if well informed, cannot make rational decisions because of their physical or psychological limitations, such as a comatose condition following a head injury. As in the case of information problems, consumers unable to make rational decisions cannot act in their own best economic interest (in other words, maximize utility).

Public Goods and Externalities

A pure **public good,** in economic theory, is a good or service that is inexhaustible (one individual may consume the good without depleting it) and nonexclusive (individuals may consume the good whether or not they pay for it). Public goods are also usually produced by the government. **Private goods** are typically produced in private markets and are exhaustible (the goods may be depleted, leading to shortages) and exclusive (consumers are expected to pay for the good or service).

For example, a new pair of eyeglasses typically represents a private good; a consumer (or his or her insurance company) is expected to pay for the glasses, and if the quantity demanded exceeds the quantity supplied, a shortage of glasses occurs. By contrast, a community's sewage disposal and treatment system is an example of a public good. Consumers of sewage disposal and treatment who reside in the community may be taxed or billed for this service, but typically the cost is spread among all resident consumers regardless of the amount of the service they use. Visitors from outside the community may use the sewage system without any requirement for payment. In addition, depletion of sewage disposal and treatment is uncommon in most communities, although expansion of this service may be required if a community experiences substantial growth.

Public goods represent the collective consumption of selected goods and services, and if a government provides a public good, all consumers have relatively free access to it. As a result, the quantity of the public good demanded depends on its utility (value to the consumer), not its price in the market, and the quantity of the public good supplied depends on the collective willingness to pay (generally through taxes or other fees levied by the government). For example, Chapter 14 discusses the values about health care access and social welfare among industrialized nations—citizens in many industrialized nations are willing to be taxed at a higher rate than in the United States to support a more comprehensive and universal level of health care benefits for all of their citizens.

One potential concern with the provision of public goods is the **free rider problem,** in which many individuals or parties benefit from a public good, but few or no individuals or parties pay for the production of the good. If no one pays for a good or service, even the "inexhaustible" public good becomes depleted or cannot be provided as the resources for production are inadequate. As a result, governments not only levy taxes and fees to pay for services but may also establish guidelines for eligibility or provision of goods and services. For example, although Medicare benefits are available as an entitlement to Americans over age 65, recipients must file applications and meet Social Security guidelines, and Medicare reimbursement for health care goods and services must meet guidelines as well.

Unlike public goods, **externalities** represent the uncompensated social consequences of producing or consuming selected goods and services. Externalities may be positive, negative, or neutral. For example, a consumer of dentistry may benefit greatly from dental care, but the externality is largely neutral—the rest of society experiences little or no benefit as a result of the individual's dental care. By contrast, a consumer obtaining a vaccination for influenza creates a positive externality, because influenza is less likely to be transmitted to other members of society when individuals obtain vaccinations. The consumption of tobacco

Public Goods vs. Externalities

Public Goods
- Collective consumption of selected goods or services made available to all
- Demand is determined by utility (value), so consequences of production are positive
- Free riders share the benefits of consumption but not the costs of production

Externalities
- Social consequences of production or consumption
- Potentially positive or negative consequences
- Costs and benefits of production or consumption are borne by different individuals

in public places creates a negative externality, as environmental tobacco smoke is harmful to persons in the smoker's vicinity. Box 1-4 compares the key features of public goods compared to externalities.

Health Care Labor Markets

The economics of health care extend to the health care labor market, made up of workers who are employed or potentially employed in health care settings, and their employers or potential employers. The supply and demand curves for the health care labor markets follow the same economic principles as for any other market, with worker wages (W) representing the price, and the number of health care professionals (RNs, OTs, PTs, and so on) willing to work (and, as required, professionally qualified to work) in the particular market representing the quantity demanded or supplied (Q).

Figure 1-7 shows the demand curve (D) for a health care labor market (such as hospital RNs), which represents the quantity of workers a specific labor market (industry, employer) demands over a specific time period for each possible wage level. The supply curve (S) represents the quantity of workers willing to work over a specific period of time for each possible wage level. The movement along the demand and supply curves is influenced by the effect of wages—as wages rise, the number of health care workers demanded decreases and supplied increases, and vice versa.

Increased wages in the labor market increase production costs, as labor is an input. With rising costs of production, producers increase the price

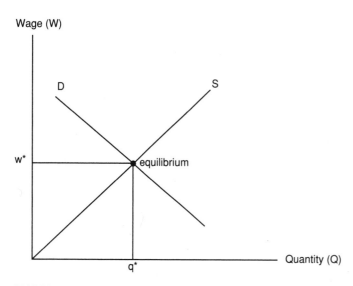

FIGURE 1.7 ■ **Effect on competitive labor market of changes in wages (W).**

charged to consumers (or payers), which reduces the quantity of health care goods or services demanded. As a result, the quantity of health care labor supplied and demanded reaches equilibrium in a competitive market, similar to the dynamics of production in competitive markets.

Health Care Labor Demand Shifters

The quantity of health care workers demanded is a **derived demand,** or the quantity of a product that is demanded for the sake of an ultimate output, not for the product itself. For example, there is a demand for hospital RNs to provide hospital care because the output desired is hospital care, not the RNs *per se*. Radiology technicians are employed because radiologic procedures are necessary. If the quantity of hospital care or radiologic procedures demanded should change, the quantity of hospital RNs or radiology technicians that are demanded will change accordingly. As a result, the expansion or contraction of a particular health care market (such as hospital care or radiologic procedures) that increases or decreases derived demand is a health care labor market demand shifter.

Another influence on the health care labor market related to derived demand is the increase or decrease in health care reimbursement or revenues. Increased reimbursement enables health care markets to expand, thus increasing the derived demand for health care workers, while decreased reimbursement contracts health care markets and reduces derived demand. In recent years, payers, including the government (for example, Medicare and Medicaid programs), insurance companies, and managed care plans, have increasingly controlled and limited reimbursement for health care goods and services. These reductions reduce the amount of resources allocated to staff health care settings, leading to reductions in staffing and in some cases layoffs.

The quantity of health care labor demanded by alternative labor markets is a demand shifter. An increase in the quantity of health care labor demanded by alternative labor markets increases the quantity of health care workers demanded, and vice versa. For example, health professionals such as RNs or PTs may be demanded by health care labor markets such as home health and outpatient clinics, in addition to hospitals, thus increasing the overall quantity of RNs or PTs demanded.

Another influence shifting the quantity demanded in the health care labor market is the **production function,** or relationship between maximum output that can be produced given any combination of labor and other inputs. In some health care settings, labor and **capital** (inputs such as equipment) can be substituted for each other to some extent. For example, the monitors in a telemetry unit are capital that serve as a partial substitute for nursing care. The **marginal product** represents the amount of change in output associated with a one-unit change in labor or capital, so in the telemetry unit it would represent the change in the number of patients who could be managed in the unit given a one-unit change in the number of RNs or monitors. Producers (in this case, hospital administrators) attempt to estimate the optimal mix or ratio of labor to capital to maximize output and profits. An increase in the use of capital compared to labor reduces the quantity of health care workers demanded, and vice versa.

Productivity (the efficiency of production) is a demand shifter influencing the health care labor market. Labor productivity improves when the units of goods or services produced increase for each hour worked. For example, if the radiologic technician can perform three diagnostic procedures per hour instead of two, then productivity is improved. Health professionals are well aware of pressures in their work settings to improve productivity. Productivity increases offset the effects of reduced staffing, as the same number of patients may be managed with fewer staff. Productivity increases also help maximize profits, as in many settings increasing the number of patients managed by the staff (without increasing staff or staff costs) increases revenues. Increased productivity reduces the quantity of health care workers demanded, and vice versa.

Factor substitutions (inputs that enhance another input) are another demand shifter in the health care labor market. For example, dental assistants perform many of the preventive procedures that dentists would otherwise perform, so they are factor substitutes. Physician assistants and nurse practitioners enhance the productivity of physicians, and nurse assistants enhance the productivity of registered RNs in acute and long-term care settings. The availability, skills, and cost of factor substitutions affect staffing and staffing decisions.

Events also may shift the quantity of health care workers demanded. For example, regulations that specify staffing standards for acute care settings increase the quantity of health care workers demanded. Changes in many areas of surgical practice from inpatient to outpatient procedures reduce the quantity of health care workers demanded.

Health Care Labor Supply Shifters

Various influences shift the quantity of health care labor supplied. The level of wages paid in alternative labor markets is a supply shifter. Increased wages in alternative labor markets decrease the quantity of health care workers supplied in the original labor market, and vice versa. For example, if the wages paid to RNs or PTs in home health or outpatient clinics increase relative to acute inpatient settings, the supply of RNs or PTs willing to work in home health or outpatient clinics increases, thus decreasing the supply available to inpatient settings.

Education and training costs also shift the quantity of health care labor supplied. Increased education and training costs decrease the quantity of health care workers supplied, and vice versa. For example, increasing the availability of scholarships and stipends increases the numbers of students enrolling in health care professional programs because they reduce education and training costs.

Events may shift the quantity of health care workers supplied up or down, depending on the effects. Changes in immigration policies that increase the numbers of foreign health care workers increase the quantity of health care workers supplied (for example, the increased immigration of RNs related to the nursing shortage in the United States). Regulations increasing barriers to entry, such as more stringent educational and training requirements for certified nursing assistants, reduce the quantity of health care workers supplied. Box 1-5 summarizes the shifters of demand and supply in health care labor markets.

Health Care Labor Market Failures

Recall that the quantity of labor supplied in a competitive market is related to wages—as wages increase for a given type of worker, so does the quantity of labor supplied. Shortages or surpluses of health care workers may be a result of health care labor market failures, or these market failures may make labor shortages or surpluses more difficult to address. Imbalances in health care labor are anticipated as future trends, discussed in Chapter 15.

In an earlier section about market failures, the situation of a monopsony (few buyers exerting market power over many suppliers) was discussed. Shortages in the supply of RNs and other health care professionals are a serious concern. One problem related to labor market failure is **wage stickiness,** a situation of persistent labor shortage in which wages do not rise to reach competitive equilibrium and end the shortage as would occur in a competitive market. The monopsony market power exerted by the hospitals gives the hospitals control over the wages, so wage stickiness persists.

For example, to maximize profits, the revenues generated by each RN added to the staff of a hospital must be greater than the cost of the RN (wages). Wage stickiness occurs as hospital administrators are willing to hire more RNs at the current wage (which is below the amount of revenue generated by an RN), but will not raise wages in order to hire more RNs (which would reduce the shortage in a competitive market). The unfilled budgeted positions (staff shortages) reflect additional RNs the hospital would hire at the current wage level but not at a higher, competitive wage.

The health care labor market in many parts of the United States faces shortages in health professionals such as pharmacists, dental hygienists, and laboratory technicians, as well as RNs. In many cases, these

---

☐ B O X 1 - 5

Demand and Supply Shifters in Health Care Labor Markets

Demand Shifters
- As derived demand increases, the quantity (Q) of health care workers demanded increases.
- As reimbursement or revenues increase, the quantity (Q) of health care workers demanded increases.
- As the demand from alternative labor markets increases, the quantity (Q) of health care workers demanded increases.
- As the substitution of capital for labor increases, the quantity (Q) of health care workers demanded decreases.
- As productivity increases, the quantity (Q) of health care workers demanded decreases.
- As the use of factor substitutions increases, the quantity (Q) of health care workers demanded decreases.
- Events may increase or decrease the quantity (Q) of health care workers demanded.

Supply Shifters
- As wages in alternative labor markets increase, the quantity (Q) of health care workers supplied in the original labor market decreases.
- As education and training costs increase, the quantity (Q) of health care workers supplied decreases.
- Events may increase or decrease the quantity (Q) of health care workers supplied.

Note: Decreases in the above economic factors operate in the reverse direction as increases.

---

situations represent **dynamic labor shortages.** The quantity of labor demanded continues to increase, but even with wage increases the quantity supplied cannot end the shortage because of barriers to entry (educational requirements for licensure) and other factors such as alternative labor markets.

For example, although their wages are relatively high, until recently there was a dynamic labor shortage of physical therapists. Barriers to entry include the requirement for a master's degree to practice as a physical therapist. Although the quantity demanded and the wages were high, the quantity supplied remained low related to the opportunity costs of the time and expense to meet the educational requirements for physical therapy. More recently, changes in reimbursement mechanisms reduced reimbursement for physical therapy services, thus reducing the quantity demanded and reducing the shortage of physical therapists.

Is Health Care "Different?"

Principles applicable to economic markets, including markets for health care and health care labor, have been presented. This concluding section reviews some of those principles in the context of examining whether, and to what extent, the health care industry differs from other industries.

In many industries, assuming a competitive market, price has the effect of increasing the quantity of a given product supplied and reducing the quantity demanded. Does price exert the same influence in health care? Economists could argue that health care is relatively inelastic with respect to price for individual consumers for several reasons. First, many consumers need health care, so they will demand a given quantity of health care goods and services regardless of price or income, if these products are necessary to sustain life or well-being. Second, consumers frequently lack sufficient information or capability to make rational economic choices about health care.

For most consumers, a large portion of their health care is paid by insurers or government programs rather than as an out-of-pocket expenditure, so that consumers are often unaware of the costs of care. Chapter 2 discusses the information problem and effect of insurance in more detail, including the elasticity with respect to out-of-pocket costs such as the price of health insurance premiums (for relatively healthy persons) and costs of care (for relatively unhealthy persons). It appears that consumers are far more sensitive to the price of out-of-pocket health care than to health care paid for by insurance plans or government programs.

In many industries, assuming a competitive market, the quantity supplied reaches a competitive equilibrium with the quantity demanded as the price approaches the marginal cost of production. Health care often takes place in a monopoly market, in which the quantity supplied does not reach the quantity demanded even though the price rises, because of barriers to entry and concentration of market power. The concentration of market power also leads to monopsony health care labor markets, so that the quantity of health care workers supplied may not meet the quantity demanded.

At the organizational level, health care economics operate in a very similar way to other industries in competitive markets. Although many hospitals and some other health care settings have nonprofit status, Chapter 10 explains in detail that both nonprofit and for-profit enterprises must maximize their profits to survive and grow. Health care organizations must be attentive to the effects of cost and price. For example, many small rural hospitals are struggling for financial survival, even though they have the advantage of holding a monopoly over acute care in the local area, because of rising costs and limited reimbursement (price).

In conclusion, it is important to consider factors such as barriers to entry and imperfect information that make health care economics differ from many other industries. On the other hand, it is essential for health professionals to understand the fundamentals of health economics, as the organizations in which they work are directly influenced by the factors that influence the quantity of health care goods and services supplied and demanded. Returning to Figure 1-1, although many producers and consumers of health care products expect high quality and ready access to health care while controlling costs, it is frequently necessary in practice to accept tradeoffs between these three expectations, as is the case in other non–health care industries.

Conclusion

This chapter introduces concepts of health economics that health professionals can apply to national trends and to their own work settings and discipline. Box 1-6 presents Internet resources for further information about health care economics.

☐ **B O X   1 - 6**

On-line Sources for Information on Health Economics

Association of Health Services Research: http://www.ahsr.org/
Centers for Medicare & Medicaid Services: http://www.cms.hhs.gov/
Health Economics Wharton: http://knowledge.wharton.upenn.edu/category.cfm?catid=6.
Health Economics—Places to Go: http://www.medecon.de/HEC.HTM
HealthEconomics.com: www.healtheconomics.com

CRITICAL THINKING EXERCISES

1. List events in your work setting (or a health care setting of interest) that shift the quantities demanded and supplied of the goods or services produced. What recent events (over the last year) appear to exert the most influence on the quantities demanded and supplied?
2. Try drawing supply and demand curves for what you believe is the labor market for your health discipline in your local area. Is the market in a competitive equilibrium—for example, are wages in balance with the quantity of health workers supplied and demanded, so neither shortages or surpluses are a problem? If there is market failure, what would you propose to return the market to competitive equilibrium?
3. What are the most important inputs for the health care goods and services you produce in your work setting (or a health care setting of interest)? How would you describe the mix of labor and capital in this setting?

REFERENCES

Centers for Medicare & Medicaid Services. (Retrieved June 15, 2002). National Health Care Expenditures Projections Tables. Baltimore, MD. Available at *http://www.hcfa.gov/stats/nhe%2Dproj/proj2001/tables/default.htm*

Chang, C. F., Price, S. A., & Pfoutz, S. K. (2000). *Economics of Nursing: Critical Professional Issues*. F. A. Davis.

Feldstein, P. J. (1993). *Health Care Economics,* 4th ed. Albany, NY: Delmar.

Folland, S., Goodman, A. C., & Stano, M. (1997). *The Economics of Health & Health Care,* 2nd ed. Upper Saddle River, NJ: Prentice Hall.

Getzen, T. E. (1997). *Health Economics: Fundamentals and Flow of Funds.* New York: John Wiley & Sons.

Gilmartin, M. J. (2001). Economic issues in health care. In Creasia, J. L., & Parker, B. (eds.), *Conceptual Foundations: The Bridge to Professional Nursing Practice,* 3rd ed. Philadelphia: Mosby, pp. 228-255.

Jacobs, P., & Rapoport, J. (2002). *The Economics of Health and Medical Care,* 5th ed. Gaithersburg, MD: Aspen.

Morris, S. (1998). *Health Economics for Nurses: An Introductory Guide.* London: Prentice Hall Europe.

Phelps, C. E. (1997). *Health Economics,* 2nd ed. New York: Addison-Wesley.

Quittman, J. E. (April 3, 1997). A brief guided tour of health care economics. Presentation to the Department of Public Management, University of San Francisco, San Francisco.

Santerre, R. F., & Neun, S. P. (1996). *Health Economics: Theory, Insights, and Industry Studies.* Chicago: Irwin.

CHAPTER 2

Fundamentals of Insurance and Managed Care

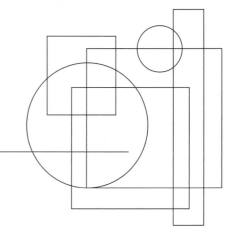

Learning Objectives

1. Compare and contrast information problems and asymmetric information from the perspectives of the patient, provider, and insurer.
2. Differentiate between deductibles, co-insurance, co-payment, and caps as strategies to control health insurance costs.
3. Explain how capitation helps control health care costs.

Key Terms

Adverse selection
Advertising
Agent
Align incentives
Asymmetric information
Benefits management
Cap
Capitation
Carve-in
Carve-out
Churning
Coinsurance
Community rating
Concurrent review
Conflict of interest

Co-payment
Creaming
Deductibles
Diagnostic related groups (DRGs)
Experience rating
Fee-for-service (FFS)
Gatekeeping
Health maintenance organization (HMO)
Incentive
Major diagnostic category (MDC)
Managed care organization (MCO)
Moral hazard

...continued

Point-of-service (POS)
Pre-authorization
Pre-existing condition clause
Preferred provider organization
  (PPO)
Principal
Prospective payment system
  (PPS)

Prospective review
Retrospective review
Risk pooling
Skimming
Stop-loss insurance
Supplier-induced demand
Third party transaction
Utilization review

This chapter introduces and discusses concepts of health insurance and managed care. One underlying theme throughout this chapter is describing how various **incentives** (rewards or reinforcements) are addressed among the major interests in health care: the provider of care, the client receiving care or care of a loved one, and the entity paying the provider for care. Incentives influence how and how well the health care expectations of cost, quality, and access are met. This chapter examines how systems of health care may or may not **align incentives** for the provider, client, and payer (in other words, reinforce the simultaneous goals of improving quality and access while reducing costs).

Financial rewards or savings are most commonly thought of as incentives in health care insurance and managed care systems. Another important incentive for consumers is to have as much free choice as possible in the selection of their physician, hospital, and other providers based on established relationships, preferences, and perceived quality. Choice is also an incentive for providers, who prefer to select procedures and schedule visits as they think best. Insurers paying for health care have incentives to limit consumer and provider choice in order to control costs.

Time is yet another incentive in health care systems. Assuming that the cost of a given health care good or service remains the same, the longer the time for the delivery of that good or service, the more costly it becomes for the consumer. The passage of time represents an opportunity cost, or alternative benefit that could be derived during that same time period using the same amount of resources. For example, if an uninsured worker must wait all day to be seen at a free clinic, there is still the "cost" of the wages that would have been earned during the day spent waiting at the clinic. Providers have incentives to have their charges paid as quickly as possible. Payers (insurers) have incentives to delay approval and payment for health care services, as they thereby decrease demand, accrue savings, and increase the time they have use of funds that would otherwise be paid out to providers.

Many of the approaches and strategies developed in managed care systems are intended to align incentives or to correct problems with the alignment of incentives. Before discussing principles of managed care, it is important to understand some fundamental principles of health insurance and historic systems of payment for health care in the United States. As managed care represents a shift from these earlier approaches, it is important to understand and compare the changes brought about by managed care systems.

Health Insurance History and Principles

The first sections of this chapter discuss the history and basic principles of health insurance to allow for better understanding and comparison between "traditional" payment systems and managed care. After a brief review of the history of health insurance, basic principles of health insurance are presented, then a discussion of incentives and the alignment of incentives.

Historic Foundations of Health Insurance

Throughout most of human history, health "insurance" existed as health care provided by one's family, within one's immediate social setting (clan, tribe, or village), and later, in Western Europe and the United States, through charitable religious groups. The concept of insurance, and its establishment as a business, developed as financial contracts for the cargo of ships at sea at the time of the Industrial Revolution. As a wage-based economy began to develop throughout the industrialized nations, factory owners or donations from workers supplied sums of money for ill or injured workers as needed, whether for medical services, disability support, or funeral expenses and care for the worker's widow and orphans.

Among some industries, such as mining, "sickness funds" began to be supplied by owners or taken up as donations among the workers in a more systematic way than in the past. In addition, some factory and other industrial owners began hiring "company doctors" for sick and injured workers and their families. Throughout the late 1800s and by the early 1900s, national health plans were instituted by governments throughout most European countries, ensuring access to medical services for workers and their families.

In the United States, the government at all levels (federal, state, and local) played a much smaller role in financing and insuring health care than in many other industrialized nations. It was not until the economic upheaval of the Great Depression during the 1930s that health insurance began to gain popularity. One early plan was the nonprofit enterprise Blue Cross, which provided health insurance plans for hospitalization. By covering populations instead of individuals, hospitalization plans could benefit from **risk pooling** (spreading the risk of health care costs across an entire population of predominantly healthy consumers paying the plan's premiums).

Hospitals benefited from hospitalization insurance plans such as Blue Cross, because rather than their historical reliance on "charity" supplied by religious groups and donors, hospital managers could now be reasonably sure that their charges would be paid in full. The 1930s represented the beginning of the use of many technologies such as improved sanitation, surgical techniques, and diagnostic equipment. Hospitalization insurance helped hospitals fund these new technologies, attract desirable physicians, and establish a role as a place to be treated and cured rather than die.

Other health insurance plans, such as Blue Shield, arose to provide coverage for physician care. Although physicians historically charged fees for their services, this greater certainty of full **fee-for-service (FFS)** reimbursement (paying all allowable costs meeting accepted standards of care) greatly enhanced both the financial status and the political power of physicians compared to other health care professionals in the United States. In addition, physicians established state and local medical societies that determined whether physicians could practice. Among other benefits, membership in medical societies enabled physicians to drive out anyone practicing medicine who challenged the FFS reimbursement system. Medical societies further increased the political and lobbying power of physicians compared to other health care professionals.

The next major event that stimulated the widespread growth of health insurance plans in the United States occurred during World War II, when the federal government enacted wage and price controls in the interest of national security. Health insurance premiums were exempted from the federal wage and price control regulations and were tax-exempt for both employees and employers. These exemptions tremendously increased the popularity of health insurance coverage among both workers and employers. In 2000, employer insurance plans accounted for about $443.9 billion, or 34.2% of all health care expenditures (Table 2-1).

A major impetus to FFS reimbursement health insurance coverage came about with President Lyndon B. Johnson's War on Poverty initiatives in the 1960s. The Social Security Acts of 1965, which established and financed the Medicare (Title XVIII) and Medicaid (Title XIX) programs, provided coverage for elderly Americans and poor American families. Table 2-1 shows that Medicare and Medicaid (state and federal) expenditures totaled $427.1 billion or 32.9% (nearly a third) of national health expenditures in 2000.

TABLE 2 - 1

National Health Expenditures, Amounts, % of Total and Average % Growth, by Funding Source, 1970 and 2000

Funding Source	1970 $ billions	% Total 1970	Average % Growth 1969–1970	2000 $ billions	% Total 2000	Average % Growth 1999–2000	Increase $ billions 1970–2000	Estimated Growth 1970–2000 (times)
Out-of-pocket consumer payments	25.1	34.3%	6.9%	194.5	15.0%	5.5%	169.4	6.7
Private health insurance	15.5	21.2%	10.2%	443.9	34.2%	8.4%	428.4	27.6
Other private funding	4.8	6.6%	14.0%	73.8	5.7%	1.5%	69.0	14.4
Private Funding	**$45.4**	**62.1%**	**8.5%**	**$712.3**	**54.8%**	**6.9%**	**$666.9**	**14.7**
Medicare	7.7	10.5%	n/a	224.4	17.3%	5.6%	216.7	28.1
Medicaid, federal	2.8	3.8%	n/a	118.4	9.1%	9.2%	115.6	41.3
Other federal	7.1	9.7%	9.6%	68.7	5.3%	7.7%	61.6	8.7
Medicaid, state	2.4	3.3%	n/a	84.3	6.5%	7.7%	81.9	34.1
Other state and local	7.6	10.4%	7.2%	91.4	7.0%	6.4%	83.8	11.0
Public Funding	**$27.6**	**37.8%**	**15.4%**	**$587.2**	**45.2%**	**7.0%**	**$559.6**	**20.3**
Total national health expenditures	**$73.1**	**100.0%**	**10.6%**	**$1,300**	**100.0%**	**6.9%**	**$1,226.4**	**16.8**

NOTE: Numbers may not add to totals because of rounding error.
SOURCE: Levit et al., 2002.

Both Medicare and Medicaid were enacted with strong provisions protecting FFS reimbursement. Related to the lack of effective utilization and cost controls for Medicare and Medicaid, U.S. publicly funded health expenditures increased by over 20 times from $27.6 billion in 1970 to $559.6 billion in 2000 (see Table 2-1). From 1970 to 2000, overall national health expenditures grew 16.8 times, from $73.1 billion to $1,226.4 billion.

In 1983, health care financing underwent a major change with the establishment of the **prospective payment system** (PPS) by Medicare, which established fixed reimbursement rates to hospitals based on **diagnostic related groups (DRGs)**. DRGs classify illnesses by **major diagnostic category** (MDC) and standardize the expected length and expense of inpatient care. PPS was an attempt to address the tremendous health care cost inflation that resulted from the retrospective FFS reimbursement system initially used by Medicare. Medicare prospective payment has now been extended to skilled nursing care and home health care as well as acute care services.

Principles of Health Insurance

Health insurance is based on principles that affect the alignment of incentives around cost, quality, and access. These principles are related to concepts such as information, predictability of risk, and ways that the demand for health care may be influenced.

Information Problems and Asymmetric Information

Some economists point out that health care differs from the provision of other goods and services because of information problems, or the inability of patients, providers, or payers to possess all the information needed for completely rational decision making (discussed in Chap. 1). Optimum rational decision making occurs under conditions of perfect information, when an individual can compare prices among various goods or services and select the optimal quantity and quality to meet preferences (or needs) within budget constraints. Under conditions of perfect information, consumers are as knowledgeable as sellers.

Many businesses approach the economic ideal of perfect information. For example, consumers can study publications and other information sources and obtain a similar level of knowledge as the car dealer when purchasing a new automobile. If perfect information were the rule in health care, then patients, providers, and payers would largely base their choices on quality and access, while controlling costs.

Probably the most obvious example of information problems concerns patients and their families, who by definition are unable to adequately diagnose and treat disorders (or they would not be seeking health care in the first place). Patients often do not even understand when they should go to a physician's office instead of an emergency room, or whether they should seek any kind of health care. Even though consumers are better educated today than ever before, information problems continue to influence their decisions.

Health care professionals also experience information problems. For example, even the most highly qualified physician may not know the disorder from which a patient suffers until the results of the appropriate diagnostic tests are available. Patients may forget or fail to inform providers about important issues such as their use of nonprescription medications or medications prescribed by another physician. Even with the dramatic advances in today's health care technologies, in many cases providers cannot accurately predict the outcomes of patient care. In other cases, providers may not be sure which intervention would be the most cost-effective. For example, a physician may not know whether extended physical therapy or surgery would be best and least costly to resolve chronic severe back pain.

Finally, insurers (payers) have information problems. The primary reason for health insurance coverage is to protect against unpredictable risk: the costs of an unexpected illness, injury, or disability. Young and relatively healthy persons may pay health insurance premiums for years before an illness or other disorder occurs. Other persons may require extensive health care at or even before birth. However, the premise is that neither the consumer nor the insurer can predict, at least on an individual basis, when and how much health care will be required, and how much it will cost.

The problem of **asymmetric information** differs from information problems in that one party possesses knowledge needed to enable rational decision making that the other party lacks. In the case of the patient–physician relationship, the patient, or **principal**, who lacks the knowledge needed for health care, delegates decision-making authority to the physician, or **agent**, who possesses the necessary knowledge. Patients rely on their physicians and other health care professionals to make informed decisions about their needs. The patient with severe back pain wants relief and trusts that the physician knows what treatment is best, so he or she allows the physician to decide between physical therapy or surgery. In other cases, otherwise rational patients are too ill to make an informed decision (for instance, a person found unconscious cannot choose a hospital).

The physician's role as an agent creates a potential for **conflict of interest** (an ethical discord between two or more desired but opposing circumstances), as the physician is not only an agent but also a provider billing for services. For example, the dual role of agent and provider invites physicians to engage in **churning**, or scheduling more office visits or procedures than may actually be necessary for the patient. The physician as an agent (a "good doctor") advises the patient to schedule the office visit or procedure, and as provider the physician benefits from additional fees.

Asymmetric information also affects physicians and other health care professionals. It is not unusual for patients to conceal lifestyle information, such as the use of illicit drugs or risky sexual practices. Patients may choose not to discuss the use of alternative health practices or nonprescription medications, or may state they are compliant with the treatment regimen when they are not. A patient's caregiver may also conceal or distort information that would be helpful to the provider.

Health insurers face asymmetric information when consumers do not disclose conditions such as diabetes, cardiovascular disorders, serious risk behaviors, or disabilities. For this reason, many health insurance plans include a **pre-existing condition clause** that requires the consumer to disclose any illnesses or conditions to the health insurance plan, and limit coverage accordingly. For example, a health plan may require consumers to disclose a diagnosis of diabetes, and use this information to deny enrollment or to charge a higher premium. The pre-existing condition clause thus reduces health plan costs related to asymmetric information.

Health insurers also face asymmetric information when they lack sufficient information about the choices and decisions of providers. Under the traditional FFS plans, insurers did not closely review a provider's charges unless there was reason to suspect fraud. Health plans today frequently require much closer scrutiny of the care a provider gives or plans to give before authorizing payment. The section on review mechanisms discusses this issue further.

A fundamental incentive related to information problems is to have more and better information available and, in the case of asymmetric information, to equalize information among all parties. Patients want better information about their provider's quality of care, and providers as well as insurers want to have as complete an understanding of the patient, patient history, and patient risk factors as possible. Insurers also want information about the provider's care and plan of care to be sure that payment is restricted to medically necessary interventions.

Setting Premiums and Rating

Health plans must make decisions about the premiums they charge. **Experience rating** is a method used by many traditional indemnity health insurance plans in which premiums are based on the utilization or claims history of the group, rather than on the characteristics of the group's population as a whole. As a result, a plan year in which a group experiences an unusual number of high-cost claims (such as AIDS cases) may result in higher premiums the following year.

Community rating is a method in which premiums are based on the population characteristic of an entire group. In many cases, community ratings are adjusted for age and sex, and sometimes other factors as well. A relatively young group (such as college students) is typically healthier, and its health plan would likely charge lower premiums than for an older group (such as an employee group). Over much of the life span, females are more costly than males, so community-rated premiums might also be sex-adjusted. In some cases, premiums might also be adjusted by industry, so that employee groups working in industries with documented health risks that predict increased utilization might be charged higher premiums.

Third Party Transactions

Health insurance represents a **third party transaction**; in other words, a provider supplies goods or services to the consumer (patient) but bills a private or government insurance entity, which is the third party. As a result, consumers typically are largely unconcerned with the costs of their care, knowing that their bills are paid by another party.

Third party transactions also remove providers from concerns about the cost of care, as they do not need to confront an ill or disabled patient covered by insurance with the charges, no matter how high. Providers also profit from an increased demand for their services because health care is more accessible to consumers. As a result, providers increase the amount of health care goods and services supplied.

Private insurers profit from third party transactions as long as they can pool the risk (so they can offset a relatively small proportion of high-cost members with a majority of low-cost members) and can increase their premiums to cover the costs that accrue. Government insurers (as with Medicare or Medicaid) benefit as long as their programs provide services of community value and are not seen as burdening the taxpayer.

Third party transactions provide incentives to patients to utilize health care goods and services that may not be necessary, as they are not sensitive to the cost of these interventions. Providers have incentives to encourage and offer health care goods and services as they know their charges will be reimbursed. As long as their costs are covered by higher, profitable premiums or taxes and public support, insurers have incentives to allow relatively unrestricted access to health care goods and services. The higher the amount of insurance coverage, the greater the access and demand for health care services, and the greater the increase in health care costs.

Deductibles, Coinsurance, Co-payment, and Caps

Deductibles represent minimum threshold payments before a plan begins to cover health care costs. For example, there may be a $100 annual deductible for prescription medications: after the beneficiary pays the first $100, the insurance plan covers the remainder of the prescription medication costs for the plan year. **Coinsurance** represents a percentage of a given health care cost that is required by the insurer to be paid by the beneficiary; by comparison, **co-payment** represents a specific dollar amount of the given health care cost required of the beneficiary. For example, a beneficiary may be required to pay a 20% coinsurance for the inpatient hospital bed rate after the fifth inpatient day, or required to pay $20 co-payment for every visit to a primary care physician's office.

Deductibles, coinsurance, and co-payments make consumers more sensitive to the cost of health care services, thereby reducing demand and access that may be unnecessary and reducing costs. Increases in deductibles, coinsurance, and co-payment rates decrease the demand for health care goods and services. In addition, sharing health care costs with the consumer via deductibles, coinsurance, and co-payment reduces the health plan's costs.

One additional way to reduce health care access and costs is for health care insurers to establish **caps**, or limits to coverage. Caps are most frequently set on either an annual or a lifetime basis. For example, a dental plan may set an annual cap of $1,500; beyond that limit, any additional dental expenses accrued must be paid by the patient until the following plan year. A lifetime cap might be a $100,000 or 90-day limit on inpatient psychiatric care.

One implication of the use of annual or lifetime caps is the role of **benefits management** as part of case management for patients with costly or long-term disorders. Benefits management involves continual monitoring of a member's benefit status for patients with frequent hospitalizations or other high-cost care. Another important function in benefits management is conserving the benefit whenever possible. One example of conserving the benefit is replacing high-cost psychiatric inpatient care with outpatient day programs whenever appropriate, or referring the patient to public sector programs. The benefits manager is also responsible for alerting the employer and the health plan of the need for extension of benefits and for educating plans and employers. Health plans may hire or contract with benefit or case managers and assign them to high-cost and potentially high-cost cases.

Consumers have incentives to reduce their utilization when they must pay for all or a portion of health care. Providers have incentives to become more informed about the rules that insurers have established if they must collect all or part of their charges from the patient rather than the insurer. Insurers are able to reduce unnecessary utilization of health care goods and services, thereby reducing their costs. Deductibles, coinsurance or copayments, and benefit caps play a role in aligning incentives.

Adverse Selection

Adverse selection is the over-selection of a health plan based on its coverage of persons likely to have high health care costs. When the consumer is more knowledgeable about the probability of illness and health care costs than the insurer (asymmetric information), the problem of adverse selection can occur.

For example, a health plan providing more generous coverage to persons with diabetes than competing health plans unknowingly attracts a greater proportion of diabetic beneficiaries than would be expected in the overall risk pool. Diabetics therefore over-select the more generous health plan, and its costs increase at a greater rate than competing health plans with less generous diabetes benefits or pre-existing condition clauses. As a result, the health plan's premiums increase, so that healthy persons are unable or unwilling to pay these higher premiums and either choose a competing, cheaper plan or become uninsured. However, even when premiums increase, the health plan generous to diabetics continues to attract and retain persons with diabetes, because the premiums are still far less than out-of-pocket diabetes care.

Adverse selection poses a serious financial threat to health insurance plans. Another effect of adverse selection is reduced access, first because fewer "healthy" consumers can afford the higher premiums, and second because "unhealthy" consumers cannot meet pre-existing condition clause requirements to obtain health insurance coverage.

In 1999, 49 million Americans were uninsured either at the time they were surveyed, or at some time during the prior 12 months—17.9% of the total population of 273 million. Over half of those reporting that they were uninsured (27 million) lacked insurance coverage for 12 months or more, 9.9% of all Americans in 1999. Although most of the uninsured tend to be young or low-income adults who do not qualify for government programs, the numbers of middle-aged and employed uninsured are rising. Only 64.7% of employed non-elderly Americans had employer-sponsored health coverage in 2001, down from 66.0% in 2000.

Persons at high risk for health problems have financial incentives to select health insurance plans that will cover their higher costs, even if the premiums are high. Healthy persons (particularly if also low-income) have incentives to select relatively inexpensive health plans or forgo health coverage altogether. Insurers have incentives to select populations at lower risk and lower cost, a process known as **skimming** or **creaming**.

Moral Hazard

Moral hazard represents a plan member's higher utilization of covered services. Unlike adverse selection, it is not that the member is primarily at higher risk for health care costs, but because these costs are covered by insurance, the member utilizes more health care goods or services than might be necessary. For example, a person with vision coverage might purchase new glasses more frequently, even if the eye examination indicates that the lens prescription has not changed.

Provider self-interest may play a role in moral hazard, as providers typically benefit from the increased numbers of patients and amount of revenue. Moral hazard, asymmetric information, and conflict of interest may lead to **supplier-induced demand**, in which agents use their knowledge and authority over the principal to influence (increase) demand. For example, a provider might continue to recommend patient visits for treatment such as massage that patients like to receive, and that may be fully covered by insurance, for far longer than clinical standards might determine are medically necessary.

A fairly recent phenomenon related to moral hazard is the preponderance of **advertising**, or mass media communication purchased by a sponsor (such as a pharmaceutical company) to persuade a target audience. Advertising differs from supplier-induced demand in that the agent–principal relationship does not exist; rather, the advertising message primarily focuses on persuasion rather than information and is prepared on behalf of the sponsor. Advertisements for prescription medicine are frequently seen on television, billboards, and the Internet and in popular magazines and newspapers. Advertising increases demand and stimulates moral hazard as it encourages patients to ask their physician for interventions that might not be entirely necessary or that might be provided by less costly alternatives. A similar phenomenon is the increasing use of the Internet by health care consumers, who then approach their physician with requests for interventions publicized on the Internet.

Patients have incentives to make maximum use of their health care insurance benefits, as they are largely insensitive to the cost of health care goods and services, other than the health plan premium. Providers have incentives to induce demand, as it increases the number of patients or procedures, is profitable, and reinforces their role as helpers and agents. Sponsors have incentives to advertise health care goods and services, thus increasing demand, sales, and profits. Insurers have incentives to compel patients and providers to reduce utilization and to select among less costly alternatives, unless premiums can be increased to maintain profitability

Capitation and Managed Care

Much of the history and background of health insurance in the United States was dominated by FFS reimbursement systems and incentives related to third party transactions. Although prepaid health plans (the forerunners of capitation and managed care) emerged at the same time as "traditional" health insurance, the dominance of capitated and other managed care systems is much more recent. The following sections review the history and some basic principles of managed care as it has developed.

Historic Foundations of Managed Care

Just as "traditional" health insurance had its foundations in the United States with the onset of the Great Depression, prepaid medical plans also began at that time. In 1929, Dr. Ross and Dr. Loos started the Ross-Loos prepaid group practice plan in Los Angeles, which covered municipal workers. Instead of charging fees to patients for each service provided, the physicians were paid a lump sum of money in advance to cover all services over an agreed time period. Dr. Ross and Dr. Loos were both subsequently expelled from the Los Angeles County Medical Society because of the opposition to their practice from the medical community. Also in 1929, Dr. Shadid established the first full-risk capitated contract at the Community Cooperative Hospital in Elk City, Oklahoma, to meet the needs of the rural poor. Dr. Shadid was expelled from the local and state medical societies and was threatened with revocation of his medical license because of his efforts. Most other similar attempts met tremendous opposition from the medical community.

In 1933, Dr. Sidney R. Garfield established a prepaid plan for construction workers in the Mojave Desert in Southern California. The industrialist Henry Kaiser then employed Dr. Garfield to create a prepaid group practice plan for construction workers at the Grand Coulee Dam, which was later extended to other Kaiser workers and their families. During World War II, the health plan covered shipyard workers in San Francisco

Bay area and other locations on the West Coast. Unlike other early prepaid health plans, Dr. Garfield's plan grew and developed into what is now called Kaiser Permanente. The term **health maintenance organization (HMO)** was coined to represent a **managed care organization (MCO)**, a managed care plan providing health care to persons voluntarily enrolled in a prepaid plan.

The growth of managed care plans continued to face prohibitive state and local regulations guarding the interests of physicians and hospitals favoring FFS reimbursement. However, by the early 1970s the largely uncontrolled costs of Medicare and other health insurance plans led to widespread interest in more cost-effective approaches. The growth of managed care was greatly stimulated by the HMO Act of 1973, which gave states the responsibility for oversight and regulation of managed care plans. By 1986, nearly all states passed regulations for licensing (therefore legalizing) HMOs.

The 1980s were a time of rapid growth of HMOs, largely related to health care inflation. Employers increasingly believed that their health care costs were spinning out of control and making American industry less competitive and profitable as a result. In addition, there was more awareness and publicity about the prevalence and potential dangers of unnecessary health care, along with increasing evidence that HMOs such as Kaiser Permanente could provide high-quality care while reducing costs.

Over the 1990s, HMOs and other MCOs continued to grow, given their success at controlling health care costs. Figure 2-1 shows the growth in HMO enrollment in the United States from 1980 to 2001, increasing from 9.1 million enrollees in 1980 to 33.0 million in 1990, and rising to 81.3 million enrollees in 1999.

HMO Enrollment in the U.S., Selected Years, 1980-2001

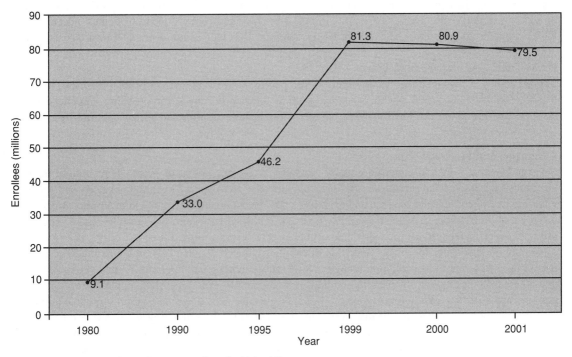

FIGURE 2.1 ■ **HMO enrollment growth in the United States.**

The 1990s were also a time of intense MCO competition, mergers and acquisitions, and new forms of managed care. Government programs such as Medicare, Medicaid, and CHAMPUS (coverage for military retirees and dependents) began contracting with HMOs and developing managed care plans in the public sector to control costs and improve access. However, despite the proliferation of managed care and mechanisms to control health costs, national health expenditures increased as a percent of gross domestic product from 7.0% in 1970 to 13.2% in 2000.

Recent Events in Managed Care and Health Expenditures

At the federal level, there has been an increased focus since the mid-to-late 1990s on Medicare fraud and abuse identification and control, which has reduced hospital, home health, and nursing home payments. Despite continued health care cost inflation, the Balanced Budget Act of 1997 (BBA) reduced Medicare expenditure increases to 0.6% for 1997–1998 and 1.5% for 1998–1999. The Balanced Budget Refinement Act of 2000 (BBRA) offset some of these cost reductions and increased Medicare expenditures by 5.6% for 1999–2000 by increasing coverage for some types of hospital, skilled nursing home, and AIDS care (see Table 2-1).

At the state as well as federal levels, the State Children's Health Insurance Program (SCHIP), part of the BBA legislation, increased Medicaid enrollment from 1999 to 2000 by increasing the coverage of eligible uninsured children. States are experimenting with strategies such as disproportionate share hospital (DSH) payments and Medicaid waivers allowing public sector managed care plans for Medicaid recipients to attempt to better control state expenditures for Medicaid while improving quality and access.

Spending for both private and public health care increased at similar rates for 1999–2000 (see Table 2-1). Private health insurance increased by 8.4% from 1999–2000, largely related to increased coverage for outpatient prescription medications (not covered by Medicare) and increased hospital costs, insurers seeking profitability, increases in enrollment, and a shift by consumers to plans offering higher-cost benefit options. Increased resistance to restrictions imposed by managed care reduced physicians' acceptance of HMO contracts and consumer selection of HMO coverage, thus increasing recent health care costs.

Principles of Managed Care

The principles of managed care were largely developed to address and correct problems related to incentives created by "traditional" health insurance, such as third party transaction problems, supplier-induced demand, and moral hazard. Ideally, managed care should enable appropriate access and high-quality care while controlling costs.

Capitation and Financial Risk

One fundamental principle underlying many managed care plans is that of prepayment. Rather than the insurance plan paying the provider's charges following the provision of health care goods and services, managed care plans typically estimate and negotiate a predicted amount, which is paid in advance. **Capitation** is a form of prepayment in which a fixed payment is established per health plan enrollee and is paid to the provider (or provider system) for a specified set of services over a specified time period.

Capitation introduces incentives that address supplier-induced demand and problems inherent in third-party transactions. In most capitation contracts, providers can keep surplus funds if they can provide care that is less than the amount of the capitation budget. For example, Pine Tree Medical Group receives a capitation contract for $5 million for the care of 10,000 HMO enrollees. If the medical group is able to provide care over the entire year of the health care plan at $4,800,000, the remaining $200,000 is retained as a bonus. On the other hand, if Pine Tree Medical Group spends $5,200,000 on this patient population over the plan year, they must accept a loss of $200,000. Capitation results in the provider sharing the financial risk of the insured population with the insurer.

As a result, the physicians in the group have financial incentives to prescribe and recommend only interventions that are medically necessary. The physicians will not want to induce demand for unnecessary visits, procedures, or other treatments, as they face financial penalties if they let their costs run above the contracted amount. Moreover, the physicians in Pine Tree Medical Group become much more sensitive to the costs of their services. Although the incentives may have shifted more from "over-care" to "under-care," hospital readmission rates, emergency room visits, and complication rates are indicators of appropriate access to medically necessary services.

Pine Tree Medical Group may face unanticipated and uncontrollable financial losses from an unusually high-cost patient (such as treating a rare carcinoma) or from unusually high losses overall. **Stop-loss insurance** coverage protects providers or managed care organizations from unusually costly cases or from overall financial losses that exceed a given percentage of the total capitation contract. However, the cost for the stop-loss premium is an additional expense that must be deducted from capitation revenues.

Gatekeeping

Gatekeeping is a requirement by MCOs that access to specialists must be authorized by a primary care provider. For example, a patient suffering from a rash would first have to see a primary care provider (usually a primary care physician) who might authorize a referral to a dermatologist, or who might diagnose and treat the rash without a referral. If the patient insisted on seeing a dermatologist without authorization, the dermatologist's claim would likely be denied and the patient would likely have to pay the costs of specialty care. Emergency care is generally exempted from gatekeeping requirements.

Some managed care plans offer a **preferred provider organization (PPO)** option, in which the plan contracts for services with independent providers at a discounted rate. The PPO option gives more generous coverage if the member selects from these "preferred providers," even without gatekeeper authorization, than if the member chooses providers outside the plan. Another option is the **point-of-service (POS)** plan (a variation of the PPO), in which the plan covers services from providers within the plan more generously than services from providers outside the plan.

Gatekeeping uses financial incentives to limit the consumer's free choice to control costs of care by more expensive specialists that could be provided at the same level of quality by a less costly primary care provider. Consumers insisting on freer choice may pay higher deductibles, co-payments, or premiums to participate in PPO or POS plans, or may go outside the plan altogether and incur out-of-pocket expenses for all or nearly all the costs of care.

Provider Reimbursement Mechanisms

Capitation is one approach to align incentives in managed care system, but a mix of reimbursement mechanisms is used in various health care settings. For example, physicians may be reimbursed by MCOs or managed care plans based on a fee schedule (such as the one devised for Medicare reimbursement) or a flat rate such as a contracted capitation amount (as in the case of the Pine Tree Medical Group).

Hospitals may be reimbursed by MCOs or managed care plans under a fee schedule, a per diem rate, or based on a patient's diagnosis and procedures (such as Medicare's prospective payment system). In cases in which the MCO or managed care plan and the hospital do not have a contract, reimbursement may be based on the hospital's own list of charges. The MCO or managed care plan has strong financial incentives to review, limit, and control provider costs whenever possible.

Review Mechanisms

Unlike the "traditional" FFS reimbursement systems that typically paid provider charges without oversight or review unless there was evidence of fraud, managed care plans use various review mechanisms to reduce unnecessary costs. **Prospective review** (or **pre-authorization**) involves reviewing a provider's plan for care prior to the intervention, and determining whether the plan will pay the costs for the intervention. For example, the Welby HMO requires prospective review for most elective surgeries, reviewing the patient's history and the treatment plan to ensure that the surgery is medically necessary.

Concurrent review (or **utilization review**) most frequently occurs during hospitalization when the reviewer evaluates the medical record and determines whether continued hospitalization is medically necessary, for each additional day of hospitalization. **Retrospective review** (or review of claims) occurs after health care is provided and the claim for reimbursement is filed. Documentation, including the claim itself, is reviewed to determine whether the intervention was medically necessary and is authorized for payment.

Review mechanisms address problems with third party transactions and supplier-induced demand. Providers must clearly support their recommendations and decisions and carefully document their treatment plan, care, and outcomes. Incentives are increased for providers to carefully think through the necessity of their interventions in advance. As a result, review mechanisms help reduce unnecessary utilization and control health care costs, although review mechanisms also generate considerable administrative costs for the managed care plan and the providers. The appeals process that frequently follows the denial of claims adds to the administrative costs of review mechanisms.

Quality Management

An increasingly systematic approach to providing, improving, and managing quality was stimulated by the growing dominance of managed care. One reason quality management is facilitated in managed care environments is the acceptance of continuous prospective, concurrent, and retrospective review of treatment plans and decisions about patient care. Another reason quality management increased in popularity was due to concerns by the public and policy-makers about the ethics of managed care, given the financial incentives for under-care.

A third reason quality management became more formalized and established was the increasing public demand for more and better information about their provider's quality of care. "Report cards" provide information to the public on the performance of managed care organizations and hospitals using quality indicators such as immunization rates. Popular news magazines publish these data annually, as do sources on the Internet.

Incentives for quality are frequently regulatory or related to reimbursement. For example, to receive reimbursement from Medicare and Medicaid and to obtain many group contracts, MCOs must obtain accreditation from entities such as the National Committee for Quality Assurance (NCQA), which establish and evaluate quality indicators such as immunization rates. The MCO also may require quality standards before contracting with providers in order to increase the quality of care provided.

Provider Networks or Panels

MCOs frequently develop and rely upon networks or panels of providers (typically physicians, but in some cases psychologists and other health care professionals) who contract to provide services at a negotiated (usually discounted) rate. Patients typically must utilize these network providers or risk paying all or part of the out-of-network costs (except in cases such as emergency care outside the network's service area). Just as gatekeeping limits choice while reducing costs, so does the provider network.

The incentive for consumers is that the network mechanism reduces cost even though it also reduces choice, keeping the insurance premiums lower. An incentive for providers is that they receive a high volume of referrals from the health plan. Insurers have financial incentives to keep costs down, but another incentive is that they can exert enough control over the provider network to establish and implement quality standards.

Specialty Managed Care

As managed care became more established and covered more lives, concerns began to increase about access to specialty care services. This section focuses on the specialty area of behavioral health (mental health and substance abuse treatment), as behavioral health represents one of the largest specialty managed care areas and illustrates many of the problems and solutions encountered in other specialty care areas (such as oncology).

Many of the concerns about behavioral health in populations covered by MCOs were related to requirements for primary care gatekeeping. Patients, families, and advocates argued that frequently the primary care provider is not the best-qualified person to determine whether a referral for behavioral health care should be authorized. In addition, concerns arose regarding confidentiality and the reluctance of many patients to discuss or divulge their problems to their primary care provider in order to see a behavioral health provider.

Medical care is oriented toward acute care and dealing with crisis situations, so that in some cases the behavioral health problems of patients are not addressed by gatekeepers until hospitalization is required. This crisis approach in the long run increased rather than reduced overall costs while reducing access and quality. Finally, many HMOs did not adequately finance behavioral heath programs, leading to further reduction in access and quality care.

Beginning in the early 1980s, these problems with specialty behavioral health care led to the establishment of managed care **carve-outs**, or specialty MCOs operating separately and independently from the HMO or other medically oriented MCO. Behavioral health carve-outs focus on specialty care and early intervention to improve access and quality while controlling costs. Typically patients and families may self-refer, often using a designated toll-free telephone number, and are put in immediate contact with a mental health professional for authorization, utilization review, and case management. Review mechanisms are employed once the patient is referred for care, with various limits on outpatient visits and inpatient days depending on the health plan (typically insuring a large employee group or a public sector population).

One problem with carve-outs is the potential difficulty of integrating medical and specialty health care. For example, a patient with severe depression following a myocardial infarction not only has at least two providers (a cardiologist and a mental health professional), but also receives care through two organizations, the HMO and the behavioral health care organization. This arrangement may make it difficult for the medical and behavioral health providers to communicate with each other and coordinate care.

One approach taken by some large MCOs is to establish behavioral health (or other specialty) **carve-ins**, or specialty MCOs operating within the larger HMO or other medically oriented MCO. Carve-ins allow the advantages of specialty care, access, and early intervention provided by carve-outs but potentially allow for greater integration of services as all of the health care providers, medical and behavioral, operate under the same umbrella organization.

Carve-outs and carve-ins increase consumer incentives to seek access for specialty care and offer financial incentives for insurers to save on acute care costs while improving access and quality. Specialty providers have incentives to join networks as they receive referrals from the carve-outs or carve-ins.

BOX 2-1

On-line Sources for Information on Health Insurance

American Association of Health Plans: www.aahp.org
Council for Affordable Health Insurance: www.cahi.org
Employee Benefit Research Institute: www.ebri.org
Health Insurance Association of America: http://www.hiaa.org/index.flash.cfm
Kaiser Family Foundation: www.kff.org

☐ **BOX 2-2**

On-line Sources for Information on Managed Care

American Managed Behavioral Health Association: http://www.ambha.org/
California Department of Managed Care: http://www.dmhc.ca.gov/
HRSA Health Services Financing & Managed Care: http://www.hrsa.gov/financeMC/
Managed Care Information Center: http://www.themcic.com/
National Committee for Quality Assurance: www.ncqa.org
National Managed Health Care Congress: http://www.nmhcc.org/

Conclusion

This chapter discussed the history and fundamental concepts of health insurance and managed care in the United States. Chapter 3 builds on these concepts using practical applications for financial reporting in managed care. Box 2-1 provides Internet resources for additional information about health insurance. Box 2-2 provides Internet resources for additional information about managed care.

■ **CRITICAL THINKING EXERCISES**

1. Request health plan information from the human resources department in your work setting. Evaluate the types of plans offered in terms of benefits and any co-insurance, co-payments, deductibles, or caps. Compare and discuss the health plans in terms of adverse selection, moral hazard, cost control, quality, and access.
2. If workplace health plan information is not available, request benefit information from your state's Medicaid program or other publicly sponsored program such as California's Healthy Families (http://www.healthyfamilies.ca.gov/Handbook/HBpg6.htm). Evaluate and compare the plans as in Exercise 1.
3. Discuss the organization and financing of your health care work setting, concealing its identity as appropriate. To what extent are there mechanisms imposed by managed care? To what extent is the setting financed by FFS mechanisms? Does a particular payer dominate, such as Medicare? How does the organization and financing of your setting affect costs, quality, and access?

■ **REFERENCES**

Bataille, G., Anderson, K., & Penner, S. (January 1995). A public–private sector venture in managed mental health: Solano County's experience. *Administration and Policy in Mental Health, 22*(3), 327–344.

Berwick, D. M., Godfrey, A. B., & Roessner, J. (1991). *Curing Health Care: New Strategies for Quality Improvement.* San Francisco: Jossey-Bass.

Bowman, L. (1999, Sept. 4). Health care takes back seat to cost. *San Francisco Examiner,* p. A-2.

Cohen, J., Cornelius, L., Hahn, B., & Levy, H. (no date, data from National Medical Expenditure Survey, 1987). *Use of Services and Expenses for the Noninstitutionalized Population Under Medicaid.* (AHCPR Pub. No. 94-0051). National Medical Expenditure Survey Research Findings 20, Agency for Health Care Policy and Research, Rockville, MD: Public Health Service.

Gabel, J., Levitt, L., Pickreign, J., Whitmore, H., Holve, E., Rowland, D., et al. (October 2001). Job-based health insurance in 2001: Inflation hits double digits, managed care retreats. *Health Affairs, 20*(5), 180–186.

Gilmartin, M. J. (2001). Economic issues in health care. In J. L. Creasia & B. Parker (eds.), *Conceptual Foundations: The Bridge to Professional Nursing Practice* (3d ed., pp. 228–255). Philadelphia: Mosby.

Goldstein, A. (1999, Oct. 4). More Americans lack health coverage. *San Francisco Chronicle,* pp. A-1, A-17.

Health Grades.com (1999–2002). http://www.healthgrades.com

Heffler, S., Smith, S., Won, G., Clemens, M. K., Keehan, S., & Zezza, M. (March/April 2002). Health spending projections for 2001–2011: The latest outlook. *Health Affairs, 21*(2), 207–218.

Hoffman, C. & Wang, M. (January, 2003). *Health Insurance Coverage in America: 2001 Data Update.* Kaiser Commission on Medicaid and the Uninsured. *www.kff.org*

Hoffman, P. B. Ethics in health care delivery. (1999). In A.R. Kovner & S. Jonas (Eds.), *Health Care Delivery in the United States* (6th ed., pp. 474–502). New York: Springer.

Jones, R. W. (1994). *The Ultimate HMO Handbook.* Albany, CA: TTM Health Publishing.

Kaegi, L. (April 1998). Managed care ethics: oxymoron or opportunity? An interview with John La Puma. *Joint Commission Journal on Quality Improvement, 24*(4), 212–217.

Kaiser Commission on Medicaid and the Uninsured. (June 2003). Lack of Coverage: a long-term problem for most uninsured. The Henry J. Kaiser Family Foundation. Fact Sheet *www.kff.org*

Kaiser Permanente Newsroom. (retrieved May 1, 2002). History. http://www.kaiserpermanente.org/newsroom/history.html, copyright 2002.

Kirk, R. (1997). *Managing Outcomes, Process, and Cost in a Managed Care Environment.* Gaithersburg, MD: Aspen.

Knight, W. (1998). *Managed Care: What It Is and How It Works.* Gaithersburg, MD: Aspen.

Kongstvedt, P. R. (1997). *Essentials of Managed Health Care* (2d ed.). Gaithersburg, MD: Aspen.

Kongstvedt, P. R. (2002). *Managed care: What it is and how it works* (2d ed.). Gaithersburg, MD: Aspen.

Kongstvedt, P. R. (2001). *The Managed Health Care Handbook* (4th ed.). Gaithersburg, MD: Aspen.

Kovner, A. R., & Jonas, S. (Eds.). (1999). *Health Care Delivery in the United States* (6th ed.). New York: Springer.

Levit, K., Smith, C., Cowan, C., Lazenby, H., & Martin, A. (January/February 2002). Inflation spurs health spending in 2000. *Health Affairs, 21*(1), 172–181.

Marks, J. S. (Spring/Summer 1997). Public health and managed care: Beyond coexistence to partnership. *Chronic Disease Notes & Reports, 10*(1), 2, 15.

Penner, M. J. (1997). *Capitation in California: A Study of Physician Organizations Managing Risk.* Chicago: Health Administration Press.

Penner, M. (1999). Administrative competencies for physician organizations with capitation. *Journal of Healthcare Management, 44*(3), 185–196.

Penner, S., Baler, S., Walkover, M., & Cohen, E. (2000). Challenges to quality management in the public sector. In G. Stricker, W. Troy, & S. Shueman (Eds.), *Handbook of Quality Management in Behavioral Health* (pp. 157–169). New York: Plenum.

Penner, S. (January 1996). Case studies in managed care clinical review. *Journal of Practical Psychiatry and Behavioral Health, 2*(1), 33–38.

Penner, S. (2000). The role of the managed care organization in ensuring quality of the service system: Maintaining the full continuum of services. In G. Stricker, W. Troy, & S. Shueman (Eds.), *Handbook of Quality Management in Behavioral Health* (pp. 129–143). New York: Plenum.

Quittman, J. E. (April 3, 1997). A brief guided tour of health care economics. Presentation to the Department of Public Management, College of Professional Studies, University of San Francisco, San Francisco.

Rognehaugh, R. (1998). *The Managed Health Care Dictionary* (2d ed.). Gaithersburg, MD: Aspen.

U.S. Census Bureau. (Jan. 17, 2002). Detailed health insurance table 2. http://www.census.gov/hhes/hlthins/hlthin00/dtable2.html

U.S. Census Bureau. (Jan. 17, 2002). Detailed health insurance table 1. http://www.census.gov/hhes/hlthins/hlthin00/dtable1.html

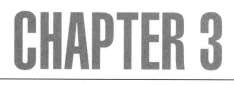

CHAPTER 3

Financial Reporting
in Managed Care Settings

Learning Objectives

1. Define and explain the application of at least two financial indicators used in managed care settings.
2. Explain why it is important for a health plan or capitated group practice to monitor the financial indicators for both primary and specialty providers.
3. Define and explain the importance of identifying outliers in a capitated population.

Key Terms

Case mix
Formulary
Generic
Incurred but not reported (IBNR)
  expense
Independent practice
  association (IPA)

Member month
Outlier
Per member per month (PMPM)
Per member per year (PMPY)
Per thousand members per year
  (PTMPY)
Profit and loss (P&L) statement

Chapter 2 presented fundamental concepts of managed care. This chapter applies many of these managed care concepts using pediatricians in a medical group practice as the case example. Based on the utilization and cost data for the medical group's pediatricians, indicators to analyze and evaluate utilization and costs in a managed care setting are calculated.

Pine Tree Medical Group

Pine Tree Medical Group is an **independent practice association (IPA)** that contracts with Welby HMO. IPAs are organizations such as physician group practices that contract with a managed care plan to provide services for a capitation rate. The following tables show examples of financial reporting for the pediatricians at Pine Tree Medical Group who serve as primary care providers (PCPs) for Welby enrollees. This section reviews and links general concepts of managed care presented in Chapter 2 with the practice patterns of Pine Tree Medical Group pediatricians and referral specialists. Data and financial indicators are discussed to help the reader understand and analyze the financial performance of Pine Tree Medical Group pediatricians.

Overall Primary Care Utilization and Financial Data

Welby HMO negotiates a capitation contract each year with Pine Tree Medical Group. Remember that managed care plans, particularly those using capitation financing, focus on population-level care. The capitation rate is adjusted by the age and sex of its members, so the capitation rate for the Pine Tree Medical Group pediatricians is somewhat lower than for PCPs of adult and elderly members.

It is important for the Pine Tree Medical Group pediatricians to know the size of the population for which they provide services. One population measure is to calculate the **member months**, or the total of all months of coverage of each health plan enrollee over the plan year. As shown in Table 3-1, for the first quarter of 2003, the member months are calculated as follows:

1st Quarter Member Months 2003 = Members
Enrolled January 2003 + Members Enrolled February 2003 + Members Enrolled March 2003

$$31,134 = 10,492 + 10,257 + 10,385$$

Table 3-2 presents indicators used in evaluating performance and calculating managed care financial indicators. The member months are reported as well as the number of total primary care visits (6,084) for Pine Tree Medical Group pediatricians in the first quarter of FY 2003. The paid charges (charges authorized by the capitation plan and used in this section as a measure of costs) include $244,702 for primary care visits.

Other primary care charges (such as lab, x-ray, and other procedures such as immunizations and pharmacy) amount to $291,232, which is a fairly high figure, partly because the pediatricians maintain a high rate of immunizations. Authorized visits to specialists are $251,580, with other specialty care charges amounting to $264,692. The Pine Tree Medical Group assumes 50% of the risk of inpatient hospitalization, so the inpatient paid charges are 50% of the total inpatient paid charges of $561,600, or $280,800. Total paid charges for the first quarter of FY 2003 are $1,333,006.

⃝ T A B L E 3 · 1	
Pine Tree Medical Group, Members with Pediatric PCP, 1st Q, FY 2003	
Month	**Members**
January	10,492
February	10,257
March	10,385
Member months (1st Q)	**31,134**

The capitation revenue is calculated at $45 multiplied by the number of member months (31,134), or $1,401,030 for the first quarter of FY 2003 (see Table 3-2). For the purposes of simplicity, all paid charges are covered by this capitation rate, including inpatient care. In many managed care settings, inpatient and some other charges are budgeted and paid separately.

A $4 co-payment is charged to the patient for each PCP visit, of which about 80% or $24,336 is collected, for a total revenue of $1,425,366 (patients are not denied access if unable to pay at the time of the visit, and about 20% of the co-pay bills are uncollected). The total revenues less paid charges result in a **profit and loss (P&L) statement** (difference between revenues and costs, or $1,425,366 minus $1,332,985) of $92,360 in profit for the first quarter of FY 2003.

Overall Primary Care Financial Indicators

In many cases, data and indicators for managed care reporting are spread over an entire fiscal year. Table 3-3 presents data from FY 2002, for

TABLE 3 · 2	
Pine Tree Medical Group, Pediatric Primary Care Services Data, 1st Q, FY 2003	
Member months (1st Q)[1]	31,134
Total primary care visits[2]	6,084
Paid Charges	
Primary care visits	$244,702
Primary care other	$291,232
Specialty care visits	$251,580
Specialty care other	$264,692
Inpatient (50% risk)	$280,800
Total paid charges	**$1,333,006**
Revenue	
Capitation revenue	$1,401,030
Co-payment revenue	$24,336
Total revenue	**$1,425,366**
P&L statement	**$92,360**

[1] Calculated as members enrolled January + February + March.

[2] Target visits = 11 wks/quarter*5days/wk*22 visits/day*5 PCPs = 6,050. 11 wks/quarter allows for holidays and vacation.

which an entire year of data are reported. The capitation revenue for FY 2002 was $5,024,600 and total paid charges (including IBNR, discussed later in this section) total $4,598,798. The P&L statement shows a profit of $425,802 for FY 2002 ($5,024,600 minus $4,598,798).

Financial indicators in managed care reporting frequently calculate charges, revenues, or utilization by membership measures to allow better comparison and understanding. One commonly used indicator is **per member per month (PMPM)**, a measure of revenue, cost, or utilization for each health plan enrollee per month, calculated by dividing the monthly revenue, cost, or utilization value by the number of members. If more than one month of data are involved, PMPM is calculated by dividing the revenue, cost, or utilization value for a specified time period by the same time period's member months.

For example, as shown in Table 3-3, total capitation revenue for the Pine Tree Medical Group pediatricians was $5,024,600 for FY 2002, and the total member months for FY 2002 was 114,848. The PMPM capitation revenue is calculated as follows:

PMPM Capitation Revenue FY 2002 = Total Capitation Revenue ÷ Total Member Months

$43.75 = $5,024,600 ÷ 114,848

The paid charges PMPM for Pine Tree Medical Group pediatricians for FY 2002 are calculated the same way, except that the total paid charges for FY 2002 are divided by the member months. Note that in Table 3-2, the $45 capitation rate is $45 PMPM, multiplied by the member months to calculate the total capitation revenue.

The **per member per year (PMPY)** represents a measure of revenue, cost, or utilization for each health plan enrollee per year, which may be calculated by multiplying the PMPM value by 12. As shown in Table

3-3, the FY 2002 capitation revenue PMPY for the Pine Tree Medical Group pediatricians is calculated as follows:

$$\text{Capitation Revenue PMPY FY 2002} = \text{Total Capitation Revenue} \div \text{Total Member Months} \times 12$$

$$\$525.00 = \$5,024,600 \div 114,848 \times 12$$

The FY 2002 paid charges PMPY ($480.51) are calculated in the same way, replacing the total capitation revenue with the total paid charges.

One additional commonly used population measure is **per thousand members per year (PTMPY)**, most frequently used as a utilization measure for services such as inpatient hospital days. PTMPY is calculated as utilization PMPY $\times$ 1,000, which makes the utilization value easier to read and interpret, as typically such values are very small. For example, as shown in Table 3-3, the inpatient utilization PTMPY for Pine Tree Medical Group pediatricians is calculated as follows:

$$\text{Inpatient Utilization PTMPY FY 2002} = \text{Total Inpatient Days} \div \text{Total Member Months} \times 1,000 \times 12$$

$$102.7 = 983 \div 114,848 \times 1,000 \times 12$$

The inpatient utilization rate of 102.7 is substantially lower than more typical rates such as 210.5 for medical groups, because the pediatric patients represent a young and relatively healthy population.

One other measure important in many managed care settings, including medical groups, is the **incurred but not reported (IBNR) expense**, which represents the estimated outstanding contracted expenses accrued near the end of an accounting period that have not been filed with the medical group. For example, the average charges for the PCPs, specialists, and inpatient facilities used by the Pine Tree Medical Group pediatricians enable a fairly accurate estimate of paid charges over a specified time period. Of these approved charges, a given percentage of services are not yet submitted to the Pine Tree Medical Group for payment by the end of the quarter or fiscal year. It is important for the Pine Tree Medical Group to have reasonable estimates for these unpaid expenses, as these bills must eventually be paid.

Table 3-3 shows the estimated IBNR charges as 30.9% of total charges. In other words, an estimated $1,421,029 (30.9% $\times$ $4,598,798) of the total paid charges of $4,598,798 accrued over FY 2003 have yet to be reported by the providers.

TABLE 3-3

Pine Tree Medical Group, Members with Pediatric PCP, Financial and Utilization Indicators, FY 2002

Indicators	
Total member months	**114,848**
Financial performance:	
Total capitation revenue	**$5,024,600**
PMPM	$43.75
PMPY	$525.00
Total paid charges	**$4,598,798**
PMPM	$40.04
PMPY	$480.51
Estimated % charges IBNR	30.9%
Utilization	
Total PCP visits	**22,511**
PMPM	0.20
PMPY	2.35
Total specialty visits	**9,094**
PMPM	0.08
PMPY	0.95
Total inpatient days	**983**
PTMPY	102.7
P&L statement	**$425,802**

TABLE 3-4

Pine Tree Medical Group, Pediatric Primary Care Visits and Costs by PCP, FY 2003

PCP	Primary Care Visits	Total Paid Charges	Average Charge per Visit
Dr. A	1,218	$47,028	$38.61
Dr. B	1,209	$47,618	$39.39
Dr. C	1,225	$49,831	$40.68
Dr. D	1,339	$57,122	$42.66
Dr. E	1,093	$43,103	$39.44
Total	**6,084**	**$244,702**	**n/a**
Average	**1,217**	**$48,940**	**$40.22**

Primary Care Utilization and Financial Data and Indicators by PCP

Tables 3-1, 3-2, and 3-3 present financial and utilization data and indicators helpful in reviewing the overall performance of the Pine Tree Medical Group pediatricians. However, it is necessary to break these data and indicators into more detail to provide insights on the practice patterns of each of the PCPs that may affect utilization and costs. Table 3-4 shows the number of visits, total paid charges for PCP visits, and average cost per PCP visit for each pediatrician in the Pine Tree Medical Group for the first quarter of FY 2003. These data allow evaluation and comparison among the pediatricians and average values for the pediatricians.

For example, Dr. A had 1,218 visits during the first quarter of FY 2003 (see Table 3-4), very close to the average number of visits (1,217). Dr. A's total paid charges are $47,028, higher than the average of $48,940. However, Dr. A's average charge per visit is $38.61, which is the lowest charge of all the physicians. Dr. D has the highest number of visits (1,339) and highest average charge per visit ($42.66). Dr. E has the lowest number of visits (1,093).

The medical director of Pine Tree Medical Group might consider further analysis to determine whether Dr. D is "churning" an unnecessarily high number of higher-cost visits. One way to evaluate Dr. D's practice patterns is a random review of patient charts and treatment plans. The medical director might also want to determine whether Dr. E is allowing sufficient access because of the low number of visits. A review of quality indicators such as ER admissions and immunization rates would help in evaluating Dr. E's practice patterns.

Table 3-5 reports other costs such as lab, x-ray, other procedures (such as immunizations), and pharmacy by each pediatric PCP in the Pine Tree Medical Group for the first quarter of FY 2003. For simplicity the lab charges are estimated at $25 per procedure, x-rays at $120 per procedure, other procedures at $100 per procedure, and pharmacy at $18 per prescription. These estimates are made for the sake of keeping this example as simple as possible. Note that Dr. C has the highest average additional cost per PCP visit ($59.75) and Dr. D has the lowest additional cost per PCP visit ($40.23), with Dr. B and Dr. E close to the average of $47.87 ($47.14 and $47.00, respectively).

The primary care services data may be broken down into even more detail; for example, in examining the utilization and costs of pharmacy by each Pine Tree Medical Group pediatrician, as shown in Table 3-6. Dr. C has the highest number of prescriptions per primary care visit (2.8), Dr. D the lowest (1.6). Dr. D also

TABLE 3 - 5

Pine Tree Medical Group, Pediatric PCPs, Other Costs per Primary Care Visit by PCP, FY 2003[1]

PCP	Primary Care Visits	Lab	Lab Charges	X-ray	X-ray Charges	Other Procedure	Other Procedure Charges	Pharmacy Rx	Pharmacy Rx Charges	Total Other Costs	Average Other Costs per PCP Visit
Dr. A	1,218	48	$1,200	26	$3,120	88	$8,800	2,372	$42,696	$55,816	$45.83
Dr. B	1,209	57	$1,425	38	$4,560	107	$10,700	2,239	$40,302	$56,987	$47.14
Dr. C	1,225	66	$1,650	22	$2,640	92	$9,200	3,317	$59,706	$73,196	$59.75
Dr. D	1,339	43	$1,075	39	$4,680	113	$11,300	2,045	$36,810	$53,865	$40.23
Dr. E	1,093	22	$550	17	$2,040	124	$12,400	2,021	$36,378	$51,368	$47.00
Total	6,084	236	5,900	142	$17,040	524	$52,400	11,994	$215,892	$291,232	n/a
Average	1,217	47	$1,180.0	28	$3,408	105	$10,480	2,399	$43,178	$58,246	$47.87

[1] Lab charges estimated as $25 per procedure; x-ray $120 per procedure; other $100 per procedure; pharmacy $18 per Rx.

○ **TABLE 3-6**

Pine Tree Medical Group, Pediatric PCP Pharmacy Utilization and Costs, 1st Q, FY 2003

PCP	Primary Care Visits	Pharmacy Rx	Rx per Visit	% Generic or Formulary	Total Pharmacy Rx Charges	Pharmacy Rx Charges per Visit
Dr. A	1,218	2,472	2.0	78.7%	$44,496	$36.53
Dr. B	1,209	2,329	1.9	85.6%	$41,922	$34.67
Dr. C	1,225	3,417	2.8	77.4%	$61,506	$50.21
Dr. D	1,339	2,146	1.6	93.1%	$38,628	$28.85
Dr. E	1,093	2,321	2.1	90.2%	$41,778	$38.22
Total	**6,084**	**12,685**	**n/a**	**n/a**	**$228,330**	**n/a**
Average	**1,217**	**2,537**	**2.1**	**85.0%**	**$45,666**	**$37.70**

prescribes the greatest (93.1%) and Dr. C the lowest (77.4%) percentage of **generic** (less costly than the equivalent brand-name drug) or **formulary** (generic or brand-name drug on an approved prescribing list for a health plan) pharmaceuticals. Generic and formulary prescriptions are lower in cost than non-formulary and brand name pharmaceuticals, so managed care plans encourage their use whenever possible.

Dr. C's pharmacy charges per PCP visit are the highest for the Pine Tree Medical Group pediatricians for the first quarter of FY 2003 ($50.21), with Dr. D the lowest ($28.85). The medical director might want to evaluate Dr. C's prescribing patterns in more detail to determine if it would be possible to lower unnecessary pharmacy charges.

Overall Specialty Care Utilization and Financial Data

Pine Tree Medical Group contracts with Welby HMO and so is at risk for specialty referral costs that come out of the capitation reimbursement. Table 3-7 presents some specialty services data and indicators for overall review and evaluation of specialty physician utilization and referral costs by the Pine Tree Medical Group pediatricians over the first quarter of FY 2003.

The total number of specialty referrals for the first quarter of FY 2003 is 1,343, and the total number of referral visits is 2,283. There are 0.07 referral visits PMPM (2,283 ÷ 31,134) and an average of 1.7 visits per specialty referral (2,283 ÷ 1,343). Specialty referral costs total $251,580, with referral costs PMPM of $8.08 ($251,580 ÷ 31,134). The average cost per referral visit is $110.19 ($251,580 ÷ 2,283) and the average cost per referral was $187.33 ($251,580 ÷ 1,343).

○ **TABLE 3-7**

Pine Tree Medical Group, Pediatric PCPs, Specialty Services Data and Financial Indicators, 1st Q, FY 2003

Member months (1st Q)	31,134
Total number of referrals	**1,343**
Total referral visits	**2,283**
Referral visits PMPM	0.07
Average visits per referral	1.7
Total referral paid charges	**$251,580**
Referral costs PMPM	$8.08
Average cost per referral visit	$110.19
Average cost per referral	$187.33

Specialty Care Data and Indicators by PCP and by Specialist

Table 3-8 breaks down the referral patterns of the pediatricians in the Pine Tree Medical Group in greater detail, by referrals, referral rates, and costs per specialty. The specialties of allergy, cardiology, ENT (ears, nose, and throat disorders), neurology, and orthopedic services are included; for the sake of simplicity in this example, other specialties are omitted. The report of referrals to specialists by PCPs helps in evaluating the PCPs' gatekeeping effectiveness. ER utilization is reported and is important to evaluate, as over-utilization of ER services may represent a lack of appropriate access to primary care services. The ER is a costly substitute for primary care.

A referral rate per 100 PCP visits is calculated for each PCP by each specialty to allow comparison between the PCPs. For example, Dr. A reported 1,218 PCP visits over the first quarter of FY 2003 and made 48 referrals to allergists. The referral rate per 100 to allergists by Dr. A is calculated as follows:

$$\text{Referral Rate per 100} = \text{Referrals} \div \text{PCP Visits} \times 100$$

$$3.9 \text{ per } 100 = 48 \div 1,218 \times 100$$

For example, as shown in Table 3-8, Dr. A's referral rate to allergists was higher than the first-quarter FY 2003 average for the Pine Tree Medical Group pediatricians (3.9 per 100 vs. 2.7 per 100). Dr. A's referral rate to cardiologists was lower than the average (0.6 per 100 vs. 1.4 per 100), a little above the average for ENT (5.3 per 100 vs. 4.2 per 100), and close to the average for neurology (0.1 per 100 vs. 0.2 per 100). The orthopedic specialty referral rate for Dr. A was close to the average (5.3 per 100 vs. 5.5 per 100). The average costs per specialty referral for Dr. A were fairly close to the overall average ($185.90 vs. $187.33). The medical director of the Pine Tree Medical Group might want to evaluate Dr. A's referrals to allergists more closely to determine whether gatekeeping is effective.

ER utilization by Dr. A's patients was well under the average (6.3 per 100 vs. 8.1 per 100), indicating the possibility that access to Dr. A is good, thus preventing unnecessary ER utilization. On the other hand, ER utilization by patients of Dr. B (11.6 per 100) and Dr. E (10.8 per 100) is higher than the average rate. Recall in the discussion of Table 3-4 that Dr. E has the lowest number of patient visits for the first quarter of FY 2003 (1,093) and that the medical director might evaluate quality indicators for Dr. E to determine if there are access problems. It is possible that some of Dr. E's patients are seeking primary care in the ER rather than from the PCP.

Table 3-9 focuses on the practice patterns and costs of the orthopedic specialists to whom the Pine Tree Medical Group pediatricians referred patients over the first quarter of FY 2003. Drs. Q through U represent orthopedic specialists. Note that the total number of referrals (335) and paid charges ($60,300) are the same as summarized for the orthopedic referrals by PCP in Table 3-8.

This closer look at referrals and referral visits by orthopedic specialist shows that Dr. U received the most referrals (132) from the Pine Tree Medical Group pediatricians over the first quarter of FY 2003, but Dr. Q scheduled the most referral visits (482), with the highest average visits per referral (5.3). Dr. T had the highest average cost per referral visit, $345.79 ($13,140 ÷ 38). A review of this report by the medical director and pediatricians of the Pine Tree Medical Group might indicate further evaluation and analysis of Dr. Q and Dr. T's practice patterns and costs, and consideration regarding further referral decisions.

Table 3-10 breaks down the other specialty costs (lab, x-ray, pharmacy, and other procedures) for the orthopedic specialists receiving referrals from Pine Tree Medical Group pediatricians over the first quarter of FY 2003. The reviewer can evaluate the utilization of other services and pharmacy for each of the orthopedic specialists.

For example, Dr. Q authorizes 2.1 lab tests per referral on average, close to the overall average (2.0). Dr. Q orders 2.2 x-rays per referral, higher than the overall average (1.5), but Dr. Q's authorization of other

TABLE 3-8

Pine Tree Medical Group, Pediatric PCPs, Referrals to Specialty Care by PCP, 1st Q, FY 2003[1]

PCP	PCP Visits	Allergy			Cardiology			ENT			Neurology		
		Referrals	Referral Rate/100 Visits	Paid Charges	Referrals	Referral Rate/100 Visits	Paid Charges	Referrals	Referral Rate/100 Visits	Paid Charges	Referrals	Referral Rate/100 Visits	Paid Charges
Dr. A	1,218	48	3.9	$8,640	7	0.6	$1,260	64	5.3	$11,520	1	0.1	$180
Dr. B	1,209	34	2.8	$6,120	12	1.0	$2,160	58	4.8	$10,440	2	0.2	$360
Dr. C	1,225	19	1.6	$3,420	25	2.0	$4,500	45	3.7	$8,100	0	—	$—
Dr. D	1,339	38	2.8	$6,840	18	1.3	$3,240	51	3.8	$9,180	4	0.3	$720
Dr. E	1,093	26	2.4	$4,680	23	2.1	$4,140	38	3.5	$6,840	3	0.3	$540
Total	**6,084**	**165**	**n/a**	**$29,700**	**85**	**n/a**	**$15,300**	**256**	**n/a**	**$46,080**	**10**	**n/a**	**$1,800**
Average	**1,217**	**33.0**	**2.7**	**$5,940**	**17.0**	**1.4**	**$3,060**	**51.2**	**4.2**	**$9,216**	**2.0**	**0.2**	**$360**

[1] Costs estimated as $120 for initial visit; $60 follow-up visit; '$200 ER visit; excluding lab, x-ray, and other added costs. Estimated 2 visits per referral per quarter except ER.

[2] ER visits indicate possible PCP access problems.

procedures is 1.0 per referral, the same as the overall average for the orthopedic specialists. Dr. Q reports an average of 2.9 prescriptions per referral, somewhat less than the overall average (3.4). Dr. Q's total other specialty costs are substantially higher than the average ($42,652 vs. $26,469), as are the average costs per referral to Dr. Q ($468.70 vs. $391.20).

As with the review of Table 3-9, a review of Table 3-10 allows for the evaluation of practice patterns and costs generated by specialists to which the Pine Tree Medical Group pediatricians send referrals. The medical director must determine whether differences in **case mix** (the combination of various disorders and their severity levels for a given provider) explain the differences in specialist costs. For example, if Dr. Q receives more referrals for more complex cases requiring more x-rays and procedures, the higher costs per referral are explained.

Inpatient Utilization and Costs by PCPs

Table 3-11 shows the utilization and costs of inpatient services by the pediatricians at the Pine Tree Medical Group over the first quarter of FY 2003. The Pine Tree Medical Group pediatricians only admit members to Welby General Hospital, and the capitated bed rate of $2,400 per patient-day is inclusive of all charges (see the note to Table 3-11).

Looking at Dr. A's inpatient services utilization and costs, the 1.7 admission rate is only slightly under the average of 2.0, and the length of stay (LOS) for Dr. A's inpatients is 1.4 days, under the overall average LOS of 2.0 days. The total cost of Dr. A's inpatients is $69,600, well under the overall average for the pediatricians of $112,320. Dr. A's average cost per inpatient admission is also less than the overall average ($3,314 vs. $4,680).

Dr. C is the Pine Tree Medical Group pediatrician with the highest average cost per inpatient admission ($6,470), much higher than the overall average of 4,680. Table 3-12 shows Dr. C's admissions in more detail, by individual patient (coded with inpatient numbers IP-1 through IP-23), so the source of the higher costs may be identified. For the first quarter of FY 2003, Dr. C admitted 12 patients with only a 1-day LOS, 6 patients with

Orthopedic			ER[2]			Total FY 2003			Average FY 2003
Referrals	Referral Rate/100 Visits	Paid Charges	ER Utilization (Visits)	ER Utilization Rate/100 Visits	Paid Charges	Referrals	Referral Rate/100 Visits	Paid Charges	Costs per Referral
64	5.3	$11,520	77	6.3	$15,400	261	21.4	$48,520	$185.90
75	6.2	$13,500	140	11.6	$28,000	321	26.6	$60,580	$188.72
42	3.4	$7,560	63	5.1	$12,600	194	15.8	$36,180	$186.49
73	5.5	$13,140	94	7.0	$18,800	278	20.8	$51,920	$186.76
81	7.4	$14,580	118	10.8	$23,600	289	26.4	$54,380	$188.17
335	**n/a**	**$60,300**	**492**	**n/a**	**$98,400**	**1,343**	**n/a**	**$251,580**	**n/a**
67.0	**5.5**	**$12,060**	**98.4**	**8.1**	**$19,680**	**268.6**	**22.1**	**$50,316**	**$187.33**

2 days LOS, and 3 patients with 3 days LOS. However, one patient (IP-10) was in the hospital for 8 days, and one patient (IP-13) was in the hospital for 21 days. At $2,400 per patient-day, these two patients alone account for a great deal of the average LOS and costs for Dr. C.

These patients illustrate the concept of **outliers** (values considerably above or below the expected range or overall average). In health care, the focus is typically on the higher values, which usually represent the cost or utilization of a provider or patient.

In the case of Dr. C, patients IP-10 and IP-13 illustrate outlier utilization and costs, as 8 days LOS and 13 days LOS are considerably higher than the overall average of 2.7 days LOS. The costs for patients IP-10 and IP-13 were $19,200 and $50,400, respectively, much higher than the overall average inpatient cost of $6,470. The medical director must analyze these unusually high LOS and high-cost admissions to determine if utilization and costs were appropriately controlled by Dr. C. By identifying outliers, the sources of the unusually high costs are recognized and may then be analyzed or addressed.

In the example given in Table 3-12, it is fairly easy to identify the outliers that

TABLE 3-9

Pine Tree Medical Group, Pediatric PCPs, Orthopedic Specialty Care Visits and Costs, 1st Q, FY 2003[1]

Orthopedic Specialists	Referrals	Referral Visits	Referral Charges	Average Visits per Referral	Average Cost per Referral Visit
Dr. Q	91	482	$11,520	5.3	$126.59
Dr. R	45	37	$13,500	0.8	$300.00
Dr. S	29	109	$7,560	3.8	$260.69
Dr. T	38	188	$13,140	4.9	$345.79
Dr. U	132	394	$14,580	3.0	$110.45
Total	**335**	**1,210**	**$60,300**	**n/a**	**n/a**
Average	**67**	**242**	**$12,060**	**3.6**	**$228.71**

[1] Charges exclude lab, x-ray, and other additional costs.

Pine Tree Medical Group, Pediatric PCPs, Orthopedic Specialty Care Other Costs, 1st Q, FY 2003[1]

Orthopedic Specialists	Referrals	Lab per Referral	Lab Charges	X-ray	X-ray Charges	Other Procedure	Other Procedure Charges	Pharmacy Rx	Pharmacy Rx Charges	Total Other Specialty Costs	Total Other Specialty Costs per Referral
Dr. Q	91	2.1	$4,778	2.2	$24,024	1.0	$9,100	2.9	$4,750	$42,652	$468.70
Dr. R	45	2.7	$3,038	1.7	$9,180	1.2	$5,400	3.8	$3,078	$20,696	$459.90
Dr. S	29	1.6	$1,160	1.2	$4,176	0.9	$2,610	3.0	$1,566	$9,512	$328.00
Dr. T	38	1.7	$1,615	1.1	$5,016	1.1	$4,180	3.6	$2,462	$13,273	$349.30
Dr. U	132	1.9	$6,270	1.3	$20,592	0.8	$10,560	3.7	$8,791	$46,213	$350.10
Total	**335**	n/a	**$16,860**	n/a	**62,988**	n/a	**$31,850**	n/a	**20,648**	**$132,346**	n/a
Average	**67.0**	**2.0**	**$3,372**	**1.5**	**$12,598**	**1.0**	**$6,370**	**3.4**	**$4,130**	**$26,469**	**$391.20**

[1] Lab charges estimated as $25 per procedure; x-ray $120 per procedure; other $100 per procedure; pharmacy $18 per Rx.

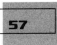

○ **TABLE 3 · 11**

Pine Tree Medical Group, Pediatric PCPs, Inpatient Care Services by PCP, 1st Q, FY 2003[1]

PCP	PCP Visits	Admissions	Admission Rate/100 Visits	ALOS	Total Days	Total Cost	Average Cost per Admission
Dr. A	1,218	21	1.7	1.4	29	$69,600	$3,314
Dr. B	1,209	30	2.5	2.1	63	$151,200	$5,040
Dr. C	1,225	23	1.9	2.7	62	$148,800	$6,470
Dr. D	1,339	17	1.3	1.3	22	$52,800	$3,106
Dr. E	1,093	29	2.7	2.0	58	$139,200	$4,800
Total	**6,084**	**120**	**n/a**	**n/a**	**234**	**$561,600**	**n/a**
Average	**1,217**	**24**	**2.0**	**2.0**	**47**	**$112,320**	**$4,680**

[1] $2,400 daily charge, including lab, x-ray, pharmacy, & all procedures.

account for Dr. C's high inpatient costs. It is possible to simply view the days and charges for each patient and notice that IP-10 and IP-13 differ from the usual range. In many situations, however, there are far more individual-level data and it is much more difficult to visually identify and analyze outlier values. For example, it would be more difficult to visually detect outliers in reviewing a data table of all inpatient admissions for all of the Pine Tree Medical Group pediatricians for an entire fiscal year.

One way to quickly identify whether one or more outlier values may be present that affect the overall indicators is to compare the overall average (calculated as the sum of the values divided by the number of the values) utilization or cost measure to the overall median (midpoint or middle value) measure (see Math Review at http://connection.lww.com/go/penner). The greater the difference between the average compared to the median, the greater the magnitude of the outlier value(s) on the average. If the average is larger than the median, the outlier(s) is substantially higher than average; if lower, the outlier(s) is substantially lower than average.

For example, Table 3-12 shows that the overall average LOS is 2.7 days and the overall average inpatient cost is $6, 470. By comparison, the median value for LOS is only 1 day and the median inpatient cost is only $2,400; in other words, half of the inpatients have 1 day LOS or less and cost $2,400 or less, and half the inpatients have LOS and costs above the median values. The substantial differences between the average of 2.7 days and the median of 1 day LOS, and the average of $6,470 and the median of $2,400, indicate that one or more unusually high individual values (outliers) are affecting the overall average value.

Although comparing the average to the median allows the reviewer to determine if outliers exist, the use of tools such as percentiles (the value below which a given percentage of measures fall, reviewed in Appendix B) helps the reviewer identify the actual outlier values. For example, Table 3-12 reports the 90th percentile, or value below which 90% of the measures fall for LOS (3 days) and inpatient costs ($7,200). Outlier values include any that are above the 90th percentile, in this case IP-10 and IP-13. The level at which the percentile is set may be higher or lower than 90, depending on the typical range of values expected in a given health care setting.

In some cases, it is helpful to evaluate the utilization or cost data with the outlier data excluded to obtain a better idea of what the overall utilization or costs are for the majority of more typical cases or situations. For example, if the Pine Tree Medical Group's medical director finds that the two outlier cases for Dr. C for the first quarter of FY 2003 (see Table 3-12) are justified as the children each had more complex, long-term acute disorders, one might recalculate the average LOS and costs, reporting that the outlier values are excluded.

When the overall values for Dr. C for the first quarter of FY 2003 are recalculated, excluding IP-10 and IP-13, the average overall LOS is only 1.6 days, substantially lower than the previous average LOS of 2.7 days and less than the overall average for all the Pine Tree Medical Group pediatricians of 2.0 days. The average inpatient cost, excluding the outliers, is $3,771 as compared to the previous average inpatient cost for Dr. C of $6,470 and less than the overall average inpatient costs for all the Pine Tree Medical Group pediatricians of $4,680 (see Tables 3-11 and 3-12).

When recalculating the average utilization or cost by excluding outlier values, it is very important to report that outliers are excluded (and if possible, to identify the outliers), so the reviewer obtains a fair idea of overall performance. Outliers should not be omitted to make the performance figures appear better than they really are, but to enable comparison of indicators including uncontrollable utilization and costs with indicators based on typical utilization and costs.

TABLE 3-12

Pine Tree Medical Group, Pediatric PCPs, Inpatient Outlier Analysis by Dr. C, PCP, 1st Q, 2003

Pt ID	Days	Charges
IP-1	1	$2,400
IP-2	1	$2,400
IP-3	2	$4,800
IP-4	2	$4,800
IP-5	2	$4,800
IP-6	2	$4,800
IP-7	1	$2,400
IP-8	3	$7,200
IP-9	1	$2,400
IP-10	8	$19,200
IP-11	1	$2,400
IP-12	1	$2,400
IP-13	21	$50,400
IP-14	3	$7,200
IP-15	1	$2,400
IP-16	1	$2,400
IP-17	2	$4,800
IP-18	1	$2,400
IP-19	1	$2,400
IP-20	2	$4,800
IP-21	1	$2,400
IP-22	3	$7,200
IP-23	1	$2,400
Total	**62**	**$148,800**
Average	**2.7**	**$6,470**
Median	**1.0**	**$2,400**
90th Percentile	**3.0**	**$7,200**
Average excluding IP-10 & IP-13	**1.6**	**$3,771**

Comparison of Data and Indicators Over Time

One additional way of evaluating and analyzing managed care data and performance indicators is to report these values over time, comparing past to present performance. Table 3-13 shows overall data and indicators for Pine Tree Medical Group pediatricians. (The FY 2002 column was previously shown in this chapter as Table 3-3.) The FY 2003 column reports data and indicators obtained for all of FY 2003.

Most of the data and indicators increased for the Pine Tree Medical Group pediatricians from FY 2002 to FY 2003. One of the largest increases was paid charges, with an increase in paid charges PMPY from $480.51 to $507.46 from FY 2002 to 2003. It is possible that the increase in paid charges is related to the increase in inpatient utilization from 102.7 to 107.8 inpatient days PTMPY. The percent of paid charges estimated as IBNR decreased from 30.9% to 27.1%, and profits decreased from $425,802 to $333,289 from FY 2002 to FY 2003.

Conclusion

This chapter builds on Chapter 2 by providing an overview of approaches to financial reporting in managed care settings. Boxes 3-1 through 3-5 summarize the overall managed care data and indicators used in IPA and medical group financial management reporting that were shown in this section discussing the performance of the pediatricians at the Pine Tree Medical Group. Box 3-1 focuses on health plan members, Box 3-2 on primary care services, Box 3-3 on specialty care services, and Box 3-4 on inpatient care services. Box 3-5 provides some Internet resources for managed care financial reporting.

TABLE 3-13

Pine Tree Medical Group, Members with Pediatric PCP, Financial and Utilization Indicators, FY 2002–2003

Indicators	FY 2002	FY 2003
Total member months	**114,848**	**122,887**
Financial performance		
Total capitation revenue	**$5,024,600**	**$5,529,931**
PMPM	$43.75	$45.00
PMPY	$525.00	$540.00
Total paid charges (including IBNR)	**$4,598,798**	**$5,196,642**
PMPM	$40.04	$42.29
PMPY	$480.51	$507.46
Estimated % charges IBNR	30.9%	27.1%
Utilization		
Total PCP visits	**22,511**	**24,199**
PMPM	0.20	0.20
PMPY	2.35	2.36
Total specialty visits	**9,094**	**9,838**
PMPM	0.08	0.08
PMPY	0.95	0.96
Total inpatient days	**983**	**1,104**
PTMPY	102.7	107.8
P&L statement	**$425,802**	**$333,289**

■ CRITICAL THINKING EXERCISES

1. Review the use of averages, medians, and percentiles in identifying outliers for inpatients of the pediatricians at the Pine Tree Medical Group (refer to Math Review at http://connection.lww.com/go/penner). Calculate median values for cost and utilization by specialty, PCP, or specialist for Table 3-8, Table 3-9, or Table 3-10 and compare the median to average values. Discuss.
2. After identifying the differences between medians and averages in Exercise 1 that indicate outlier value(s), calculate percentiles to identify the outlier value(s) and discuss. How would you advise the medical director of the Pine Tree Medical Group to evaluate the outliers further?

Medical Group and IPA Cost and Utilization Data and Financial Indicators by Health Plan Member

- ■ Average capitation per member month
  - Total Capitation Revenue ÷ Member Months
- ■ Average cost PMPM
  - Total Paid Charges ÷ Member Months
- ■ PCP visits per member per year
  - Primary Care Visits ÷ Member Months × 12
- ■ Specialty referral visits per member per year
  - Referral Visits ÷ Member Months × 12
- ■ Specialty care costs PMPM
  - Total Specialty Referral Costs ÷ Member Months
- ■ Inpatient care costs PMPM
  - Total Inpatient Costs ÷ Member Months
- ■ Inpatient admissions per 1,000 members per year (PTMPY)
  - Total Admissions ÷ Member Months × 12 × 1,000
- ■ Inpatient days per 1,000 members per year
  - Total Inpatient Days ÷ Member Months × 12 × 1,000

Medical Group and IPA Cost and Utilization Data and Financial Indicators by Primary Care Services (PCP)

- ■ Primary care visits by PCP
- ■ Paid charges by PCP
- ■ Other primary care paid charges by PCP
- ■ Average cost per primary care visit
  - Paid Charges by PCP ÷ PCP Visits

Medical Group and IPA Cost and Utilization Data and Financial Indicators by Specialty Care Services

- ■ Referral costs by specialty, by PCP and by specialist
- ■ Total number of referrals and referral rates per 100 (or 1,000) PCP visits by PCP
  - Referral Rate = Referrals ÷ PCP visits × 100 (or 1,000)
- ■ Referral visits per referral by specialist
  - Referral Visits for each Specialist ÷ Total Authorized Referrals for each Specialist
- ■ Referral visits per referral by each specialty
- ■ Average referral cost by PCP
  - Total Referral Costs ÷ Referrals by PCP
- ■ Average cost per visit by specialist
  - Referral Costs by Individual Specialist ÷ Referral Visits by Individual Specialist

◻ **B O X   3 - 4**

Medical Group and IPA Cost and Utilization Data and Financial Indicators by Inpatient Care Services

■ Inpatient costs by PCP
■ Admissions and admission rates per 100 (or 1,000) PCP visits by PCP
  ● Admission Rate = Admissions ÷ PCP Visits × 100 (or 1,000)
■ Inpatient LOS and inpatient days by PCP
■ Average inpatient LOS
  ● Total Inpatient Days ÷ Total Admissions
■ Average cost per admission by PCP
  ● Inpatient Costs ÷ Admissions by PCP

◻ **B O X   3 - 5**

On-line Sources for Information on Managed Care Financial Reporting

AMA Office of Group Practice Liaison: http://www.ama-assn.org/ama/pub/category/1736.html
American College of Healthcare Executives: http://www.ache.org/
Healthcare Financial Management Association: http://www.hfma.org/
Medical Group Management Association: http://www.mgma.com/

3. Using your knowledge of your or a selected clinical discipline (such as nursing or physical therapy), create a report for a group practice or clinic using the financial indicators presented in this chapter to present utilization and cost data for nursing, physical therapy, or your selected clinical discipline.

■ R E F E R E N C E S

Getzen, T. E. (1997). *Health Economics: Fundamentals and Flow of Funds*. New York: John Wiley & Sons.
Harris-Shapiro, J., & Greenstein, M. (July/August 1999). Reducing risk under capitation: Use of analytical tools, sound actuarial analysis can help prevent financial disaster. *TIPS on Managed Care, 3*(3), 13–15.
Jacobs, P., & Rapoport, J. (2002). *The Economics of Health and Medical Care*, 5th ed. Gaithersburg, MD: Aspen.
Kirk, R. (1997). *Managing Outcomes, Process, and Cost in a Managed Care Environment*. Gaithersburg, MD: Aspen.
Knight, W. (1998). *Managed Care: What It Is and How It Works*. Gaithersburg, MD: Aspen.
Kongstvedt, P. R. (1997). *Essentials of Managed Health Care*, 2nd ed. Gaithersburg, MD: Aspen.
Kongstvedt, P. R. (2002). *Managed Care: What It Is and How It Works*, 2nd ed. Gaithersburg, MD: Aspen.
Kongstvedt, P. R. (2001). *The Managed Health Care Handbook*, 4th ed. Gaithersburg, MD: Aspen.
Penner, M. J. (1997). *Capitation in California: A Study of Physician Organizations Managing Risk*. Chicago: Health Administration Press.
Penner, M. (1999). Administrative competencies for physician organizations with capitation. *Journal of Healthcare Management, 44*(3), 185–196.
Rognehaugh, R. (1998). *The Managed Health Care Dictionary*, 2nd ed. Gaithersburg, MD: Aspen.
Senn, G. F. (May 1998). Clinical buy-in is key to benchmarking success. *Health Care Financial Management*, pp. 46–50.
Sides, R. W., & Roberts, M. A. (2000). *Accounting Handbook for Medical Practices*. New York: John Wiley & Sons.
Tinsley, R. (September/October 2001). Making the most of management tools and reporting. *TIPS on Managed Care, 5*(4), 24–27.

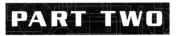

PART TWO

Budgets, Budget Monitoring, and Budget Preparation

CHAPTER 4

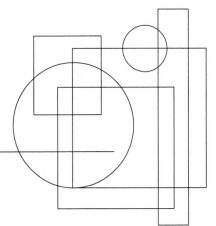

Types and Components of Budgets

☐ Learning Objectives

1. Describe the types of budgets used in health care settings and their purposes.
2. Provide examples of measures for volume in health care settings.
3. Explain the importance of monitoring cash flow in health care organizations.

◯ Key Terms

Allowable costs
Average daily census (ADC)
Average length of stay (ALOS)
Bad debt
Budget year
Capital budget
Cash flow budget (cash budget)
Charge
Charge-based reimbursement
Charity care
Cost-based reimbursement
Direct costs
Discounted charge
DRG (diagnostic related category)
Ending cash balance
Expense budget

Expense
Fiscal year (FY)
Fixed budget (static budget)
Flexible budget
Full-time equivalent (FTE)
Gross revenue
Indirect cost
Job position
Lagged value
Line item
Negotiated charge
Net revenue
Non-personnel expenses
Non-service revenue
  (non-operating revenue)
Occupancy rate
Operating budget

...continued

What comes to mind when hearing the word "budget" in health care settings? Many health care professionals think of budgets in terms of cutbacks and limits, rather than choices and possibilities. A budget is a way to review, monitor, and plan the production of goods and services. Budgets have three important managerial and financial functions: description, monitoring, and planning for inputs (financial and non-financial resources), outputs (service units such as the number of clients served), and revenues. Figure 4-1 illustrates the three major functions of budgets and also shows that these functions are interconnected. Chapter 4 focuses on the descriptive function of various types of budgets commonly encountered and reviewed in health care settings. Chapter 5 shows how budgets are used in monitoring resource use, and Chapter 6 discusses how budgets are used in planning for the future and in preparing budgets for the following year or more. Chapter 9 discusses cost allocation and cost finding, concepts used in budgeting indirect as well as direct costs.

This chapter describes and discusses elements included in typical budget reports and identifies various types of budgets seen in health care settings. The setting used throughout Chapters 4, 5, 6, and 7 is Freeston ElderCare, which provides 42 skilled nursing facility (SNF) beds, 83 intermediate care beds, and 50 assisted living units. Freeston ElderCare is one of a chain of long-term care facilities owned by XYZ Health Corporation. Marie Phillips, RN, MSN, is the administrator for Freeston ElderCare, with responsibilities for review, monitoring, and preparation of the annual operating, capital, and cash flow budgets.

The Freeston ElderCare budgets that are examined in the most detail include departments providing direct patient services: nursing services, rehabilitation, and ancillary services (laboratory and

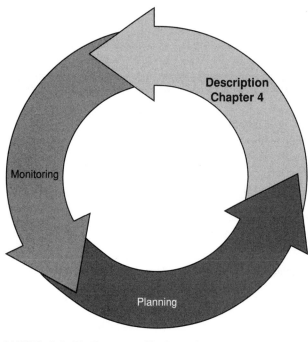

FIGURE 4.1 ■ Functions of budgets: description, monitoring, and planning.

> **BOX 4-1**
>
> **What Budgets Describe**
>
> ■ Amount and sources of volume, expense, or revenue
> ■ Decisions about resource allocation
> ■ Trends in volume, expense, or revenue
> ■ Adherence to budget guidelines, standards, and targets (budget monitoring—Chap. 5)
> ■ Plans and projections about volume, expense, and revenue (budget preparation—Chap. 6)

pharmacy). The sample budgets created in this text are often simplified for introductory applications. In many cases only the first 3 months of the fiscal year, the first-quarter totals, and the fiscal year totals are reported. The complete budget tables with all 12 calendar months reported for all Freeston ElderCare departments are in the "Supplemental Tables and Displays" section of the Back-of-Book CD-ROM.

This chapter presents key fundamental concepts required in understanding budgetary review in acute and non-acute health settings. However, it is important to learn the budget policies and practices that apply in each work setting, as they will likely differ somewhat from this text and from setting to setting. It is also essential to maintain current knowledge about changes in reimbursement (such as Medicare guidelines), staffing, and other factors affecting budgets and budgeting.

Budgets as Descriptions

The focus of this chapter is on reviewing budgets; in other words, on focusing on budgets as descriptions. Budgets describe the amount and sources of **volume**, or the numbers of clients or units of a good or service representing outputs. Budgets also describe the amount and sources of **expenses**, also referred to as inputs or costs incurred in the process of producing goods and services. Another financial activity that budgets describe is the amount and sources of **revenue**, or income derived from the reimbursement provided or the price paid for goods and services. Some types of budgets focus on volume, other budgets on expenses or revenue, and some budgets report and link all three.

Most types of budgets describe decisions about resource allocation. For example, in most health care settings personnel costs represent the greatest expense. The budget describes whether the setting allocates its personnel resources to employ a higher proportion of more costly professional staff, a higher proportion of less costly paraprofessional staff supervised by professionals, or some mix of professional and paraprofessional staff. In other situations, budgets may describe allocation of resources to purchase equipment or to develop a new program.

Trends in volume, expenses, and revenue are also described by budgets. For example, some health care settings show seasonal increases or decreases in the amount of volume, expenses, or revenue, such as increased hospital admissions for respiratory disorders during winter months when influenza and pneumonia are more prevalent. Other settings may show increases or decreases in volume, expenses, or revenue continuing over time.

Budgets describe adherence to financial goals (discussed in Chap. 5) in relation to budget monitoring. Budgets also present plans and projections about volume, expenses, and revenue (discussed in Chap. 6) related to budget preparation. Box 4-1 summarizes what health care budgets typically describe.

Budget Components

Most budgets encountered in health care contain certain elements or components. The specific sources and types of budget items listed in each line (row) of the budget are an important component to examine in

TABLE 4-1

Freeston ElderCare Rehabilitation Operating Expense Budget, 1st Quarter 2003

7300	Rehabilitation Department	FTE	Amount	Type	January Budget	February Budget	March Budget	Q1 Budget	FY 2003 Budget
001	Rehabilitation Dir./Physical Therapist	1.0	$4,992	Monthly	$4,992	$4,992	$4,992	$14,976	$59,904
002	Occupational Therapist	0.5	$4,866	Monthly	$2,433	$2,433	$2,433	$7,299	$29,196
003	PT Aide	1.0	$2,993	Monthly	$2,993	$2,993	$2,993	$8,979	$35,916
004	OT Aide	0.5	$2,888	Monthly	$1,444	$1,444	$1,444	$4,332	$17,328
110	**Rehabilitation Payroll**				**$11,862**	**$11,862**	**$11,862**	**$35,586**	**$142,344**
120	Benefits		25% of Payroll		$2,966	$2,966	$2,966	$8,898	$35,586
200	**Rehabilitation Personnel**				**$14,828**	**$14,828**	**$14,828**	**$44,484**	**$177,930**
220	Medical Supplies		$585	Monthly	$585	$585	$585	$1,755	$7,020
230	Medical Equipment		$193	Monthly	$193	$193	$193	$579	$2,316
290	Other Non-Personnel		$78	Monthly	$78	$78	$78	$234	$936
300	**Rehabilitation Non-Personnel**				**$856**	**$856**	**$856**	**$2,568**	**$10,272**
	Total Rehabilitation				**$15,684**	**$15,684**	**$15,684**	**$47,052**	**$188,202**

reviewing budgets. Another important component is information on the calculation of budget amounts, including subtotals and totals of budget line items. The time period specified in the budget is a third budget component required of all budgets.

Line Items

The specific types of items in each line (or row) of the budget are known as **line items**. Line items represent categories of volume, expense, or revenue defined and coded by the institution as a way to organize the budget. Codes are frequently used to identify groups of line items as well as individual line items, followed by a brief description that defines the line item. Table 4-1 presents examples of line item coding and description for expense budget items reported by the Rehabilitation Department at Freeston ElderCare.

The group code identifies the overall source of volume, expense, or revenue, such as a department or cost center (discussed in Chap. 7). The Rehabilitation Department is coded as 7300, so that any item of expense generated by the Rehabilitation Department falls under the group code 7300, which is included with the department name in the header line of Table 4-1. In this way, the source of expenses for items such as personnel benefits or medical supplies may immediately be traced to the Rehabilitation Department.

The line item code identifies the associated line item. Two major categories of line items include **personnel expenses** (costs for employee salaries, wages, and benefits) and **non-personnel expenses** (non-employee costs for items such as supplies, some equipment, and contracted services). Budgets reporting both personnel and non-personnel expenses usually separate personnel and non-personnel items. Many health care settings report personnel budgets in somewhat more detail than non-personnel budgets because the largest source of cost is typically for personnel.

Line items and their associated codes may be specific or may represent summarized information. Table 4-1 shows that at Freeston ElderCare, specific line items for the Rehabilitation Department end with an integer from 1 to 9, while summarized line items end in 0 or 00. For example, the line items for personnel employed in the Rehabilitation Department are coded from 001 (the director and physical therapist) to 004 (occupational therapy aide). The summary line item for hourly payroll for all the Rehabilitation Department employees is 110, and the summary line item for all personnel expenses is 200. In other words, the 7300-200 code represents all salary and benefits expenses for all of the personnel employed in the Rehabilitation Department at Freeston ElderCare.

The non-personnel expenses in the Rehabilitation Department are coded according to a similar logic, as shown in Table 4-1. Medical supplies (items such as adhesive tape and splints) are grouped under the code number 220. Medical equipment, which includes items such as walkers and crutches, is grouped under the code number 230. The code number specific to walkers is 221 and to crutches is 222, and the code summarizing all Rehabilitation Department non-personnel expense items is 300.

Coding systems differ among health care settings but are likely to identify specific budget items and groups of budget items. Detailed line items enable the reviewer to look very closely at amounts and sources of volume, revenue, and expense and obtain a more precise understanding of the financial activities in the setting. Summary line items contain less detail but provide the reviewer a general, overall understanding. Further uses of both detailed and summarized line items for budget monitoring and planning are provided in Chapters 5 and 6.

Budget Calculations

After identifying the line items and their coding, a next step in reviewing a budget is to determine how the amounts entered in budget lines are reported and calculated. To understand budget reports, it is important to understand what the budgeted amounts represent. This discussion focuses on knowing the calculation of budget amounts in order to review a budget. Concepts required for making estimates and preparing a new budget are presented in Chapter 6.

Looking at the Freeston ElderCare Rehabilitation Department expense budget (see Table 4-1), the group and line item code for the department director (also the physical therapist) is shown. The next column indicates the **full-time equivalent (FTE)**, which represents 40 hours of work per week (weekends excluded), multiplied by 52 weeks for a year, resulting in 2,080 work hours per year, as shown in the formula:

$$FTE = 40 \text{ hours per week} \times 52 \text{ weeks}$$

$$FTE = 2,080 \text{ hours/year}$$

When reporting personnel budget items in health care settings, FTEs are typically reported instead of the number of employees. **Job positions** specify how many full-time (one FTE) or part-time (portion of an FTE) employees may be hired; for example, two job positions of 0.5 FTE each equals one job position of 1.0 FTE. FTEs are a more accurate measure of personnel resource use in many health care settings than a count of employees or job positions. Table 4-1 shows that there is one full-time (1.0 FTE) director and physical therapist, a part-time occupational therapist working half-time (0.5 FTE), a full-time physical therapy aide, and a half-time occupational therapy aide.

Table 4-1 then shows a column for budget amounts. The monthly salary is indicated for one FTE for each of the positions in the Rehabilitation Department expense budget. To find the monthly salary for each of the budgeted positions, it is necessary to multiply the monthly salary by the FTE. For example, the monthly salary for the half-time occupational therapist is calculated as follows:

$$Budgeted \text{ OT Monthly Salary} = OT \text{ Monthly Salary} \times OT \text{ FTE}$$

$$\$2,433 = \$4,866 \times 0.5$$

In other words, the half-time occupational therapist earns half the occupational therapist salary budgeted for 1.0 FTE, as indicated in the monthly budgeted amounts for this line item. In the section on flexible personnel budgeting, budget calculations using FTEs are discussed further.

Although the types of budget calculations differ among health care settings, most budgets include subtotals and total calculations.

Following the salary amounts for the personnel line items, Table 4-1 shows the calculation of benefits for the Rehabilitation Department. The summary of benefits (including health insurance, pension, and worker's compensation insurance) amounts to 25% of the monthly payroll, so is calculated by multiplying the total monthly payroll by 25%. For January 2003, benefits amount to 25% of $11,862, or $2,966. The personnel expense budget subtotal amounts of $11,862 for total monthly payroll and $2,966 for benefits are then added, for a total monthly personnel expense of $14,828 for January 2003. Note that the budgeted amounts for the remaining months of FY 2003 are the same as for January.

The non-personnel section of the expense budget for the Freeston ElderCare Rehabilitation Department is also shown in Table 4-1. Summary line items are shown in the non-personnel part of the expense budget, with medical supplies budgeted at $585 per month, medical equipment at $193 per month, and other non-personnel expenses (such as subscriptions and office supplies) at $78 per month. The total Rehabilitation Department non-personnel expense budget totals $856 per month ($585 + $193 + $78). The subtotals for the Rehabilitation Department personnel expenses ($14,828) and non-personnel expenses ($856) are then added to calculate the total monthly Rehabilitation Department expenses of $15,684.

Budgeting Time Period

Budgets describe volume, revenues, and expenses as calculated over specified time periods. Most budgets, particularly those used at the department or program level, are prepared over a calendar year (January 1 through December 31) or **fiscal year (FY)**, a 12-month period designated by organizational policy for financial reporting.

In some settings, the fiscal year is referred to as the **budget year**. July 1 through June 30 is frequently selected as a fiscal year, although the time frame selection may differ based on the organization's cycles of funding or financial activity. Institutional level budgets may extend to a time frame of 2, 5, or 10 years, frequently reflecting planning and projections into the future as well as comparison with the previous years' performance.

As in the case of line items, the budget's time frame may be reported at various levels of detail. Most budgets used at the department or program level are reported monthly; in some cases, when closer review is required, weekly budget reports may be provided. Quarterly reports (prepared every 3 months) provide summaries of budgets throughout the fiscal year. Table 4-1 shows monthly, quarterly, and annual subtotals and totals. The total quarterly budget for the Rehabilitation Department represents the sum of the total budget amounts for January, February and March, or $47,052 ($15,684 + $15,684 + $15,684). Annual expense budget amounts are calculated as the sum of all 12 months in FY 2003. The total budget for the Freeston ElderCare Rehabilitation Department for FY 2003 amounts to $188,202.

Types of Budgets

Various types of budgets are commonly seen in health care settings, each serving a specific purpose. The annual statistics budget, operating budget, and capital budget are discussed in detail, as they are the budgets most frequently reviewed. The cash flow budget is also presented in detail, as it helps in understanding the importance of adequate cash flow to the financial health of institutions. Other budgets introduced in this chapter include the product line budget and the special purpose budget. The various aspects or approaches to budgets and budgeting may differ from one work setting to another, and from the conventions used in this text.

Statistics Budget

The **statistics budget** presents an estimate or forecast of the volume of service units (such as goods sold, procedures completed, or patients) over the fiscal year. The statistics budget provides a basis for the estimates used in the operating and cash flow budgets. A statistics budget is particularly helpful in **flexible budgeting** (discussed in the operating budget section), in which budgeted revenues and expenses are linked to volume. Table 4-2 presents the statistics budget for the SNF unit at Freeston ElderCare. Each SNF bed type is itemized in the statistics budget by a group number (indicating the level of care), line number (indicating payor source), and a brief description. Volume is reported in several ways, as is common in most 24-hour health care settings.

The basis for volume reporting is the use of **patient days**, or the number of days a patient occupies a 24-hour bed over a specified time period. Monthly reports of patient days are calculated by adding the daily patient census figures for all the days of that month. Table 4-2 shows that the patient days for private pay SNF patients for January 2003 are 217. Patient days for private pay SNF patients for the first quarter of FY 2003 are 512 (a total of all daily census amounts for the quarter) and for FY 2003 are 1,887.

The monthly **average daily census (ADC)** is calculated by dividing the number of patient days for a specific time period by the number of days in that time period. The ADC informs the reviewer about the number of patients, on average, occupying a 24-hour bed on any given day of a specified time period. Table 4-2 shows that the budgeted ADC for private pay SNF patients for January 2003 is 7 (217 patient days ÷ 31 days in January). The ADC for private pay SNF patients for the first quarter of 2003 is 5.7 (512 patient days ÷ 90 days in the quarter), and for FY 2003 is 5.2.

The number of admissions, or patients entering a 24-hour facility, is another measure of volume. Table 4-2 shows that there are eight budgeted admissions for private pay SNF patients for January 2003. For the first quarter, 21 admissions are budgeted, and 69 for FY 2003. Using patient days and admissions, the

○ TABLE 4-2

Freeston ElderCare, SNF Unit Statistics Budget, 2003

Line #	4511 SNF Revenue Item	FY 2003 Budget ALOS	January Budget	February Budget	March Budget	Q1 2003 Budget	FY 2003 Budget
501	Private Pay SNF Patient Days		217	140	155	512	1,887
	Private Pay SNF ADC		7	5	5	5.7	5.2
	Private Pay SNF Admissions	27.3	8	7	6	21	69
551	Managed Care SNF Patient Days		341	308	341	990	4,015
	Managed Care SNF ADC		11	11	11	11.0	11.0
	Managed Care SNF Admissions	33.5	12	11	10	33	120
555	Medicaid SNF Patient Days		217	196	248	661	3,136
	Medicaid SNF ADC		7	7	8	7.3	8.6
	Medicaid SNF Admissions	39.2	8	7	7	22	80
557	Medicare SNF Patient Days		217	196	217	630	3,106
	Medicare SNF ADC		7	7	7	7.0	8.5
	Medicare SNF Admissions	30.8	9	10	9	101	101
565	Managed Care Hospice Patient Days		62	56	62	180	730
	Managed Care Hospice ADC		2	2	2	2.0	2.0
	Managed Care Hospice Admissions	60.8	2	0	2	4	12
	Total SNF Patient Days		**1,054**	**896**	**1,023**	**2,973**	**12,874**
	SNF Average Daily Census		**34**	**32**	**33**	**33.0**	**35.3**
	SNF Admissions	**33.7**	**39**	**35**	**34**	**108**	**382**
	SNF Occupancy Rate (42 beds)		**81.0%**	**76.2%**	**78.6%**	**78.7%**	**84.0%**
	Calendar Days		31	28	31	90	365

average length of stay (ALOS) may be calculated, which reports the number of days, on average, a patient occupies a 24-hour bed. ALOS is typically calculated on an annual basis. For FY 2003, the ALOS for private pay SNF patients is calculated as follows:

$$\text{ALOS Private Pay SNF FY 2003} = \text{Patient Days} \div \text{Admissions}$$

$$27.3 = 1,887 \div 69$$

In other words, on average, a private pay SNF patient is budgeted to occupy a bed for 27.3 days in FY 2003. Some settings calculate ALOS by dividing the number of patient days by the number of discharges rather than the number of admissions.

One additional volume measure commonly used in health care settings providing 24-hour care is the **occupancy rate**, which reports the percentage of 24-hour beds to which patients are assigned over a specified time period. The occupancy rate is calculated by dividing the ADC by the number of beds available in a facility, department, or program. For example, Table 4-2 shows that for January 2003 the occupancy rate for the SNF at Freeston ElderCare is 81.0% (ADC of 34÷42 beds available). In Table 4-2, subtotals are calculated for SNF bed types, then total figures for the entire SNF unit are presented.

Box 4-2 summarizes items commonly described by a 24-hour care statistics budget. Statistics budget settings such as an outpatient clinic use volume measures such as the number of patient visits or the number of laboratory tests. Some settings, such as surgery departments, measure the volume of procedures. Other settings measure the volume of health care goods, such as prescription medications or medical equipment.

☐ B O X   4 - 2

What 24-hour Care Statistics Budgets Describe

■ Patient days for a specified unit or bed type over a specified time period
■ Average daily census (patient days ÷ days in specified time period) for a specified unit or bed type
■ Average length of stay (patient days ÷ admissions) for a specified unit or bed type over a fiscal year
■ Occupancy rate (occupied beds ÷ available beds) for a specified unit or bed type over a specified time period

---

Freeston ElderCare Statistics Budget
The complete FY 2003 statistics budget for the SNF, intermediate care, and assisted living units at Freeston ElderCare is found in the "Supplemental Tables and Documents" section of the Back-of-Book CD-ROM. This statistics budget reports patient days, ADC, ALOS, and occupancy rate as volume measures. Note the volume varies from month to month for each of these units.

Operating Budget
The **operating budget** is an itemized summary of the revenues and expenses generated by a program, department, or institution over a specified period of time (usually a fiscal year) related to the generation of goods or services (operations). The following sections describe and discuss the expense and revenue sections of the operating budget in detail, as they are among the most frequently used reports for financial activities in health care settings. Note that data summarized from the statistics budget (such as patient days) are included as a line in many operating budgets and are used in many of the operating budget calculations. The operating expense budget is discussed, then the operating revenue budget.

Operating Expense Budget
The operating **expense budget** includes all of the line items and their dollar estimates associated with the operating costs. In other words, the operating expense budget represents the "expense" side of the operating budget. The two major components of the operating expense budget are personnel expenses and non-personnel expenses. Operating expense budgets largely represent **direct costs**, which are incurred in the provision of health care goods or services. Nursing personnel and medical supplies are examples of direct costs.

In some cases, operating expense budgets may include a budget line for **indirect costs** (also referred to as administrative costs) that include the costs of operating the institution as a whole, or costs incurred indirectly in the provision of health care goods or services. Laundry and housekeeping are examples of indirect costs. This textbook defines **overhead** as a specified amount or rate of indirect costs that are included as a line in the operating expense budget per organizational policy (the terms "indirect costs," "administrative costs," and "overhead" are often used interchangeably).

Marie Phillips, the administrator for Freeston ElderCare, is not required to add overhead to the nursing services or other department or program budgets. However, the operating expense budgets for departments at Freeston ElderCare such as administration, laundry, housekeeping, and plant operations represent indirect costs. Chapter 7 discusses these indirect costs in more detail, and presents reports accounting for indirect costs.

Fixed and Flexible Budgets. Before reviewing the components of an operating budget, it is important to discuss two approaches to budgeting for operations frequently encountered in health care settings. The **fixed budget** (also referred to as a static budget) itemizes expenses (or revenues, discussed in the operating revenue budget section) for an unchanging (fixed) volume of service units. Over the course of a fiscal year, a fixed budget is expected to remain the same regardless of volume.

For example, the FY 2003 budget for the Rehabilitation Department at Freeston ElderCare is a fixed budget (see Table 4-1). The personnel (physical therapist, occupational therapist, and aides) are hired on a permanent basis to work their scheduled FTEs over FY 2003 regardless of any changes in volume. The budget amounts for personnel remain unchanged (fixed) from month to month. The Rehabilitation Department non-personnel budget is also fixed, with the same amounts budgeted for items such as supplies and equipment from month to month.

Flexible budgeting adjusts the operating expense budget based on variation in volume, which changes the costs required to provide goods or services. Volume variation also changes revenues, which is further explained in the section discussing the operating revenue budget. In many health care settings, including hospitals and other 24-hour care facilities, volume varies from day to day. The difference in volume between time periods, or **volume variance**, changes personnel and non-personnel expenses that are closely related to volume. For example, personnel expenses based on hours of direct care per patient day are expected to increase as volume increases and decrease as volume decreases. These variable expenses represent costs that are expected to vary given volume variance over the fiscal year.

Flexible Budgeting for Personnel Expenses. Table 4-3 presents a personnel budget worksheet for the 24-hour nursing services units (SNF and intermediate care) at Freeston ElderCare. The overall group (department or cost center) code is 7200 for Nursing Services, with subgroup numbers of 7210 for the SNF unit and 7220 for the Intermediate Care Unit. This enables the review of Nursing Services as a whole, or of each of its service units. Each unit provides 3.6 total direct hours of care per patient day (PPD), with fewer direct hours assigned to RNs and LPNs compared to CNAs. The hours are allocated differently for the SNF unit compared to the intermediate care unit.

The first line reports the SNF budgeted patient days (see the statistics budget, Table 4-2). This information on volume is important because it provides the basis for flexible budgeting and scheduling of direct care nursing staff. The line following the SNF patient days reports the RN direct hours (hours of nursing care directly provided to patients). RNs in the SNF unit are budgeted to provide 0.2 hours of direct care PPD. For January 2003, there are 1,054 SNF patient days, so the monthly direct hours are calculated as follows:

$$\text{RN Direct Hours January 2003} = \text{Direct Hours PPD} \times \text{Patient Days}$$
$$211 = 0.2 \times 1,054$$

In other words, 211 hours of RN direct care staff are budgeted for January 2003 (direct hours are rounded to the nearest hour). LPNs in the SNF unit are budgeted to provide 1.0 hour of direct care PPD, so they are scheduled for 1,054 hours, and CNAs are budgeted to provide 2.4 direct hours PPD, so they are scheduled for 2,530 hours for January 2003.

Nursing Services direct care personnel expenses are then calculated in the line following the SNF unit RN direct hours by multiplying the RN direct hours by the average hourly wage. In the column for FTE the direct care staff are designated as "var," or variable staff, because their scheduling varies (as indicated in the flexible budget) based on volume. An average hourly wage is used for simplicity, but in most work settings, each employee's hourly wage differs based on seniority and other factors, so it is calculated individually and then totaled. For January 2003, RN direct care personnel expenses are calculated as follows:

$$\text{January 2003 RN Expense} = \text{RN Direct Hours} \times \text{Average Hourly RN Wage}$$
$$\$6,181 = 211 \times \$29.32$$

The RN direct care personnel expense for the SNF unit for January 2003 is $6,181. The direct care personnel expense for LPNs is $19,394 and for CNAs is $27,117, totaling $52,692 in direct care nursing staff hourly wages for January 2003.

TABLE 4-3

Freeston ElderCare Nursing Services Direct Hours Worksheet and Personnel Expense Budget, 2003

Line #	7200 Nursing Services Item	FTE	Amount	Type	January Budget	February Budget	March Budget	Q1 Budget	FY 2003 Budget
010	Director of Nursing	1.0	$5,433	Monthly	$5,433	$5,433	$5,433	$16,299	$65,196
008	N.S. Clerical	1.0	$2,598	Monthly	$2,598	$2,598	$2,598	$7,794	$31,176
120	Benefits		25%	of Salaries	$2,008	$2,008	$2,008	$6,023	$24,093
130	**Nursing Administration Personnel**				**$10,039**	**$10,039**	**$10,039**	**$30,116**	**$120,465**
	7210 SNF Patient Days				**1,054**	**896**	**1,023**	**2,973**	**12,874**
	RN Direct Hours	0.2		Direct Care Hours PPD	211	179	205	595	2,575
001	RN Expense	var	$29.32	Wage	$6,181	$5,254	$5,999	$17,434	$75,493
	LPN Direct Hours	1.0		Direct Care Hours PPD	1,054	896	1,023	2,973	12,874
002	LPN Expense	var	$18.40	Wage	$19,394	$16,486	$18,823	$54,703	$236,882
	CNA Direct Hours	2.4		Direct Care Hours PPD	2,530	2,150	2,455	7,135	30,898
003	CNA Expense	var	$10.72	Wage	$27,117	$23,052	$26,320	$76,489	$331,222
110	**SNF Direct Care Wages**				**$52,692**	**$44,793**	**$51,142**	**$148,626**	**$643,597**
115	Overtime (150% of hourly wage)		4%	of Direct Care Hours	$3,161	$2,688	$3,069	$8,918	$38,616
120	Benefits		25%	of Wages	$13,173	$11,198	$12,785	$37,157	$160,899
130	**Total SNF Personnel**				**$69,026**	**$58,679**	**$66,996**	**$194,700**	**$843,112**
	SNF PPD				$65.50	$65.50	$65.50	$65.50	$65.50

(table continues on page 74)

TABLE 4 - 3 (continued)

Freeston ElderCare Nursing Services Direct Hours Worksheet and Personnel Expense Budget, 2003

Line #	7200 Nursing Services Item	FTE	Amount	Type	January Budget	February Budget	March Budget	Q1 Budget	FY 2003 Budget
	7,220 Intermediate Care Patient Days				**2,139**	**1,960**	**2,170**	**6,269**	**26,254**
	RN Direct Hours			Direct Care Hours PPD	214	196	217	627	2,625
001	RN Expense	var	$29.32	Wage	$6,272	$5,747	$6,362	$18,381	$76,977
	LPN Direct Hours			Direct Care Hours PPD	1,070	980	1,085	3,135	13,127
002	LPN Expense	var	$18.40	Wage	$19,679	$18,032	$19,964	$57,675	$241,537
	CNA Direct Hours			Direct Care Hours PPD	6,417	5,880	6,510	18,807	78,762
003	CNA Expense	var	$10.72	Wage	$68,790	$63,034	$69,787	$201,611	$844,329
110	**Intermediate Care Unit Direct Care Wages**				**$94,741**	**$86,812**	**$96,114**	**$277,667**	**$1,162,842**
115	Overtime (150% of hourly wage)		3%	of Direct Care Hours	$4,263	$3,907	$4,325	$12,495	$52,328
120	Benefits		25%	of Wages	$23,685	$21,703	$24,028	$69,417	$290,711
130	**Total Intermediate Care Unit Personnel**				**$122,689**	**$112,422**	**$124,467**	**$359,578**	**$1,505,881**
	Intermediate Care Unit PPD				$57.40	$57.40	$57.40	$57.40	$57.40
200	**Total Nursing Services Personnel**				**$201,754**	**$181,139**	**$201,502**	**$584,395**	**$2,469,458**

The direct hours and personnel expenses for SNF nursing staff vary between January, February, and March 2003. Although the budgeted direct hours PPD and hourly wages remain the same, the direct hours and budgeted personnel expenses increase or decrease with the patient days. The budget is flexible, varying based on volume variance. As a result, the SNF budgeted hourly wages of $52,692 for January is not "over budget" compared to February ($44,792), but reflects that the budgeted patient days for January are higher than for February (1,054 vs. 896).

Following the line for the SNF direct care wages, the amount of overtime is budgeted as 4% of the total SNF direct care hours, with an hourly wage 50% higher than the standard hourly wage. To calculate overtime averaged across all the SNF staff levels, 4% of the total SNF direct care wages are multiplied by 1.5, as follows:

$$\text{SNF Overtime} = 4\% \text{ of SNF Direct Care Wages} \times \text{Overtime Hourly Wage Increase}$$

$$\$3,161 = 0.04 \times \$52,692 \times 1.5$$

The budgeted overtime for the Freeston ElderCare SNF unit for January 2003 is $3,161. Note that for simplification overtime is calculated across all staff levels, but in many settings overtime would be budgeted separately for RNs and other levels of staff, and thus would be calculated separately for each staff level, then totaled.

Benefits are calculated for the SNF hourly nursing staff as 25% of direct care wages. Although in many settings some benefits would be added to the overtime wages, it is not done in this example for simplicity. Therefore, the benefits for the hourly SNF nursing staff for January is $13,173 (25% × $52,692). Budgeted direct care wages, overtime wages, and benefits total $69,026 for the Freeston ElderCare SNF nursing staff for January 2003.

The final line of the budget worksheet shown in Table 4-3 is a calculation of SNF personnel expenses PPD. Depending on the work setting, budget reports may or may not include this calculation, which is the total personnel expense divided by the number of patient days. The PPD expense for January 2003 is calculated as follows:

$$\text{SNF Unit Personnel Expense PPD} = \text{Total SNF Unit Personnel Expense} \div \text{SNF Patient Days}$$

$$\$65.50 = \$69,026 \div 1,054$$

The SNF PPD personnel expense represents the average personnel expense PPD.

Direct hours and personnel expenses of intermediate care nursing staff are calculated in the same way as for the SNF staff, with $94,741 direct care wages for January 2003 and total intermediate care unit personnel expenses of $122,689. Many 24-hour settings use this or a similar approach to report budgeted direct hours and personnel expenses. The total budgeted costs for Nursing Services personnel are $201,754 for January, $584,395 for the first quarter, and $2,469,458 for FY 2003.

Flexible Budgeting for Non-Personnel Expenses. Table 4-4 shows the non-personnel expense budget for Nursing Services at Freeston ElderCare. For simplicity, the non-personnel budget combines items used by the SNF and intermediate care units, as well as Nursing Administration. The non-personnel expense budget shows a mix of fixed and flexible budget lines. The two lines of the budget following the line for patient days are flexible budget items, medical supplies and medical waste disposal. The costs for flexible budget non-personnel items are directly tied to volume, so that for medical supplies expenses budgeted at $13.82 PPD, the budgeted expense for January 2003 is $44,127 ($13.82 × 3,162). As volume changes from January through March, the expenses for flexible budget items change accordingly.

Nursing Services also includes fixed budget items as expenses, such as a budget line for medical equipment (the purchase of five wheelchairs) at $205 per month. The total Nursing Services non-personnel expense budget is $48,088 for January, $139,238 for the first quarter, and $589,158 for FY 2003.

TABLE 4 - 4

Freeston ElderCare Nursing Services Non-Personnel Expense Budget, 2003

Line #	Items	Amount	Type	January Budget	February Budget	March Budget	Q1 Budget	FY 2003 Budget
7200	**Total SNF & Intermediate Care Patient Days**			**3,193**	**2,856**	**3,193**	**9,242**	**39,128**
220	Medical Supplies	$13.82	PPD	$44,127	$39,470	$44,127	$127,724	$540,749
215	Medical Waste	$1.09	PPD	$3,480	$3,113	$3,480	$10,074	$42,650
230	Medical Equipment	$205	Monthly	$205	$205	$205	$615	$2,460
210	Education & Training	$155	Monthly	$155	$155	$155	$465	$1,860
270	Copy & Printing	$75	Monthly	$75	$75	$75	$225	$900
280	Office Supplies	$45	Monthly	$45	$45	$45	$135	$540
300	**Nursing Services Non-Personnel**			**$48,088**	**$43,063**	**$48,088**	**$139,238**	**$589,158**

Freeston ElderCare Operating Expense Budget. The Freeston ElderCare operating expense budget, including all of the departments and major expense items, is in the "Supplemental Tables and Documents" section of the Back-of-Book CD-ROM. Using the concepts and calculations provided throughout this section, the reader should be able to review the budget and identify fixed and flexible budgeting approaches. For simplicity, it is assumed there are 50 individual assisted living units, although in some settings two persons (such as a married couple) occupy an assisted living unit. The budget line for depreciation is discussed in Chapter 10.

Operating Revenue Budget

The **revenue budget** is a budget within the operating budget that represents all of the income generated by the health care setting for which the budget is prepared over a specified period of time. The revenue budget may also be referred to as the revenue side of the operating budget. Various types of revenue may be included in revenue budgets used in health care settings.

Service revenue, also referred to as patient care revenue or operating revenue, represents income derived from the primary goods or services provided in health care settings. Examples include directly providing health care, as in bedside nursing care or performing a laboratory test, and providing products for direct care such as pharmaceuticals or medical equipment. Operating revenue represents the revenue per unit multiplied by the units of volume. **Non-service revenue** or non-operating revenue is income generated from providing goods and services that are not the primary source of income or are not linked with providing direct care. For example, vending machine income and investment income represent non-service revenue.

In this text, **total revenue** is defined as operating revenue plus non-operating revenue, when a non-operating revenue line is present in the financial or budget report. However, in some settings total revenue may refer only to the total operating revenue. It is important to learn how total revenue is defined in one's own health care setting.

Most health care settings also classify revenues as either gross or net. **Gross revenue** represents the total amount charged for goods or services before any reductions are applied. **Net revenue** is revenue after reductions are applied (in other words, gross revenue less reductions). For example, assuming Freeston ElderCare charges $298 per diem for a SNF patient bed, and that there are 1,054 SNF patient days for January 2003, gross SNF revenue is calculated as follows:

$$\text{Gross Revenue} = \text{Revenue per Unit} \times \text{Volume}$$

$$\$314,092 = \$298 \times 1,054$$

Therefore, one would expect Freeston ElderCare's SNF gross revenues to total $314,092 in January 2003, prior to any reductions.

Before discussing net revenue, it is important to understand more about charges and reimbursement practices. Capitation revenue is explained in Chapter 3 as another approach to managing revenue.

Charges. The **charge**, also referred to as the list or published price, represents the full price used in calculating gross revenue before any reductions are applied. It is important to distinguish between charges, costs, and reimbursement. The charge represents the price set by the provider for a good or service, and the cost represents the expense the provider must pay to produce the good or service. **Reimbursement** represents the payment for the good or service; the **payor** or the source of reimbursement or payment is either the patient or patient's family (also referred to as private pay or self-pay) or a **third party payor**. As explained in Chapter 2, government third party payors include the Medicare and Medicaid programs, while major sources of non-governmental third party reimbursement include commercial health insurance and managed care contracts.

There are various approaches to reimbursement among payors for health care. One of the first approaches was **charge-based reimbursement**, in which the provider bills the payor for the full charges the provider establishes for the good or service. The charge-based reimbursement system is similar to many other purchases people might make, such as for groceries. A similar approach is **cost-based reimbursement**, in which the payor agrees to pay **allowable costs**, or costs directly related to the services provided. As this approach does not allow for controlling excessive charges or unnecessary costs in health care, most payors today use other reimbursement approaches. Freeston ElderCare's SNF bed charge of $298 per diem is rarely reimbursed in full.

An increasingly popular reimbursement approach is to use **negotiated charges**, in which the payor, frequently a managed care plan, negotiates a reduced rate that is less than the charge, or an enhanced level of care for the rate reimbursed to the provider. The managed care contracts at Freeston ElderCare for SNF ($248 per diem) and hospice ($235 per diem) are examples of negotiated charges. The managed care hospice contract was just negotiated for FY 2003, a new venture for Freeston ElderCare.

A **discounted charge** differs from a negotiated charge because it is a non-negotiated flat fee reimbursed by the payor that is less than the provider's full charge. The Medicaid SNF reimbursement of $215 per diem is an example of discounting. Freeston ElderCare accepts the discounted fee and attempts to control costs accordingly. (Actual Medicaid rates may vary from this example.)

Prospective payment, discussed in Chapter 2, is the reimbursement approach used by Medicare and some non-government insurance companies. The $262 per diem reimbursement Medicare provides for Freeston ElderCare's SNF beds represents a standard expectation of ALOS and expense based on **DRG (diagnostic related category)**, amount of nursing care required, and other factors. (Actual Medicare rates may vary from this example.)

Fixed and Flexible Revenue. Fixed and flexible budgets were explained in the section on operating expense budgets. Revenues may also be budgeted as fixed or flexible. For example, the vending machine revenue for Freeston ElderCare for FY 2003 is budgeted at $175 per month and is expected to remain stable regardless of patient volume. The revenues based on bed rates are budgeted using a flexible approach, varying with the number of budgeted patient days per month.

The SNF unit revenue budget shown in Table 4-5 is a flexible budget. For the first line, SNF private pay, the per diem bed rate is $185. With 217 patient days for private pay SNF beds in January 2003, the revenue is $40,145. Budgeted revenues for managed care SNF, Medicaid SNF, Medicare SNF, and managed care hospice are calculated in the same way, with total SNF unit revenues $242,792 for January 2003. First-quarter SNF revenues are $689,715 and FY 2003 SNF revenues are $3,004,377.

Pro Forma P&L Statement

Table 4-6 presents the last three lines of the complete operating revenue budget for Freeston ElderCare for the first 3 months, first quarter, and total FY 2003. By subtracting budgeted operating expenses from budgeted operating revenues, the **pro forma P&L**, a preliminary estimate of profit or loss, is obtained. Freeston ElderCare's budget reflects an unusually profitable facility, or a very profitable fiscal year, as profits for FY 2003 are $1,190,845, 14% of net revenue, higher than the budgeted target of $860,600 (10% of net revenue).

Freeston ElderCare Revenue Budget. The entire Freeston ElderCare revenue budget for FY 2003, including the intermediate care and assisted living units as well as other service and non-service revenues, is in the "Supplemental Tables and Documents" section of the Back-of-Book CD-ROM. All of the per diem bed rates reflect net revenues (negotiated, discounted, or prospective pay charges). The following lines report budgeted monthly service revenues for direct care items that are charged to private pay patients and budgeted monthly sources of non-service revenues such as vending machines. Investment income, another source of Freeston ElderCare's non-service revenues, is included as a revenue budget line.

A line is included for uncollectible revenue, which at Freeston ElderCare is budgeted as 25% of revenue not collected within 90 days. An explanation of uncollectible revenue is provided in the section discussing the cash flow budget. Uncollectible revenue is subtracted from the service and non-service revenue to obtain the net revenue. Investment income is added to net revenue to obtain total revenue. The pro forma P&L is the last line of the operating revenue budget, indicating the overall profitability of Freeston ElderCare.

TABLE 4-5

Freeston ElderCare SNF Unit Revenue Budget, 2003

Line #	4511 SNF Revenue Item	Amount	Type	January Budget	February Budget	March Budget	Q1 Budget	FY 2003 Budget
501	SNF Private Pay	$185	Per Diem	$40,145	$25,900	$28,675	$94,720	$349,095
	SNF Private Pay Patient Days			217	140	155	512	1,887
551	Managed Care SNF	$248	Per Diem	$84,568	$76,384	$84,568	$245,520	$995,720
	Managed Care SNF Patient Days			341	308	341	990	4,015
555	Medicaid SNF	$215	Per Diem	$46,655	$42,140	$53,320	$142,115	$674,240
	Medicaid SNF Patient Days			217	196	248	661	3,136
557	Medicare SNF	$262	Per Diem	$56,854	$51,352	$56,854	$165,060	$813,772
	Medicare SNF Patient Days			217	196	217	630	3,106
565	Managed Care Hospice	$235	Per Diem	$14,570	$13,160	$14,570	$42,300	$171,550
	Managed Care Hospice Patient Days			62	56	62	180	730
	Total SNF Revenue			**$242,792**	**$208,936**	**$237,987**	**$689,715**	**$3,004,377**
	SNF Patient Days			**1,054**	**896**	**1,023**	**2,973**	**12,874**

○ **TABLE 4-6**

Freeston ElderCare Pro Forma Profit & Loss Statement, 2003

Item	January Budget	February Budget	March Budget	Q1 Budget	FY 2003 Budget
Net Operating Revenue	$709,710	$632,705	$708,412	$2,050,826	$8,605,981
Total Operating Expense	$612,614	$562,198	$599,576	$1,798,372	$7,415,137
Pro Forma Operating P&L	**$97,096**	**$70,507**	**$108,835**	**$252,454**	**$1,190,845**

Box 4-3 summarizes the items commonly described by operating budgets, including volume, expenses, revenue, and a pro forma P&L.

Capital Budget

The **capital budget** is a budget for long-term investments that are often high in cost. Capital budgets may focus on items as large and complex as the construction of a new building, with millions of dollars of expense and decades of useful life. Smaller capital budgets include lines for maintenance and repair costs, or the purchase of equipment. By definition, an item's cost does not determine its inclusion in the capital budget, but its useful life beyond the operating budget year. Capital budgets are reported separately from operating budgets because only a portion of the expense (useful life) of a capital asset is used over any one year, and only a portion of the revenues generated by a capital asset are received over any one year. The capital budget is entered as a line in the cash flow budget, as it represents cash expenditures over the fiscal year.

In practice, many health care settings do not include relatively low-cost items of equipment in the capital budget. Frequently, policies are established with a dollar value specified as the limit for equipment purchases as non-capital items to include in the operating budget, even if the equipment's useful life exceeds 1 year. For example, the Freeston ElderCare policy is that departments may budget for patient care equipment not to exceed a total of $2,500 per year. The Rehabilitation Department operating expense budget for 2003 (see Table 4-1) includes $193 per month to purchase walkers, canes, and a treatment table, for a total of $2,316. The Nursing Services operating non-personnel expense budget (see Table 4-4) includes $205 per month to

☐ **BOX 4-3**

What Operating Budgets Describe

■ Sources, estimated amounts, and trends in volume
■ Operating expenses
  ● Sources, dollar amounts, and trends in direct vs. indirect expenses
  ● Sources, dollar amounts, and trends in personnel and non-personnel expenses
  ● Fixed and flexible (volume-based) personnel and non-personnel expenses
■ Operating revenues
  ● Sources, dollar amounts, and trends in service and non-service revenues
  ● Fixed and flexible (volume-based) revenue sources
  ● Dollar amounts and trends in uncollectible revenues and investment income
  ● Dollar amounts and trends in profit or loss (pro forma P&L)

purchase five wheelchairs, for a total of $2,460 for FY 2003.

Table 4-7 presents Freeston ElderCare's capital budget for FY 2003. Note that some capital budget items are per-unit costs and others represent total item costs. For example, the shelves in the linen room must be replaced, budgeted at $125 each for five shelves, so the total capital expense for the linen room shelves is $125 multiplied by 5, or $625. On the other hand, the estimate for

◯ T A B L E 4 - 7			
Freeston ElderCare Capital Budget, 2003			
Item or Project	**Unit Cost**	**No. Units**	**Total Expense**
Replace Linen Room Shelves	$125	5	$625
Exterior Painting	$14,320	1	$14,320
Interior Painting North Hall	$4,325	1	$4,325
Replace Dishwasher	$1,150	1	$1,150
Recarpet Activity Room	$1,375	1	$1,375
Repair Parking Lot Lighting	$375	4	$1,500
Total Capital Expense Budget			**$23,295**

painting the North Hall section of Freeston ElderCare is $4,325 total. The capital budget items total $23,295 for FY 2003, or $1,941 monthly (not in Table 4-7).

Cash Flow Budget

The **cash flow budget** or cash budget estimates the flow of money in and out of the institution, helping managers understand and anticipate whether there may be a substantial cash shortfall (negative cash balance) or surplus (positive cash balance). One purpose of the cash flow budget is to anticipate and plan for periods when cash inflows are low, thus enabling the institution to pay salaries and other bills and to avoid bankruptcy. Another purpose of the cash flow budget is to estimate the extent of surplus funding available for investing, replenishing the inventory, or expanding operations.

Cash flow budgets are often not reported at department or unit levels within a facility. However, it is important for health professionals to recognize the importance of adequate cash flow to the fiscal health of the overall institution. If nothing else, each work unit or department providing health care services contributes to the cash inflows (revenues) and outflows (expenses) incorporated in the cash flow budget.

When cash shortfalls occur, institutions may borrow money, but within some strict limits. Lending institutions look critically at institutions that appear to rely on loans to meet their day-to-day expenditures. At the same time, legal regulations protecting employees require that employers pay out all salaries and wages when they are due. Suppliers and other creditors also expect bills to be paid when they come due. It is quite possible for a profitable venture to go bankrupt because it cannot borrow the money to pay salaries and bills over a period of cash shortfalls. Therefore, estimating and budgeting the cash flow is important to ensure that salaries and bills are paid on schedule, and to protect the institution from bankruptcy.

Cash surpluses must be planned for and managed as well. It is poor financial management to hold onto surplus cash and allow it to sit idle rather than drawing investment interest or contributing to operations. A cash flow budget enables decisions to be made about when and how much to invest or spend any surplus cash. In some settings, periods of surplus cash flow may be used to replenish inventory and supplies. Budgeting the cash surplus also enables the institution to expand its programs or increase its services.

For various reasons, considerable time may pass before payments are made to health care providers. Laws and regulations may also limit the extent that health care settings may require advance payments, as well. Private pay patients may delay or default on their payments. Third party payors may implement extensive utilization review procedures or from denials of payment that require considerable time to appeal and resolve. Because of the anticipated delay in actual payment of net revenues, the cash flow budget differs from the operating budget in two ways. First, the budget uses both current and **lagged values**, budget figures that reflect prior financial activities for specified periods of time. These lagged values enable the manager to estimate when revenues are actually received as cash inflow. Second, given that delay is anticipated in the receipt of various revenues, the budgeted cash inflow is less than the budgeted operating net revenue. Some patients or payors fail to pay their bills within the 90-day lag time, and some do not pay their bills or do not pay them in full (**bad debt**). Facilities may budget to cover expenses for some patients who cannot pay their bills (**charity care**). In addition, some payments may be denied by insurance companies or other payors (denials). These uncollectibles result in cash flow budget figures that are less than the revenue budget figures.

The Freeston ElderCare cash flow budget for the first 3 months of FY 2003 is presented in Table 4-8. This section explains the components of the cash flow budget and the calculation of subtotals and totals, but the preparation of a cash flow budget is discussed in Chapter 6.

Cash Flow Budget Cash Inflows

Cash flow budgets are usually prepared on a monthly basis over an entire year. The first 3 months of FY 2003 are shown in Table 4-8 for Freeston ElderCare. The cash flow budget typically begins with the **starting cash balance**, or the amount of cash on hand at the beginning of the cash flow budget month. At Freeston ElderCare, the budgeted amount of the starting cash balance is $15,500; in other words, Marie, the administrator, budgets to have at least $15,500 cash available at the beginning of each month.

The next lines of the cash flow budget for Freeston ElderCare FY 2003 are expected sources of cash inflows (revenues). Note that these amounts do not match the service revenue estimates in the revenue budget. For January 2003, the total patient care revenue budgeted as collected over the past 90 days is $651,226, and over the last 91 to 360 days it is $35,750. When the total budgeted non-service revenue of $1,011 is added,

TABLE 4-8

Freeston ElderCare Cash Flow Budget, January–March 2003

Items	January	February	March
Beginning Cash Balance	**$15,500**	**$15,500**	**$15,500**
Total Patient Care Revenue Collected within 90 Days	$651,226	$633,691	$613,880
Total Patient Care Revenue Collected within 91–360 Days	$35,750	$6,014	$53,773
Total Non-Service Revenue	$1,011	$1,011	$1,011
Total Receivables	**$687,986**	**$640,716**	**$668,664**
Investment Income	$31,500	$31,500	$31,500
Total Cash Inflows	**$719,486**	**$672,216**	**$700,164**
Total Cash on Hand	**$734,986**	**$687,716**	**$715,664**
Total Personnel Expenses	$430,320	$385,594	$417,283
Non-Personnel Operating Expenses	$126,835	$111,866	$124,013
Lease	$100,000	$100,000	$100,000
Taxes	$3,841	$3,841	$3,841
Depreciation	$25,743	$25,743	$25,743
Other Property Expenses	$40,158	$40,158	$40,158
Capital Improvement Expenses	$1,941	$1,941	$1,941
Total Cash Outflows	**$728,839**	**$669,144**	**$712,979**
Ending Cash Balance	**$6,148**	**$18,572**	**$2,685**
Investments or Borrowings	**$(9,352)**	**$3,072**	**$(12,815)**

the total receivables for January 2003 total $687,986. This amount is less than the $709,710 net operating revenue for January 2003 as reported in the operating budget (Please see "Supplemental Tables and Documents" of the Back-of-Book CD-ROM) or pro forma P&L (see Table 4-6).

Most health care institutions have financial reserve policies. A cash reserve of $630,000 is held in an investment account by Freeston ElderCare to cover salaries and other operating expenses for a 1-month period should the institution need to close its operations. This money earns 5% interest, or $31,500 per month, budgeted as investment income (see Table 4-8). When the $31,500 in investment income is added to the total receivables, Freeston ElderCare has a budgeted $719,486 cash inflow for January 2003. This subtotal is added to the $15,500 budgeted beginning cash balance to estimate a total of $734,986 cash on hand over January 2003, which represents all the cash available for January 2003 to pay salaries and other cash expenses.

Cash Flow Budget Cash Outflows

Budgeted monthly cash expenses are then entered. Personnel expenses (including all salaries, hourly wages, payroll benefits, and overtime) total $430,320 for January 2003 (see Table 4-8). Non-personnel operating expenses ($126,835), the lease ($100,000), and other monthly expenses are then entered, including the monthly capital improvement expenses of $1,941. These cash outflows total $728,839 for January 2003.

Cash Flow Budget Cash Balance

The next-to-last line of Table 4-8 shows that the total cash outflows are subtracted from the total cash inflows to determine the **ending cash balance**, or the amount of money left at the end of January 2003 after Freeston ElderCare has paid out all its cash expenses, which amount to $6,148. This ending cash balance is less than the budgeted starting cash balance of $15,500, representing a cash shortfall of $9,409, recorded on the final line of the cash flow budget. In other words, $9,352 must be borrowed (or budgeted from cash surpluses) to cover all the budgeted cash requirements for January 2003. By comparison, February 2003 reports a $3,072 cash surplus, which may be invested.

In reviewing the cash flow budget for Freeston ElderCare for the first 3 months of FY 2003, note how changes in revenues and expenses change the ending cash balance from month to month. To determine overall annual cash flow, all of the amounts for investment or borrowings are added, resulting in an investment of $946 (not shown in Table 4-8). This indicates that there is no overall loss in cash flow, but that it balances fairly closely with the beginning balance of $15,500 for January 2004 (the beginning of the next fiscal year). The cash flow budget for the entire FY 2003 is in the "Supplemental Tables and Documents" section in the Back-of-Book CD-ROM.

Box 4-4 summarizes the components of the cash flow budget.

Other Budgets

The **product line budget** and special purpose budget are additional budgets managers may encounter in health care settings. The product line budget is similar to the operating budget illustrated by Freeston ElderCare, except that the focus is on a clinical specialty or on selected groups of patients with same or very similar diagnoses, rather than bed types based on revenues and reimbursement. For example, recall that the managed care hospice contract is a new venture for both the managed care payor and Freeston ElderCare. In negotiating the hospice contract, the administrator, Marie, had very little historical data or other good information on which to base the negotiated per diem bed rate of $235. Moreover, the managed care company that agreed to pay the $235 bed rate wants to re-examine the costs for care and renegotiate the contract for next year. Marie must carefully track the level of care and associated costs for the hospice patients over FY 2003 and prepare for a possible renegotiation (and reduction) of the managed care hospice rate. Marie could prepare a product line budget estimating the hours of direct nursing care and other care costs attributed to the managed care hospice patients to determine if the $235 per diem bed rate is reasonable.

The **special purpose budget** is prepared for any purpose for which the health care setting requires a plan that has not been included in any of the other budgets. Budgets prepared for business plans proposing new

---

BOX 4-4

Components of the Cash Flow Budget

1. Cash inflows
   a. Beginning cash balance
   b. Total service revenue collected within specified time period(s)
   c. Total other service and non-service revenue sources
   d. Total receivables
   e. Investment income
   f. Subtotal of total cash inflows
   g. Total cash on hand
2. Cash outflows
   a. Personnel expenses
   b. Non-personnel operating expenses
   c. Lease
   d. Taxes
   e. Depreciation
   f. Other property expenses
   g. Subtotal of total cash outflows
3. Total ending cash balance (cash inflows − cash outflows)
4. Investments or borrowings (ending cash balance − beginning cash balance)

---

ventures or substantial changes in existing programs are examples of special purpose budgets. The budget prepared to plan for the new activities program at Freeston ElderCare in Chapter 6 is an example of a special purpose budget.

Conclusion

This chapter describes types of budgets used in health care settings, and the elements that make up these budgets. Chapter 5 builds on these concepts by presenting approaches to monitoring and controlling budgets. Box 4-5 provides a summary of the types and purposes of the budgets presented in this chapter.

BOX 4-5

Types of Budgets and Their Purpose

- Statistics budget—estimate volume as basis for operating budget
- Operating budget—estimate revenues and expenses over budget period
- Capital budget—estimate capital equipment or capital improvement expenses
- Cash flow budget—estimate and forecast cash shortfalls and cash surpluses
- Product line budget—operating budget based on clinical specialty area, similar diagnoses, or other similar outputs rather than organizational departments
- Special purpose budget—estimate revenues and expenses for new ventures or any other purpose not included in other budgets

■ CRITICAL THINKING EXERCISES

1. Using the same formulas as used in calculating monthly nursing services FTEs, calculate the monthly budgeted FTEs for the cooks and dietary aides for FY 2003. Show how these FTE calculations are applied to calculate the budgeted monthly expenses for cooks and dietary aides.
2. Recalculate the SNF unit personnel expense budget for 3 consecutive months, changing the direct hours per staff PPD or the monthly volume. Discus the impact of this change on total personnel expenses.
3. If available, obtain copies of budgets from your own health care setting, concealing the setting's identity as appropriate. Explain the types of budgets and their uses. Exchange budgets and compare how they are constructed and used.

■ REFERENCES

Baker, J. J., & Baker, R. W. (2000). *Health Care Finance: Basic Tools for Nonfinancial Managers*. Gaithersburg, MD: Aspen.

Cleverley, W. O., & Cameron, A. E. (2002). *Essentials of Health Care Finance*, 5th ed. Gaithersburg, MD: Aspen.

Finkler, S. A., & Kovner, C. T. (2000). *Financial Management for Nurse Managers and Executives*, 2nd ed. Philadelphia: W. B. Saunders.

Gapenski, L. C. (2002). *Healthcare Finance: An Introduction to Accounting and Financial Management*, 2nd ed. Chicago: Health Administration Press.

Herkimer, A. G. (1988). *Understanding Health Care Budgeting*. Gaithersburg, MD: Aspen.

McGuffin, J. (1999). *The Nurse's Guide to Successful Management: A Desk Reference*. St. Louis, MO: Mosby.

Neumann, B. R., Suber, J. D., & Zelman, W. N. (1988). *Financial Management: Concepts and Applications for Health Care Providers*, 2d ed. Owings Mills, MD: National Health Publishing.

Nowicki, M. (2001). *The Financial Management of Hospitals and Healthcare Organizations*. Chicago: Health Administration Press.

Sullivan, E. J., & Decker, P. J. (2001). *Effective Leadership and Management in Nursing*, 5th ed. Upper Saddle River, NJ: Prentice Hall.

CHAPTER 5

Budget Monitoring and Control

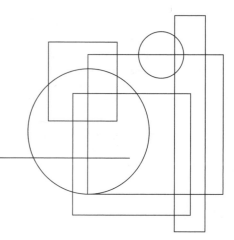

Learning Objectives

1. Explain and differentiate between budget monitoring, investigation, and control.
2. Demonstrate the calculation of budget variance, percent variance, adjusted variance, and adjusted percent variance, with an example of the application of each.
3. Describe at least two sources of budget variance and how these sources might be monitored, investigated and controlled.

Key Terms

Adjusted percent variance
Adjusted variance
Adjustment authority
Annualize
Balance the budget
Benchmark
Budget control
Budget investigation
Budget monitoring
Budget variance
Efficiency variance
Episode
Expense variance

Favorable budget variance
Line item flexibility
Percent variance
Performance target
Price variance
Profit variance
Quantity variance
Rate variance
Revenue variance
Total variance
Unfavorable budget variance
Variance analysis
YTD (year to date)

Figure 5-1 shows the functions of budgets as descriptions, monitoring devices, and planning tools. This chapter focuses on monitoring budgets to identify performance problems, investigate their sources, and, when possible, take corrective action. The FY 2003 budget reports for Freeston ElderCare are used as examples.

Budgets are used to monitor performance in several ways, first of all by comparing budgeted to actual volume, expenses, or revenues. Undesired, unexpected, or unusual performance is identified by budget monitoring, allowing for investigation of the source of performance problems. Budget monitoring enables the comparison of current financial performance to performance over the prior fiscal year. Adherence to budget guidelines, standards, and targets is also identified and compared with budget monitoring. Box 5-1 summarizes the monitoring function of budgets.

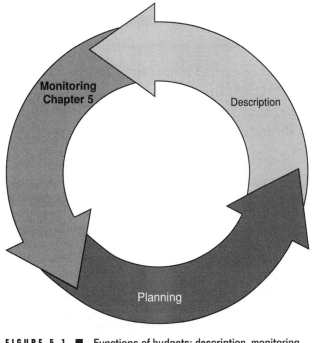

FIGURE 5.1 ■ Functions of budgets: description, monitoring, and planning.

Monitoring Budgets

Budgets are tools for evaluating and improving performance. Budget figures represent **performance targets**, or indicators that specify whether a performance standard is reached in actual practice. **Budget monitoring** identifies performance problems requiring investigation. **Budget investigation** identifies the source or sources of performance problems and determines whether the problems can be controlled. **Budget control** uses management strategies to correct performance and meet budget targets. Box 5-2 summarizes the functions of budget monitoring, investigation, and control. Each of these functions is discussed in this chapter.

Monitoring and controlling budgets are explained in the section on **variance analysis** (systematic comparison of budget and actual financial performance). Chapter 7 discusses reporting and monitoring of indirect expenses. Although all budgets are monitored, much of the discussion in this chapter focuses on expense

---

□ BOX 5-1

What Budgets Monitor

- ■ Actual compared to budgeted performance
- ■ Undesired performance and trends in volume, expense, or revenue
- ■ Unexpected or unusual performance in volume, expense, or revenue
- ■ Financial performance compared to prior budget YTD performance
- ■ Adherence to budget guidelines, standards, and targets

BOX 5-2

Budget Monitoring, Investigation, and Control

- ■ Monitoring identifies performance problems requiring investigation
- ■ Investigation:
  - ● Identifies the source(s) of performance problems
  - ● Determines whether the performance problems are controllable
- ■ Control uses management strategies to correct performance problems and meet budget targets

---

budgets, for several reasons. First, the same methods for monitoring expense budgets may be applied to other types of budgets in most situations. Second, in most health care settings, it is possible to exercise closer monitoring and greater control over budget expenses, as many of the sources of expenses are internal. For example, laboratory technician overtime expenses can be closely monitored, and it is possible to adjust laboratory technician positions and supervise their productivity to reduce excessive overtime. By contrast, decisions of physicians to order laboratory tests for patients, which affect volume and revenues, may be monitored but are external events that are difficult or impossible to control within the laboratory setting.

A third reason this chapter focuses on expense budgets compared to revenue budgets is that many of the methods effective in controlling expense budgets are effective in controlling other budgets as well. For example, if laboratory technician overtime expenses are controlled by increasing productivity, these more productive personnel may also be able to process a higher volume of tests, thus increasing revenues.

Variance Analysis

A tool often used to monitor budgets is variance analysis, which helps the reviewer identify the extent and source of differences between budget and actual performance. A fundamental purpose of budgets, particularly for revenue-generating work settings, is to report estimated profit or loss. Therefore, an important purpose of variance analysis is to monitor, investigate, and, if possible, control **profit variance** (the difference between budget and actual profit).

Profit is usually an overall institutional indicator, so it is important to analyze volume, expense, and revenue budgets in detail to determine whether profit variances are related to excessive expenses or revenue deficits. More detailed variance reports also help the reviewer understand whether the profit variance represents a long-term trend or a single, isolated incident that is now under control. This section discusses methods to analyze variance in volume, expenses, and revenues.

The time period of a variance analysis may be a month, quarter, year, or any specified time period that is appropriate to the situation. Budget variance reports frequently include **YTD (year to date)** budget figures for financial performance over the entire fiscal year up to the end of the most recent budget month. Flexible budgeting adjusts budget values based on volume variance, so that as volume changes, it is expected that direct care revenues and expenses will change accordingly. Other sources of variance besides volume are discussed later in this chapter.

Budget variance is the amount of difference between the budget and actual amount of volume, revenue, or expense. Consistent with the financial practices of many health care settings, this chapter calculates variance by subtracting the budget value from the actual value. For example, if a budget amount is $10,000 and the actual value is $12,000, the variance is reported as $2,000 ($12,000−$10,000). If both the budget and actual values are $10,000, then the variance is $0, although it is rare in practice to have budget and actual values precisely match.

Some health care settings calculate budget variance (for both revenues and expenses) by subtracting the actual value from the budget value. This method reverses the reporting of the values, so if the budget amount is $10,000 and the actual value is $12,000, the budget variance is reported as ($2,000) rather than $2,000. It is important to know how variance is calculated in the health care setting of interest and to be consistent in calculations and in reporting to avoid confusion. Whether the budget value is subtracted from the actual value or the actual value subtracted from the budget value, the focus of variance analysis is the difference between the two values. As long as the calculations, reporting, and interpretation are clear and accurate, either method for calculating and interpreting budget variance may be used.

Tables reporting budget variance are titled "variance report" rather than "budget" to specify that both budget and actual figures are reported. The variance reports in Chapter 5 include January and February 2003 as well as YTD 2003 and YTD 2002 variances. The January and YTD 2002 variances are favorable, with examples of unfavorable variances included in February 2003 and YTD 2003 for comparison and illustration of concepts.

Table 5-1 presents the Freeston ElderCare skilled nursing facility (SNF) unit statistics variance report for January and February 2003. Instead of one monthly budget column, there are three columns of budget figures per month and for YTD 2003 and YTD 2002. The first column represents the 2003 statistics budget (as presented in Chapter 4, Table 4-2). For January 2003 the budgeted number of SNF private pay patient days is 217.

The second column of budget figures in Table 5-1 reports the comparison of budget and actual performance for budget monitoring using variance analysis. For January 2003 the budget number and the actual number of SNF private pay patient days are 217. As shown in the third column, the variance is $0 (217 - 217)$. In February 2003, the budget number of SNF private pay patient days is 140 with 121 actual patient days, for a variance of 19 patient days under budget $(121 - 140)$.

The variances shown in Table 5-1 represent volume variance, or the difference between budget and actual volume. Reporting the amount of variance between the budget and actual figures enables comparison of budget to actual performance, in this case whether the actual patient days, census, admissions, and length of stay are meeting the budget targets. Most variance reports show the amount of variance between budget and actual performance as seen in Table 5-1.

When reporting budget variances (assuming the budget value is subtracted from the actual value as indicated above), a positive value indicates the variance is over budget and a negative value (designated by parentheses, a minus sign, or red ink) indicates the variance is under budget. This text designates negative variance amounts by enclosing the values in parentheses, consistent with standard spreadsheet formatting. For example, private pay SNF admissions are 1 less than budgeted (one under budget) for January 2003.

Favorable budget variance is a desirable difference between budget and actual amounts. Favorable variance may be positive, as when actual revenues exceed budget revenues, or negative, as when actual expenses are less than budgeted. **Unfavorable budget variance** is an undesirable difference between budget and actual values, as when revenues are less than budgeted or expenses are higher than budgeted. Although being "over budget" may be commonly thought of as undesirable and "under budget" as desirable, it is important to distinguish between favorable and unfavorable variances. Budget variances must be analyzed in context. For example, a flexible budget's actual revenues are likely to fall below the budgeted amount when volume decreases, but if expenses are controlled, the lower revenues may be acceptable. On the other hand, actual expenses that are below budget may indicate organizational problems, such as the failure to order equipment and supplies needed for a project on deadline, or inadequate staffing. Effective budget monitoring requires looking beyond the budget figures and understanding the context in which the financial performance takes place.

○ TABLE 5-1

Freeston ElderCare SNF Unit Statistics Variance Report, January–February 2003

Line #	SNF Unit #4511 Revenue Item	January			February			YTD 2003			YTD 2002		
		Budget	Actual	Variance	Budget	Actual	Variance	Budget	Actual	Variance	Budget	Actual	Variance
501	**Private Pay SNF Patient Days**	**217**	**217**	**0**	**140**	**121**	**(19)**	**357**	**338**	**(19)**	**393**	**399**	**6**
	Private Pay SNF ADC	7.0	7.0	0.0	5.0	4.3	(0.7)	6.1	5.7	(0.3)	6.7	6.8	0.1
	Private Pay SNF Admissions	8	8	0	7	4	(3)	15	12	(3)	13	11	(2)
	Private Pay SNF ALOS	27.3	27.1	(0.2)	27.3	30.3	2.9	27.3	28.2	0.8	30.2	36.3	6.0
551	**Managed Care SNF Patient Days**	**341**	**359**	**18**	**308**	**310**	**2**	**649**	**669**	**20**	**562**	**576**	**14**
	Managed Care SNF ADC	11.0	11.6	0.6	11.0	11.1	0.1	11.0	11.3	0.3	9.5	9.8	0.2
	Managed Care SNF Admissions	12	11	(1)	11	8	(3)	23	19	(4)	16	17	1
	Managed Care SNF ALOS	33.5	32.6	(0.8)	33.5	38.8	5.3	33.5	35.2	1.8	35.1	33.9	(1.2)
555	**Medicaid SNF Patient Days**	**217**	**236**	**19**	**196**	**164**	**(32)**	**413**	**400**	**(13)**	**407**	**423**	**16**
	Medicaid SNF ADC	7.0	7.6	0.6	7.0	5.9	(1.1)	7.0	6.8	(0.2)	6.9	7.2	0.3
	Medicaid SNF Admissions	8	6	(2)	7	4	(3)	15	10	(5)	10	9	(1)
	Medicaid SNF ALOS	39.2	39.3	0.1	39.2	41.0	1.8	39.2	40.0	0.8	40.7	47.0	6.3

Medicare SNF Patient Days **557**	217	248	31	196	159	(37)	413	407	(6)	446	458	12
Medicare SNF ADC	7.0	8.0	1.0	7.0	5.7	(1.3)	7.0	6.9	(0.1)	7.6	7.8	0.2
Medicare SNF Admissions	9	8	(1)	10	5	(5)	19	13	(6)	14	15	1
Medicare SNF ALOS	30.8	31.0	0.2	30.8	31.8	1.0	30.8	31.3	0.6	31.9	30.5	(1.3)
Managed Care Hospice Patient Days **565**	62	61	(1)	56	63	7	118	124	6	—	—	—
Managed Care Hospice ADC	2.0	2.0	(0.0)	2.0	2.3	0.3	2.0	2.1	0.1	—	—	—
Managed Care Hospice Admissions	2	1	(1)	0	1	1	2	2	0	—	—	—
Managed Care Hospice ALOS	60.8	61.0	0.2	60.8	63.0	2.2	60.8	62.0	1.2	—	—	—
Total SNF Patient Days	1,054	1,121	67	896	817	(79)	1,950	1,938	(12)	1,808	1,856	48
SNF Average Daily Census	34.0	36.2	2.2	32.0	29.2	(2.8)	33.1	32.8	(0.2)	30.6	31.5	0.8
SNF Admissions	39	34	(5)	35	22	(13)	74	56	(18)	53	52	(1)
SNF Occupancy Rate (42 beds)	81.0%	86.1%	5.1%	76.2%	69.5%	-6.7%	78.7%	78.2%	-0.5%	73.0%	74.9%	1.9%

Budget variance may be controllable or uncontrollable. For example, in some situations it may be possible to control expenses for supplies by making bulk purchases. In other situations, there may not be purchasing authority or adequate storage space to control expenses by bulk purchasing. Sources of budget variances may be internal or external to the health care setting, with external sources of variance frequently more difficult to control. Purchasing decisions and personnel supervision are examples of internal sources of variance over which considerable control may be exercised. Epidemics, disasters, supply failures, shortages, strikes, unemployment, and new governmental regulations are examples of external sources of variance over which there is often little or no control.

Variances Requiring Investigation

In practice, there is nearly always some variance between budget and actual amounts. It is therefore important to determine the level of budget variance that is not only unfavorable, but of enough concern to require further attention. A monthly budget variance report may present many variances. Strategies and guidelines are needed to pinpoint the variances that require further investigation and control, as these activities take time. Strategies and guidelines for identifying variances that require attention differ among health care settings, and there is no single rule or set of rules to apply in all situations when budget variances are reported.

An important and frequently overlooked step in reviewing budget variances that appear unusual or excessive is to recheck the data and calculations for possible data entry or computational errors. Budget figures may be provided from a finance department or may be recorded and computed by a department director or other staff. In either case, checking data sources and calculations when unusual or unfavorable variances are noticed may save considerable effort and frustration.

Most of the budget monitoring examples focus on unfavorable variances, because in practice favorable variances require little attention. Reports of unbudgeted expenses often require follow-up, as these expenses were not planned or justified at the beginning of the fiscal year. Any unexpected or unusual variance may also be investigated, such as revenues decreasing when volumes increase within a flexible budget.

The larger the amount or percent of unfavorable variance, the more likely it will require follow-up. The calculation and application of percents and adjustments for volume used in variance analysis are discussed later in this chapter to help in determining whether a variance is large enough to investigate. In some settings there are administrative policies setting an arbitrary threshold for the investigation and control of line items or budgets. For example, if the supplies expenses exceed a threshold of $500, or if patient days fall by more than 10% for a given month, budget investigation might be required. Continued increases in variance also indicate a need for further attention (for example, if an actual expense line item exceeds the budget by $500 one month, $750 the following month, and $1,000 the third month).

Another indicator for investigation is the duration of the variance. The longer the variance persists, the more likely it requires further attention. Some settings have policies to investigate unfavorable budget variances if they exceed a specified amount for a specified time period, such as $1,000 per month over 3 months. Another approach is to identify whether the variance would be considered excessive if carried monthly over an entire year. For example, if a monthly expense for a line item is $1,000 over budget, it would total $12,000 over budget for the fiscal year, which might be considered excessive and require investigation. Other guidelines or a combination of these rules and approaches may be applied.

In many cases, with or without organizational policies and guidelines regarding the investigation and control of variances, it is essential to learn by experience and develop one's own approaches. Knowledge of the particular setting and the types of volume, expenses, and revenues it generates is essential, as is knowledge of the processes, technology, and staffing. Health care professionals with budgetary responsibilities are ultimately accountable for excessive unfavorable variances, so they must apply and, if necessary, develop

---

☐ B O X   5 - 3

Reasons to Investigate Budget Variance

- ■ Possible data entry or calculation error
- ■ Loss—expenses exceed revenues
- ■ Unbudgeted expenses
- ■ Unexpected or unusual variances
- ■ Amount, percent, or adjusted percent of variance
- ■ Continual increase in variance (trend)
- ■ Duration of variance
- ■ Institutional policies or guidelines, such as dollar limits
- ■ Extent of concern if the variance were to continue the entire fiscal year
- ■ Personal knowledge and experience

---

effective approaches for variance analysis. Box 5-3 summarizes the reasons for investigating budget variance discussed in this section.

Averages and Percents in Variance Analysis

Several calculations are useful in identifying whether budget variances require further investigation. If average, percent, or adjusted variances are not included in existing budget variance reports, they may be calculated by hand or by using spreadsheet software. Average, percent, or adjusted variances may be compared to internal performance targets or external **benchmarks** (target indicators that represent an industry standard).

Budget Averages and Per-Unit Averages. The average is calculated by adding up all of the budgeted monthly values for a line item or total of line items and dividing this total by the number of budget values (see the Math Review at http://connection.lww.com/go/penner). Averages are useful as a target for comparison to actual values. Fixed budgets often reflect the use of average monthly budget values, or the total fiscal year budget for a given line item divided by 12 months in the year.

Budgets may also report overall fiscal year averages that are used as budget targets. For example, Table 5-1 shows that the average length of stay (ALOS) budgeted for each Freeston ElderCare SNF unit bed type for FY 2003 is an overall annual average used as a budget target for each month, so that 27.3 ALOS is the monthly budget target for private pay SNF beds (corresponding to Table 4-2 in Chap. 4). For February 2003 the ALOS for private pay SNF beds is 2.9 days over budget (30.3 − 27.3 with rounding error).

Another use of the average is to determine the revenue or expense averaged by service unit, or the per-unit average. In many settings it may be helpful to calculate the average revenues or expenses per unit of volume as a method of monitoring budgets. The per-unit average may also be used to calculate overhead rates, as explained in Chapter 7. Table 5-2 shows the Freeston ElderCare SNF unit RN personnel variance report for January and February 2003. The variances reported in Table 5-2 are examples of **expense variance** (difference between budget and actual expenses).

In Table 5-2 the RN expense per patient day is budgeted to average $7.68 for January, February, and YTD 2003. This average is calculated by dividing the total RN personnel expenses by the total number of patient days for each month or specified time period. The actual RN personnel expense per patient day is $11.23, or $3.55 over budget for February 2003.

Averages and Annualizing. Calculations of averages are also useful in **annualizing** (converting YTD budget or actual figures to 12 months). YTD budget or actual figures are annualized by averaging them,

○ TABLE 5-2

Freeston Eldercare, SNF Unit RN Personnel Variance Report

Line #	7210 SNF Personnel	Amount		Type	January Budget	Actual	Variance	% Var.	Adj. % Var.
	SNF Patient Days				1,054	1,121	67	6.4%	—
	RN Direct Hours	0.2		Direct Care Hours PPD	211	224	13	6.4%	0.0%
001	RN Expense	var	$29.32	Wage	$6,181	$6,574	$393	6.4%	0.0%
	RN Overtime	4%		of Direct Care Hours	8.4	0	(8.4)	−100.0%	−106.4%
101	RN Overtime Expense	150%		of Wage	$371	$0	$(371)	−100.0%	−106.4%
120	Benefits	25%		of Wages	$1,545	$1,643	$98	6.4%	0.0%
130	**Total SNF RN Personnel**				**$8,097**	**$8,217**	**$120**	**1.5%**	**−4.9%**
	Average SNF RN PPD				**$7.68**	**$7.33**	**$(0.35)**	**−4.6%**	**−10.9%**

and using the average for each of the 12 months of the fiscal year. The monthly annualized figure may be multiplied by 12 to obtain the FY annualized amount. Annualizing is frequently applied to flexible budgets, which vary in amount from month to month based on volume variance. It is also useful to apply annualizing to fixed budgets when they require revision. The calculations used in annualizing are discussed here; further applications of annualizing are discussed in the section on budget authority and line item transfers.

Table 5-3 provides an example of annualizing using the SNF and intermediate care unit budget and actual patient days for January through June 2003. The FY 2003 budgeted patient days, which are estimated as a flexible budget, are annualized monthly by dividing the FY 2003 total by the months in the year (39,128 ÷ 12) to obtain 3,261 patient days per month. This annualized amount also represents the average number of budgeted patient days per month over the fiscal year. The YTD 2003 budgeted patient days total 18,827, or the sum of budgeted patient days for January through June.

The actual budget figures shown in Table 5-3 are annualized by first summing the actual patient days for January through June (6 months), as shown in the column for YTD 2003, for a total of 19,527 patient days. At the time of the report, July 2003, the actual patient days for July through December 2003 are not available.

○ TABLE 5-3

Freeston ElderCare SNF & Intermediate Care Units, Annualized Patient Days, 2003

	January	February	March	April	May	June	YTD 2003	Annualized Monthly	FY 2003
Budget	3,193	2,856	3,193	3,150	3,255	3,180	18,827	3,261	39,128
Actual*	3,224	2,703	3,367	3,351	3,478	3,404	19,527	3,255	39,054
Variance	31	(153)	174	201	223	224	700	(6)	(74)
% Var.	1.0%	−5.4%	5.4%	6.4%	6.9%	7.0%	3.7%	−0.2%	−0.2%

* FY 2003 annualized based on January–June figures

February					YTD 2003					YTD 2002				
Budget	Actual	Variance	% Var.	Adj. % Var.	Budget	Actual	Variance	% Var.	Adj. % Var.	Budget	Actual	Variance	% Var.	Adj. % Var.
896	817	(79)	−8.8%	—	1,950	1,938	(12)	−0.6%	—	1,808	1,856	48	2.7%	—
179	238	59	32.8%	41.6%	390	462	72	18.5%	19.1%	362	379	17	4.8%	2.2%
$5,254	$6,978	$1,724	32.8%	41.6%	$11,435	$13,552	$2,117	18.5%	19.1%	$10,072	$10,557	$485	4.8%	2.2%
7.2	10.3	3.1	43.7%	52.5%	15.6	10.3	(5.3)	−34.0%	−33.4%	14.5	11.2	(3.3)	−22.6%	−25.2%
$315	$453	$138	43.7%	52.5%	$686	$453	$(233)	−34.0%	−33.4%	$611	$468	$(143)	−23.4%	−26.0%
$1,314	$1,745	$431	32.8%	41.6%	$2,859	$3,388	$529	18.5%	19.1%	$2,518	$2,639	$121	4.8%	2.2%
$6,883	$9,176	$2,293	33.3%	42.1%	$14,980	$17,393	$2,413	16.1%	16.7%	$13,201	$13,664	$463	3.5%	0.9%
$7.68	$11.23	$3.55	46.2%	55.0%	$7.68	$8.97	$1.29	16.8%	17.4%	$7.30	$7.36	$0.06	0.8%	−1.8%

The annualized monthly amount of patient days for YTD 2003 is calculated as follows:

$$\text{Annualized Monthly Amount} = \text{YTD Total} \div \text{Months YTD}$$

$$3,255 = 19,527 \div 6$$

Based on January through June performance, it is estimated that there will be 3,255 patient days per month for July through December 2003. The annualized amount for FY 2003 is then calculated as follows:

$$\text{Annualized FY Amount} = \text{Annualized Monthly Amount} \times 12$$

$$39,054 = 3,255 \times 12$$

Based on January through June performance, it is estimated that there will be 39,054 total patient days for FY 2003. This estimate is used in the section on budget authority and line item transfers later in the chapter.

Percent Variance. Calculating the percent of budget variance (**percent variance**) is another method useful and frequently employed in variance analysis. The percent variance is the percent of difference between budget and actual amounts of volume, expenses, or revenues, calculated by dividing the budget variance by the budget value for the same time period. Table 5-2 shows that Freeston ElderCare SNF unit patient days for January 2003 are budgeted at 1,054 but actually reached 1,121, or 67 patient days over budget. The percent variance for SNF patient days in January 2003 is calculated as follows:

$$\text{Percent Variance} = \text{Budget Variance} \div \text{Budget Value}$$

$$6.4\% = 67 \div 1,054$$

In other words, the actual SNF days for January 2003 are 6.4% higher than budgeted. This text designates a negative percent variance with a minus sign, consistent with spreadsheet formatting. Positive variance in patient days is a favorable variance, as revenues are generated by volume.

One reason percents are useful in making decisions about investigating budget variances is that percents allow for a greater range of comparison (see Math Review at http://connection.lww.com/go/penner). For example, an expense budget item is $1,000 over budget for the month. A fundamental question to ask is,

"This budget variance is excessive, but compared to what?" By converting the variance amount to a percent variance, comparisons are possible. For example, if the $1,000 variance represents an 11% increase over budget, when previous reports have never shown more than a 5% increase in this line item, then the variance is unusual and requires investigation. By contrast, if the $1,000 variance represents less than a 1% increase, it may not raise the same level of concern.

Percent variances can be compared to prior performance patterns, such as over the past year, past quarters, or the past months. For example, Table 5-2 shows YTD 2003 and YTD 2002 percent variances for RN direct hours and expense. The YTD 2003 percent variance is 18.5% over budget compared to only 4.8% over budget for YTD 2002. An unfavorable percent variance can be monitored to determine whether it continues to increase or decrease over a specified time period. One might also compare the percent variances for RN staff to the percent variances for LPNs and CNAs within the SNF unit.

Percent variances may be compared to similar internal work units. For example, the variance report shown in Table 5-2 could be compared to a variance report for RNs over the same time period in the Freeston ElderCare intermediate care unit. If the two work units show similar percent variances, it indicates that the source of the variances may be external to the work units. For example, both the SNF and Intermediate Care Units show similar unfavorable percent variances, then the entire Nursing Services department may be experiencing RN staffing and scheduling problems. If the percent variances are more favorable for the intermediate care unit than for the SNF unit, then the source of the unfavorable variances is more likely to be found within the SNF unit, or it may represent an external source that only affects the SNF unit.

Comparisons can also be made with percent variances used as performance targets or benchmarks. For example, the Nursing Services SNF overtime target is 4% of direct care hours, as reported in the budget. The Nursing Services SNF percent variance for overtime could be compared to an SNF industry benchmark.

The calculation of percent variances helps in analyzing flexible budgets, because the percent of volume variance is often calculated and reported with the percent variances for other line items. The closer the line item or budget variance is to the percent volume variance, the more likely it is that volume variance is the source of the budget variance. For example, Table 5-2 shows that for January 2003, the percent variance in volume (patient days) is 6.4%. The percent variance for RN direct hours (and expenses) is also 6.4%, indicating that the increase in RN direct hours is likely the result of increased volume rather than staffing problems.

One other observation may be made about percent variances. When calculated for YTD or annual time periods, the percent variance "smooths out" or averages monthly performance. For example, Table 5-2 reports the SNF unit patient days percent variance as 6.4% for January and −8.8% for February. The YTD 2003 percent variance is calculated by dividing the total variances YTD by the total budgeted SNF unit patient days YTD, resulting in −0.6% variance for January and February combined. The YTD percent variance always falls between the highest and lowest percent variances included in the YTD calculations, so −0.6% is between 6.4% and −8.8% (see Math Review at http://connection.lww.com/go/penner).

Adjusted Percent Variance. It is possible to adjust the percent variance for volume variance, as shown in Table 5-2. The **adjusted percent variance** may not routinely be included in variance reports, but may be calculated in situations in which the percent variance figures require further analysis. By adjusting the percent variance, flexible budgets may be monitored for sources of variance other than volume.

The adjusted percent variance is calculated by subtracting the percent volume variance from the percent variance. For example, based on Table 5-2, the adjusted percent variance for RN direct care hours for February 2003 is calculated as follows:

$$\text{Adjusted Percent Variance} = \text{Percent Variance} - \text{Percent Volume Variance}$$

$$41.6\% = 32.8\% - (-8.8\%)$$

Note that a negative number is subtracted from the percent variance, because the February 2003 SNF unit volume is 8.8% under budget. It is therefore likely that 41.6% of the variance between the budget and actual RN direct care hours is not related to volume variance, but to other sources of variance. The YTD adjusted percent variance "smooths" or averages the adjusted percent variances for the months included in the YTD calculation. For example, the YTD adjusted percent variance for RN direct hours is 19.1%, falling between 0.0% for January and 41.6% for February 2003.

Adjusted Variance. In some cases, it is helpful to know the amount of budget variance adjusted for volume variance (**adjusted variance**) rather than the adjusted percent variance. Table 5-4 shows monthly and YTD columns for budgeted, actual, variance, percent variance, adjusted percent variance, and adjusted variance for the non-personnel ancillary department budget at Freeston ElderCare. Adjusted percent variances and adjusted variances are calculated only for flexible budget line items. Most variance reports do not include all of these calculations within the same report, but they are included here to demonstrate the calculations and applications.

The adjusted variance is calculated by multiplying the budget value by the adjusted percent variance. Table 5-4 shows the calculation of the adjusted variance for pharmaceuticals for January 2003 is as follows:

$$\text{Adjusted Variance} = \text{Budget Value} \times \text{Adjusted Percent Variance}$$

$$\$144 = \$12,708 \times 1.1\%$$

Adjusting for volume, pharmaceuticals are $144 over budget for January and $627 over budget for February 2003.

Revenue Variance Analysis

Revenue variance is the difference between budget and actual revenues over a specified time period. Box 5-4 summarizes the calculations and applications of averages and percents in variance analysis. All of these methods may be applied in identifying unfavorable revenue variances, usually reported as revenue deficits or shortfalls. Revenue variance reports are similar in format to expense variance reports, with the revenue line items analyzed for the amount and percent variance, which may be adjusted for volume.

Investigating Budget Variance

Budget investigation identifies the possible source or sources of unfavorable variances and determines whether the variance can be controlled. Investigation frequently requires reviewing budgets in more and more detail to allow for the identification of the source or sources of unfavorable variances. For example, if an institution's pro forma P&L statement indicates that profits are below target levels, then it is first necessary to analyze the institution-level expense and revenue budgets to identify whether the profit variance is related to excessive expenses or revenue shortfalls. It then is necessary to analyze the budgets of all departments, then work units, and then line items until the source or sources of variance are located. It may also be necessary to analyze the budget in detail regarding the time period, analyzing annual and quarterly variance reports, then monthly and weekly reports to identify the time frame or patterns in possible sources of variance.

Probably the most important element in budget investigation is knowledge about the work setting, staff, and goods and services that are provided in the setting for which the budget is reported. For example, understanding the system for scheduling staff is essential in investigating possible sources of unfavorable personnel expense variances. Another element is including, as needed, input from financial analysts, managers, staff, and vendors to investigate variances and identify their sources.

The following sections discuss investigation of volume, expense, and revenue variance. Investigation of expense variance is presented in more detail, as sources of expense variance are frequently more controllable than volume or revenue variance. However, the concepts used in investigating expense variance are

○ T A B L E 5 - 4

Freeston Eldercare Ancillary Department Non-Personnel Expense Variance Report

Line # / 7400 Expense Items	Amount	Type	January						February					
			Budget	Actual	Variance	% Var.	Adj. % Var.	Adj. Var.	Budget	Actual	Variance	% Var.	Adj. % Var.	Adj. Var.
SNF & Intermediate Care Patient Days														
			3,193	**3,224**	**31**	**1.0%**	—	—	**2,856**	**2,703**	**(153)**	**-5.4%**	—	—
240 Pharmaceuticals	$3.98	PPD	$12,708	$12,976	$268	2.1%	1.1%	$144	$11,367	$11,385	$18	0.2%	5.5%	$627
250 Laboratory	$0.54	PPD	$1,724	$1,761	$37	2.1%	1.2%	$20	$1,542	$1,771	$228	14.8%	20.2%	$311
260 Radiology	$0.17	PPD	$543	$539	$(4)	-0.7%	-1.7%	$(9)	$486	$629	$143	29.6%	34.9%	$169
230 Medical Equipment	$150	Monthly	$150	$150	$0	0.0%	—	—	$150	$185	$35	23.3%	—	—
245 IV Supplies & Solutions	$993	Monthly	$993	$1,008	$15	1.5%	—	—	$993	$1,141	$148	14.9%	—	—
246 Enteral Supplies & Formula	$1,642	Monthly	$1,642	$1,660	$18	1.1%	—	—	$1,642	$1,603	$(39)	-2.4%	—	—
270 Oxygen & Oxygen Supplies	$674	Monthly	$674	$678	$4	0.6%	—	—	$674	$632	$(42)	-6.2%	—	—
300 Ancillary Non-Personnel			**$18,434**	**$18,772**	**$338**	**1.8%**	—	—	**$16,854**	**$17,346**	**$492**	**$0**	—	—
Average Ancillary Non-Personnel PPD			**$5.77**	**$5.82**	**$0.05**	**0.9%**	—	—	**$5.90**	**$6.42**	**$0.52**	**8.7%**	—	—

Freeston Eldercare Ancillary Department Non-Personnel Expense Variance Report

Line #	7400 Expense Items	Amount	Type	YTD 2003						YTD 2002					
				Budget	Actual	Variance	% Var.	Adj. % Var.	Adj. Var.	Budget	Actual	Variance	% Var.	Adj. % Var.	Adj. Var.
	SNF & Intermediate Care Patient Days			**6,049**	**5,927**	**(122)**	**-2.0%**	—	—	**5,932**	**6,046**	**114**	**1.9%**	—	—
240	Pharmaceuticals	$3.98	PPD	$24,075	$24,361	$286	1.2%	3.2%	$772	$22,245	$22,776	$531	2.4%	0.5%	$104
250	Laboratory	$0.54	PPD	$3,266	$3,532	$265	8.1%	10.1%	$331	$3,025	$3,077	$52	1.7%	-0.2%	$(6)
260	Radiology	$0.17	PPD	$1,028	$1,168	$140	13.6%	15.6%	$160	$919	$908	$(11)	-1.2%	-3.2%	$(29)
230	Medical Equipment	$150	Monthly	$300	$335	$35	11.7%	—	—	$121	$0	$(121)	-100.0%	—	—
245	IV Supplies & Solutions	$993	Monthly	$1,986	$2,149	$163	8.2%	10.2%	—	$1,867	$1,901	$34	1.8%	-0.1%	—
246	Enteral Supplies & Formula	$1,642	Monthly	$3,284	$3,263	$(21)	-0.6%	1.4%	—	$3,084	$3,107	$23	0.8%	-1.2%	—
270	Oxygen & Oxygen Supplies	$674	Monthly	$1,348	$1,310	$(38)	-2.8%	-0.8%	—	$1,252	$1,265	$13	1.0%	-0.9%	—
300	**Ancillary Non-Personnel**			**$35,288**	**$36,118**	**$830**	**2.4%**	—	—	**$32,514**	**$33,034**	**$520**	**1.6%**	—	—
	Average Ancillary Non-Personnel PPD	**$5.83**			**$6.09**	**$0.26**	**4.5%**	—	**$5.48**	**$5.46**	**$(0.02)**	**-0.3%**	—	—	—

BOX 5-4

Calculations and Applications for Variance Analysis

1. Budget variance
   a. Budget variance = actual value − budgeted value
   b. Identify favorable and unfavorable variances
   c. Compare to variance thresholds for investigation
2. Percent variance
   a. Percent variance = budget variance ÷ budget value
   b. YTD percent variance is an average percent variance
   c. Compare to prior performance patterns
   d. Compare over time—increasing or decreasing
   e. Compare to similar internal work units
   f. Compare to internal performance targets
   g. Compare to external benchmarks
3. Adjusted percent variance
   a. Percent budget variance – percent volume variance
   b. Adjusts for volume variance
   c. The more adjusted actual and budgeted percent variances differ, the more likely the variance requires investigation
4. Adjusted variance amount
   a. Budget value × adjusted percent variance
   b. Adjusts for volume variance
5. Average budget amount
   a. Monthly budget average = FY total budget ÷ 12 months
   b. Compare average budget amount to actual amount for same time period
   c. Useful as an overall target for fixed budgets
6. Average amount per unit of volume
   a. Sum of a set of budget values ÷ number of units of volume over same time period
   b. Use budgeted average amount per unit of volume as target
   c. Useful in analyzing flexible budgets
   d. Compare actual with budgeted average amount per unit of volume
   e. The more actual and budgeted average amounts per unit differ, the more likely source(s) of variance other than volume require investigation
7. Averages used to annualize
   a. Annualized monthly amount = YTD total ÷ months YTD
   b. Annualized FY amount = annualized YTD monthly amount × 12
   c. Useful in estimating or revising the budget during the FY

---

largely applicable to both volume and revenue variance. Budget investigation policies and methods differ from one work setting to another and may differ from the approach used in this text. It is important to learn how unfavorable budget variances are investigated in one's own work setting.

Types and Sources of Variance. This section discusses major types and sources of variance that lead to variance in profits, expenses, and revenues. The sources of variance are among the most frequently encountered in health care settings and identified in budget investigation. Some of the sources of variance discussed in this section are controllable; others are not.

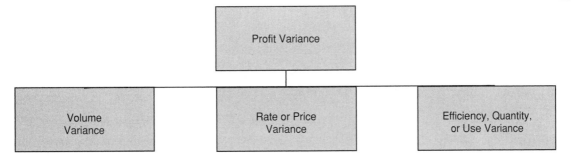

FIGURE 5.2 ■ Types of budget variance.

Figure 5-2 illustrates four major types of budget variance. Profit variance, mentioned earlier in this chapter, is the difference between revenues and expenses, as reported in the pro forma P&L statement. The investigation of profit variance requires the analysis of three types of budget variance that contribute to profit variance.

The first type of budget variance is volume variance. Change in the number of service units, such as patient days or patient visits, is the most common source of volume variance. This source of volume variance is typically based on external factors such as disease rates, so is difficult to control. Flexible budgeting adjusts for variance in the number of service units, so that other possible sources of variance in expenses or revenues may be identified.

In capitated managed care systems, change in the size of the enrolled population (also referred to as enrollment variance) is a source of volume variance. Larger populations are expected to generate a higher volume of health care goods and services than smaller populations, assuming that the population characteristics are the same. It may be possible to control volume if the population size or volume of services is negotiated as part of the contract.

Change in utilization or the amount of services provided is another source of volume variance. For example, if the duration of a patient's illness (**episode**) or the length of inpatient stay changes, it results in volume variance as measured by patient visits, patient days, or other service units. Utilization is also influenced by factors such as complication or readmission rates, as well as the characteristics of the population served, such as age and sex. Again, the most important element in most variance investigations is knowledge about the work setting, staff, and goods and services that are provided.

Some sources of volume variance related to utilization are more controllable than others. The implementation of clinical guidelines and quality improvement strategies may make it possible to reduce inpatient length of stay as well as complications and readmissions. Population characteristics are external to the health care setting, so are typically not controllable.

Rate or Price Variance. Rate variance (also referred to as **price variance**) is the difference between the budget and actual cost of personnel or non-personnel items in an expense budget report. Rate variance may be identified in both fixed and flexible budgets. In fixed budgets, changes in fixed costs (such as a mid-year increase in the lease or the loss of a fixed personnel position) are sources of rate variance.

In flexible budgets, a change in the price of supplies per service unit is a source of rate variance (also referred to as supplies variance). A change in the hourly wage rate is another source of rate variance (also referred to as staffing rate variance). For example, the use of higher-cost overtime or registry hourly wages for nursing care instead of the scheduled hourly wages is a source of staffing rate variance.

Sources of fixed cost variance may be difficult to control. For example, if utility or lease costs increase over the fiscal year, it is generally not feasible to change utility providers or relocate to another space.

Sources of supplies expenses may be controllable if it is possible to obtain supplies at a lower price by negotiating discounts or switching to another vendor.

Rate variance also represents the difference between the budget and actual amount of reimbursement in a revenue budget report. A change in the per diem bed rate paid by third party payors is a source of revenue rate variance. Changes in reimbursement denials by third party payors are another source of revenue rate variance. It is difficult to control these sources of revenue rate variance, as they are external to the health care setting.

Quantity or Efficiency Variance. Quantity variance (also referred to as **efficiency variance** or use variance) is the difference between the budget and actual amounts of non-personnel or personnel inputs used per time period or service unit. Chapter 1 discusses that efficiency is achieved by maximizing the production of goods or services while minimizing the resources required. Quantity variance therefore also represents efficiency variance, because the amount of inputs not only reflects a quantity but also the extent to which these inputs produce health care goods or services.

A change in the amount of fixed budget supplies or the amount of supplies used per service unit in flexible budgets is a source of quantity variance. A change in the amount of direct care hours provided per patient day is another source of quantity variance. In many cases, the sources of quantity variance are controllable. Staff training and supervision can reduce waste or other excessive use of supplies (including damage or theft) leading to quantity variance. Improving the efficiency of scheduling helps control personnel efficiency variance.

Quantity variance occurs in revenues as well as expenses. One source of revenue quantity variance is a change in the overall efficiency of billing and collecting reimbursement. Change in the amount of reimbursement collected over a given time period is also a source of revenue quantity variance. As discussed in Chapter 4, the longer it takes to collect reimbursement, the more likely a portion of that reimbursement will become uncollectible.

These sources of revenue quantity variance are controllable to some extent by improving the billing and collection functions of the health care institution. However, the increased use of review and denial mechanisms by third party payors is an external source of revenue quantity variance that is not controllable. Late payments and bad debt are additional sources of revenue quantity variance over which control is limited.

Total Variance. Any mix of volume, rate, or quantity variance may be combined to calculate **total variance**, which simultaneously accounts for variances in volume, price, and quantity. Total variance calculations are complex and beyond the scope of this text. Most health care settings using such complex variance reporting have finance departments with the expertise to produce such reports. A more common approach is to apply knowledge and experience about the context of personnel and non-personnel expenses to identify the source of any remaining variance after adjusting for volume. Box 5-5 summarizes types and sources of budget variance.

Budget Control

Some issues related to budget control were discussed in the section on the types and sources of variances. This section further develops concepts about budget control after monitoring and investigating unfavorable budget variances. In practice, the steps of budget monitoring, investigation, and control occur continuously and often nearly simultaneously. Many unfavorable variances that are controllable may be addressed as soon as they are identified.

One important factor in budget control, described and discussed in the previous section, is the ability to identify controllable sources of variance. As experience and knowledge of the work setting increases, it is possible to refine one's focus to monitor and investigate most closely the areas of the budget that raise the greatest financial concern and allow the most control. For example, the Nursing Services personnel budget

◻ **B O X   5 - 5**

Types and Sources of Budget Variance

■ Volume variance
  ● Change in the number of service units generating expenses or revenues
  ● Change in the incidence or prevalence of disease
  ● Change in the size of an enrolled population served by a capitated health plan
  ● Change in utilization or amount of services provided
    ● Duration of episode or length of inpatient stay
    ● Rate of complications or readmissions
    ● Population characteristics
■ Rate or price variance
  ● Change in the price of fixed or flexible budget supplies
  ● Change in salary or wage rate of flexible budget personnel
  ● Change in the reimbursement rate
■ Quantity or efficiency variance
  ● Change in the amount of supplies used
    ● Fixed (total amount) or flexible budget (per service unit)
    ● Supplies used related to waste, damage, or theft
  ● Change in direct care hours (staffing efficiency)
  ● Change in the amount of revenues
    ● Efficiency of billing and collecting reimbursement
    ● Amount of reimbursement collected over specified time period

involves a great amount of expense and the potential for considerable unfavorable variances. Although some sources of expense variance in the Nursing Services budget may not be controllable, such as volume, other sources, such as scheduling, may be controllable.

Experience and knowledge about the work setting are important in identifying sources of variance that are controllable. Sources of variance that are internal to the organization (such as scheduling, purchasing, and admissions policies) are typically more controllable than external sources of variance (such as new laws, weather or other events, and the general economy). Management authority to adjust staffing, supervise the productivity of employees, and make purchasing decisions also increases the ability to control variances.

Negotiated Contracts
One way to control both volume and revenue rate variance is through negotiated contracts for a specified volume at a predetermined price. Freeston ElderCare's contract with Zeta Health Systems (a managed care company) for managed care SNF beds is an example. A specified estimated volume of patient days with pre-set limits on length of stay is negotiated for each fiscal year, at a specified per diem bed rate. Zeta Health Systems covers a large population of elderly enrollees, so can ensure providing the contracted volume of patients. The preset bed rate is paid in full except when patient LOS exceeds the 31-day limit. By providing thorough patient assessment and rehabilitation services, Freeston ElderCare is able to control patient LOS in most cases and collect the entire revenue amount.

Management Strategies and Feedback
In many situations, budget control depends on management strategies such as closer staff supervision or instruction. For example, recall that in Table 5-4 laboratory expenses for February increased by 20.2% or

$311, adjusting for volume variance. The reason for this unfavorable variance was that nursing staff were using poor techniques in collecting specimens, so many laboratory tests had to be repeated. Controlling this unfavorable variance requires closer supervision and instruction of nursing staff. Donna Strand, the director of nursing at Freeston ElderCare, therefore works more closely with the nursing staff to improve the collection of laboratory specimens. The number of repeat laboratory tests falls as a result, and the unfavorable variance decreases accordingly over the rest of FY 2003 (not shown in Table 5-4).

Variance reports provide feedback regarding the effectiveness of management strategies. Donna will continue to closely monitor the Nursing Services non-personnel budget as well as the ancillary department laboratory line item to determine if the budget items of concern remain controlled.

Budget Adjustment Authority

Related to budget variance control is the authority to adjust the budget over the course of the fiscal year. **Adjustment authority** is addressed in organizational policies and refers to the power or permission to change the budget mid-year (in contrast to budget accountability, or responsibility for performance). The manager who has adjustment authority is allowed to revise the budget over the course of the fiscal year to correct for the difference between budget and actual in price or quantity variances that are expected to continue for the remaining part of the fiscal year. Typically, department directors or other staff accountable for budgets must present budget reports for approval of mid-year budget changes.

Line Item Flexibility. One example of budget adjustment authority is **line item flexibility**, or the authority of a manager to transfer funds from one line item to another line item, within specified policy limits. In most settings, the line items must be within the same category of personnel or non-personnel expenses, and in some settings may require additional budget justification or approval.

Line item flexibility and adjustment authority are usually exercised so the manager may **balance the budget**, applying budget control to adjust budget values to better fit the actual values, or to adjust the budget so that revenues equal or exceed expenses. There is no single formula or approach for all situations, but the following example provides insights on how managers exercise line item flexibility and budget adjustment authority.

Table 5-5 presents a report of line item transfers made by Donna, the Director of Nursing at Freeston ElderCare. Donna prepared this budget report after reviewing the June 2003 Nursing Services non-personnel variance report (not shown). An unexpected expense of $1,370 for nursing staff training required under new regulations occurred after the education and training budget of $1,860 was spent. Using budget authority, Donna looks for line items that are under budget that might allow the transfer of funds to cover the $1,370 budget shortfall for education and training.

In monitoring the budget, Donna observed that the actual medical waste expenses average about $32 per month under budget, annualized as $384 for FY 2003 (this is also indicated as the adjusted variance amount in Table 5-5). As there are only 6 months remaining in FY 2003, this budget surplus is annualized monthly at $64 ($384 ÷ 6) and authorized to be transferred monthly to the education and training budget for July through December. The revised FY 2003 budget for medical waste of $42,185 reflects the budget surplus of $384.

Donna also has the budget authority to cancel the purchase of two of the five wheelchairs budgeted as medical equipment for FY 2003 (see Table 5-5). As of June, $1,230 has been paid toward the remaining three wheelchairs ($205 × 6), leaving a final payment of $246 that will be made in July. The canceled purchase of two wheelchairs results in a budget surplus of $984 (shown as a favorable budget variance), which is annualized monthly at $164 ($984 ÷ 6) and transferred to the education and training budget for July through December. The revised FY 2003 medical equipment budget is therefore $1,476.

The transfers to education and training to meet the $1,370 deficit are indicated in the column for revised monthly amount in Table 5-5. The revised amount budgeted for education and training as of July 2003,

Freeston Eldercare Nursing Services Non-Personnel Line Item Transfers, July 2003

Line #	Items	Amount	Revised Amount[1]	Type	July Revised Budget	August Revised Budget	September Revised Budget	October Revised Budget	November Revised Budget	December Revised Budget	FY 2003 Budget	FY 2003 Revised Budget	FY 2003 Variance	FY 2003 % Var.	FY 2003 Adj. % Var.	FY 2003 Adj. Var.
7200	**Total SNF & Intermediate Care Patient Days[2]**				**3,348**	**3,379**	**3,270**	**3,441**	**3,360**	**3,503**	**39,128**	**3,9054**	**(74)**	**-0.2%**	—	—
220	Medical Supplies	$13.82	—	PPD	$46,269	$46,698	$45,191	$47,555	$46,435	$48,411	$540,749	$539,761	$(988)	-0.2%	0.0%	$35
215	Medical Waste	$1.09	See note[3]	PPD	$3,649	$3,683	$3,564	$3,751	$3,662	$3,818	$42,650	$42,185	$(465)	-1.1%	-0.9%	$(384)
230	Medical Equipment	$205	$246[4]	Monthly	$205	$205	$205	$205	$205	$205	$2,460	$1,476	$(984)	-40.0%	—	—
210	Education & Training	$155	$228[5]	Monthly	$155	$155	$155	$155	$155	$155	$1,860	$3,230	$1,370	73.7%	—	—
270	Copy & Printing	$75	—	Monthly	$75	$75	$75	$75	$75	$75	$900	$892	$(8)	-0.9%	—	—
280	Office Supplies	$45	—	Monthly	$45	$45	$45	$45	$45	$45	$540	$502	$(38)	-7.0%	—	—
300	**Nursing Services Non-Personnel**				**$50,399**	**$50,861**	**$49,236**	**$51,785**	**$50,578**	**$52,710**	**$589,158**	**$588,046**	**$(1,112)**	**-0.2%**	—	—

[1] Budget revisions effective July 15, 2003, applied to July budget.

[2] Revised budget FY 2003 patient days annualized based on January–June actual performance.

[3] Medical waste averages $32 under budget January–June so $64 per month transferred to education & training July–December.

[4] Purchase of 2 wheelchairs cancelled, final payment of $246 in July for $984 surplus transferred to education & training at $164 per month July–December.

[5] New training required at $1,370 after budget spent in June; transfers from medical waste & medical equipment July–December to meet deficit.

$228, is the sum of the $64 monthly transfer from the medical waste expense surplus and the $164 monthly transfer from the medical equipment expense surplus. The revised FY 2003 budget for education and training is $3,230. The budget is therefore balanced, with the shortfall of $1,370 in education and training covered by transfers of funds from medical waste and medical equipment.

The lines for medical supplies, copy and printing, and office supplies are within budget and included in Table 5-5 only because they are the remaining items in the non-personnel budget. A dash is inserted for each of these items in the column for revised budget amounts as there is no change in the expense allocations. Notes explaining budget revisions and transfers are included at the bottom of Table 5-5. The 39,054 revised budgeted patient days for FY 2003 are annualized from actual performance for January through June, as shown in Table 5-3.

Budget authority and line item flexibility policies and procedures may vary in other health care settings from what is indicated in the Table 5-5. Some settings might not permit the transfer of medical expenses to staff education, or might set dollar limits on the amount of funds that may be transferred. However, this example shows how budget shortfalls and surpluses might be controlled using annualization calculations and the application of budget authority and line item transfers.

Budget Justification. In some cases, the source of an unfavorable budget variance is an unexpected event that affects expenses or revenues, or an expense that is not budgeted. An example of an unusual event is an accident or other catastrophe. For example, if a fire caused the closure of Freeston ElderCare's SNF unit, the sudden unexpected reduction in capacity would result in revenues lost during the closure, and unbudgeted expenses for repairing or replacing the unit. In other cases, line items in a fixed budget might be found to vary with volume, resulting in unfavorable variances.

In many settings, a written budget justification report is prepared as part of the request for budget revisions or increases. Although these reports are longer and more detailed than the budget notes indicated in Table 5-5, they are usually relatively brief. Frequently the report is presented in a memo of one to five pages, depending on the extent and complexity of the budget concern. Box 5-6 presents some components that may be included in budget justification reports. These components are elements in the process of budget monitoring and control, so the manager uses monitoring and control information to prepare the budget justification. A sample budget justification report for budget increases related to the new managed care contract for hospice services at Freeston ElderCare is in the "Supplemental Tables and Documents" section of the Back-of-Book CD-ROM.

Box 5-7 summarizes the factors to consider in budget control discussed in this section.

☐ BOX 5-6

Components of a Budget Justification

- Budget line item(s) requiring justification
- Category and type of line item (revenue vs. expense, direct vs. indirect, fixed vs. flexible)
- Variance amounts, averages, and percents
- Adjusted variance, if applicable
- Frequency, duration, and trend of variance
- Variance source or sources
- Source identified as controllable or uncontrollable
- Control steps taken and results, if applicable
- Potential impact on revenue
- Effect on profits (if revenues are generated)
- Revised budget table with explanatory notes

□ **BOX 5-7**

Factors in Budget Control

1. Focus on controllable sources of variance
2. Negotiated contracts for a specified volume
3. Management strategy implementation and feedback to evaluate budget control efforts
4. Budget adjustment authority
   a. Line item flexibility
   b. Justification of unexpected and unbudgeted expenses or variances

Conclusion

This chapter presents concepts important in monitoring budgets, investigating budget variances, and controlling unfavorable budget variances, especially in operating expenses. Chapter 6 builds on these concepts by discussing concepts and approaches to budget preparation.

■ CRITICAL THINKING EXERCISES

1. If available, obtain copies of revenue and expense budgets from your own health care setting, concealing the setting's identity as appropriate. Practice calculating the variance, percent variance, adjusted percent variance, and adjusted variance. Think about possible sources of undesirable variance and whether they can be controlled. Discuss.
2. If budgets from health settings are not available, use information from the operating expense or operating revenue budgets for Freeston ElderCare in the "Supplemental Tables and Documents" section of the Back-of-Book CD-ROM to create a quarterly expense budget variance report for monitoring, investigation, and control. Practice calculations, consider sources of undesirable variance, and discuss as in Exercise 1.
3. Use the operating revenue budget for Freeston ElderCare in the "Supplemental Tables and Documents" section of the Back-of-Book CD-ROM to create a quarterly revenue budget variance report. Compare and contrast to the analysis of expense budgets. Identify whether variances can be controlled. Discuss.

■ REFERENCES

Baker, J. J., & Baker, R. W. (2000). *Health Care Finance: Basic Tools for Nonfinancial Managers*. Gaithersburg, MD: Aspen.

Cleverley, W. O., & Cameron, A. E. (2002). *Essentials of Health Care Finance*, 5th ed. Gaithersburg, MD: Aspen.

Eichenberger, J. (1998). Project Management, Part III: Budgets for Projects. *AAOHN Journal, 46*(5), 268–270.

Finkler, S. A., & Kovner, C. T. (2000). *Financial Management for Nurse Managers and Executives*, 2nd ed. Philadelphia: W. B. Saunders.

Gapenski, L. C. (2002). *Healthcare Finance: An Introduction to Accounting and Financial Management*, 2nd ed. Chicago: Health Administration Press.

Herkimer, A. G. (1988). *Understanding Health Care Budgeting*. Gaithersburg, MD: Aspen.

Neumann, B. R., Suber, J. D., & Zelman, W. N. (1988). *Financial Management: Concepts and Applications for Health Care Providers*, 2nd ed. Owings Mills, MD: National Health Publishing.

Nowicki, M. (2001). *The Financial Management of Hospitals and Healthcare Organizations*. Chicago: Health Administration Press.

CHAPTER 6

Budget Preparation

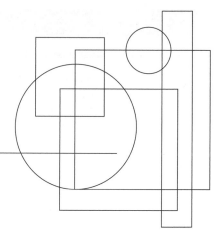

- ● **Factors in Budget Preparation**
  Budget Cycle and Strategic Plan
- ● **Operating Budget Preparation**
  Incremental Budgeting
  Forecasting
  Variance Analysis and Budget
    Preparation
  Fixed and Flexible Non-Personnel
    Expenses
  Fixed and Flexible Personnel Expenses
  Revenue Budgeting and Budget
    Balancers
  Budgeting for New Line Items
- ● **Preparing the Capital Budget**
- ● **Preparing the Cash Flow Budget**
- ● **Additional Budget Preparation**
  Concepts
  "What-If" Calculations
  Step-Fixed FTEs and Budgeting
  Zero-Base Budgeting
  Closing a Program
- ● **Conclusion**

■ Learning Objectives

1. Explain the purpose of linking the statistics budget, operating budget, capital budget and cash flow budget in sequence in budget preparation.
2. Describe and evaluate at least two approaches to making budget estimates in preparing an operating expense budget.
3. Differentiate between fixed and flexible approaches in preparing an operating expense budget, and discuss the purpose of each approach.

○ Key Terms

Acuity
Adjusted FTE
Assumption
Budget balancer
Budget cycle
Fixed staff
Forecasting
Goal
Incremental budgeting
Master budget
Objective
Profit target
Priority

Prospective forecasting
Qualitative forecasting
Quantitative forecasting
Retrospective forecasting
Staff mix
Staffing
Step-fixed staff
Strategic plan
Trend line
Variable staff
What-if calculation
Zero-base budgeting

Chapter 4 discusses how budgets describe and report financial activities, and Chapter 5 presents concepts for using budgets to monitor financial activities in health care settings. Another important function of a budget is to serve as a financial plan for the future, which is the focus of this chapter (Fig. 6-1).

Budget planning involves making predictions for future time periods, often the next fiscal year, and the resulting budget is a plan for financial performance that establishes targets for volume, revenues, and expenses. Budget planning anticipates change over the fiscal year and from year to year. Finally, budget preparation is a way to introduce and reinforce budget control by setting financial targets that require efficient management and performance.

Budget preparation is also important in developing business plans and health program grant proposals for launching a new program or service. Chapter 12 dis-

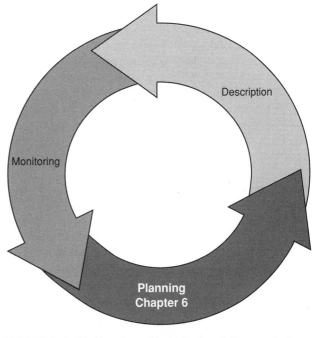

FIGURE 6.1 ■ Functions of budgets: description, monitoring, and planning.

cusses budget estimates for a business plan, and Chapter 13 discusses budget estimates for health program grant proposals.

This chapter first discusses scheduling and deadlines for budget preparation, then presents concepts relevant to budget preparation for operating and capital budgets. Considerations in preparing a cash flow budget are introduced, as well as additional concepts such as **zero-base budgeting**, or preparing a continuing budget as if it were intended for a new program or service in order to improve accuracy and control.

Freeston ElderCare continues as the setting for most of the budget examples. FY 2003 is designated as the "current year," FY 2004 is "next year," and FY 2002 is "last year" in referring to time periods for budgets discussed in this chapter. Indirect and overhead costs are discussed in Chapter 7.

Factors in Budget Preparation

A number of factors are worth considering in approaching the budget preparation process. Among these factors are the budget cycle and schedule of budgeting activities in the health care setting. The assumptions, priorities, goals, objectives, and performance targets set by the organizational leadership for the next fiscal year are other factors. Forecasting and estimating the volume, revenues, and expenses for the next fiscal year is another factor. Line items that were not currently budgeted but are reported as actual revenues or expenses, and new line items anticipated for the next fiscal year are factors in budget preparation. Decisions to offer new programs, products, or services are factors, as are directives to use zero-base budgeting approaches and needs to balance the budget to achieve the desired level of profit. Each of these sets of factors that affect budget preparation are discussed in more detail in the following sections.

Budget Cycle and Strategic Plan

Although budgeting is a continuous managerial activity, most organizations establish a **budget cycle** (a specified schedule and deadlines for budget preparation, negotiation, approval, and implementation). As with other aspects of budgeting, organizations differ in their policies for establishing the budget cycle. In many settings, a calendar that schedules deadlines for assignments such as budget reports, proposals, final budgets, and budget justification is distributed.

In many settings, an important element of the budget cycle is the **strategic plan** (a financial report that presents a plan for organizational financial management and performance for a longer time period than the next fiscal year). The strategic plan is generally prepared by the organization's executive leadership with input from department directors and financial officers. For example, Freeston ElderCare's administrator, Marie, prepares the strategic plan for FY 2004–2007 with assistance and input from the department directors, then presents the plan to executives at XYZ Health Corporation, the health system that owns Freeston ElderCare and other similar facilities.

The strategic plan often begins by reporting an intensive internal and external environmental assessment of actual and potential situations or changes that may be favorable or unfavorable to the institution. For example, improvements in uncomplicated hip replacement surgery reduced the length of stay (LOS) for SNF patients, which affected Medicare requirements regarding the intensity of rehabilitation services, as well as LOS limits. Other actual or potential changes include new third party payor regulations, consumer preferences, or technology. These and other situations or changes may enhance or threaten the organization's financial performance over the strategic plan's time period. The anticipation and analysis of actual or potential threats or opportunities over the next fiscal years enables the organizational leadership to take a proactive approach to manage these situations.

For example, Marie analyzed the expansion of Zeta Health Systems in the local area and learned they are focusing on cancer treatment as part of their "centers of excellence" mission. She anticipates a small but steady demand for hospice placement and began negotiating and contracting for providing hospice services as a result.

Based on the environmental assessment and analysis, the strategic plan then presents the mission statement and vision for what the organization is desired or expected to look like in the projected fiscal years. Assumptions, priorities, goals, objectives, and performance targets are developed from the environmental analyses, mission statement, and vision. **Assumptions** represent expectations or beliefs about the internal or external environment that influence administrative and financial decision making. For example, Marie assumes there will be increasing payor and consumer concern about the quality of life in long-term care facilities such as Freeston ElderCare, based on increased regulation, news media reports, articles in the long-term care literature, and other information sources. **Priorities** are organizational activities or issues that are believed to be of the most importance for profitability or survival. Based on Marie's assumption, one priority is for Freeston ElderCare to develop programs that improve the patient's quality of life by addressing individual preferences and needs.

Goals are broad statements describing what is to be accomplished over the long or short term. Given Marie's priority of better addressing the individual preferences and needs of Freeston ElderCare residents to enhance quality of life, one's goal is to provide patients with recreation resources appropriate to their age, culture, and health status. **Objectives** represent clearly stated, measurable tasks intended to achieve a goal within a specific time frame. For example, one of Marie's objectives is to submit a budget proposal by the scheduled deadline of Oct. 22, 2003, for an activities program at Freeston ElderCare to be implemented over FY 2004.

Performance targets are measurable indicators for evaluating the achievement of objectives. The approval of the proposed activity program's budget is one example of a performance target; another example would be the actual implementation of the activity program on schedule over FY 2004. Budget amounts are also performance targets that are compared to actual revenues or expenses over the fiscal year in budget monitoring (see Chap. 5).

Proposals for new programs and for existing program expansion or reduction are then presented in the strategic plan. Plans for major investments and projections of operating revenues and expenses are included. These plans, projections, and associated budgets are usually summarized to indicate overall estimates of volume, revenue, expenses, and profitability, and are reported in more detail when implemented and reviewed over a fiscal year. This section of the strategic plan is based on the assumptions, priorities, goals, objectives, and performance targets that were developed out of the environmental analysis, mission statement, and vision. The purpose of the proposals, plans, projections, and their associated budgets is to enable the organization to achieve its mission and vision within the environment anticipated over the next fiscal years.

Following the development of the strategic plan, department directors (often assisted by their staff) prepare and submit departmental and other work unit budget proposals. These proposals include budgets for new programs, substantial changes in programs, or extensive capital improvements. Department directors also prepare the operating and capital budgets for continuing programs and services. If responsible for cash flow management, department directors prepare and submit the cash flow budgets. After submission of these budgets, there is a schedule of review, negotiation, and approval or denial of the budgets by upper-level administration. Budgets may need to be revised and resubmitted for final approval.

For example, XYZ Health Corporation exercises close oversight over the profitability of Freeston Elder-Care and denied Marie's budgeting of a 3% raise for administrative staff and department directors for FY 2004. Marie revised the operating expense budget accordingly, leaving administrative and department director salaries the same as for FY 2003. On the other hand, during budget negotiations with XYZ executives, Marie was able to justify the proposed activities program budget expenses and obtain approval without major revisions.

After all of the budgets are prepared, submitted, negotiated, revised, and approved, budget worksheets and guidelines are distributed to implement the budget for the next fiscal year. In addition, many organizations develop a **master budget**, a budget report that combines the organization's strategic plan, long-range budget, operating budget(s), capital budget(s), cash flow budget(s), and budget proposals into one document to present the financial plan over the long term linked to planning for the next fiscal year. The master budget is presented to Freeston ElderCare's Board of Directors and serves as a general reference for the goals, objectives, and performance targets for the entire organization and each of its departments for FY 2004.

Box 6-1 summarizes elements of the budget cycle.

Budget Calendar

Table 6-1 presents the budget preparation calendar used at Freeston ElderCare. The new budget cycle begins Oct. 1, 2003, with the presentation of the FY 2004–2007 strategic plan, with any revisions completed and approval scheduled the following week.

On Oct. 15, 2003, the administration sends out packets of information to all the department directors with worksheets for preparing the FY 2004 budget. The budget worksheets (as shown in subsequent budget tables in this chapter) allow directors to report past and current year budget performance as well as their FY 2004 budget estimates. The information packet also includes the short-term strategic plan outlining the assumptions, priorities, goals, objectives, and performance targets for FY 2004 as established for Freeston ElderCare. Directors must submit budget proposals (in other words, budgets for new programs, program expansion, or extensive capital improvement) to the administration office by the following week. For example, Marie submits a budget proposal for a new activities program.

BOX 6-1

Elements of the Budget Cycle

- Calendar with schedule and assignments for budget preparation
- Communication of the organization's assumptions, priorities, goals, objectives, and performance targets for the next budget year as part of the strategic plan
- Preparation of budget proposals, followed by the operating and capital budgets, then the cash budget
- Budget negotiation, revision, and final approval
- Preparation, presentation, and approval of the master budget
- Distribution of the next budget year budget worksheets and guidelines to begin budget implementation, monitoring, and control
- Evaluation of performance over the completed budget year

TABLE 6-1

Freeston ElderCare Budget Calendar for FY 2004 Preparation

Date	Activity/Assignment	Accountability
10/1/03	Presentation & negotiation of preliminary strategic plan for FY 2004–2007	Dept. Directors & Administration
10/8/03	Final strategic plan approval	Administration
10/15/03	Budget packets with Q4 2002–Q3 2003 budget reports, FY 2004 worksheets & strategic plan for FY 2004–2007 sent to all dept. directors	Administration
10/22/03	Budget proposals (new programs, program expansions, major capital improvements) for FY 2004 due	Dept. Directors & Administration
10/29/03	Preliminary FY 2004 operating & capital budgets due	Dept. Directors & Administration
11/1/03	Preliminary FY 2004 cash budget due	Administration
11/5/03	Budget justification & negotiation for budget proposals & preliminary budgets	Dept. Directors & Administration
11/8/03	Budget justification & negotiation for the cash budget	Administration
11/12/03	Final FY 2004 budget proposals, operating budgets, capital budgets, & cash budget due	Dept. Directors & Administration
11/19/03	Presentation of strategic plan for FY 2004–2007 and master budget for FY 2004 to the Board of Directors	Administration
12/3/03	FY 2004 budget approval or denial	Administration
12/10/03	Revisions of denied budgets due	Dept. Directors & Administration
12/17/03	FY 2004 budget worksheets & guidelines sent to all dept. directors	Administration
1/21/04	Complete FY 2003 budget reports to all Dept. directors	Administration
1/28/04	Performance reports for evaluation of achieving FY 2003 priorities, goals, objectives, & targets due	Dept. Directors & Administration

Preliminary operating budgets and capital budgets must then be submitted by department directors and administrators, then justified and negotiated in budget meetings until the final budget targets are agreed upon. Marie submits and negotiates the cash flow budget. The strategic plan and master budget are then submitted to and reviewed by Freeston ElderCare's Board of Directors. Final approval or denial of budgets then occurs, with a deadline for budget revision for budgets or budget items receiving administrative denial. Budget implementation then begins with the distribution of FY 2004 worksheets and reporting guidelines. The complete budget figures for FY 2003 are available early in 2004, with the assignment for departmental directors and administrators to review their FY 2003 budget reports and evaluate how well their department met organizational priorities, goals, objectives, and performance targets. This evaluation is used as performance feedback.

Linkage

A concept useful in budget preparation is linkage of budgets so that one budget logically builds on another. Remember that the strategic plan establishes overall assumptions, goals, priorities, and objectives for the next fiscal year. The statistics budget that estimates volume over the next budget year is typically prepared before the operating budget, because revenues and expenses based on volume require statistics budget estimates. The operating and cash flow budgets are then prepared. The capital budget is often closely linked to the strategic plan, because major purchases or renovations require long-term financial investment and are expected to generate revenues over the long term.

Another aspect to linkage is that when preparing the budget, it is important to be aware of budget policies, guidelines, and targets. For example, requirements for direct care hours must be addressed in an hourly personnel budget, and a pro forma P&L statement should be estimated if a **profit target** (specified amount or percent of profit) must be met.

Operating Budget Preparation

Most of this chapter focuses on the preparation of the operating budget, with a focus on the operating expense budget. As mentioned in Chapter 5, budget authority is most often extended to reviewing and monitoring the operating expense budget, and this is the case for budget preparation as well. Considerable attention is given to the preparation of the personnel expense budget, as it is frequently the most costly and the most complex part of an operating expense budget.

Incremental Budgeting

A relatively simple and frequently used approach to budget preparation is **incremental budgeting**, in which the current year's budget is used as the base for the next year's budget, making additions or reductions or keeping the base the same. These incremental changes to the budget usually depend on administrative guidelines communicated during the budget preparation part of the budget cycle. Administrative guidelines might require either a given dollar amount or a percent of incremental change in the current budget for the new budget.

In some situations, particularly in smaller settings with less formal administrative procedures, incremental budget changes might be based on assumptions and budget variances. For example, if a clinic's volume of patient visits is 5% less than budgeted, a clinic director might assume the same performance the following fiscal year, and reduce budgeted revenues and flexible budget expense items such as medical supplies by 5%.

Table 6-2 shows the Freeston ElderCare Rehabilitation Department's incremental budget worksheet for FY 2004. Budget worksheets vary from one setting to another, and it is important to learn the format of budgets and budget worksheets used in one's own setting. The budget worksheet in Table 6-2 and in most

○ TABLE 6-2

Freeston ElderCare Rehabilitation Department, Incremental Budget Worksheet FY 2004

				FY 2002 Variance			
Items	FTE	Amount	Type	Budget	Actual	Variance	% Var.
SNF Patient Days	—	—	—	**12,387**	**12,592**	**205**	**1.7%**
Rehabilitation Dir./PT	1.0	$4,842	Monthly	$58,107	$58,107	$0	0.0%
Occupational Therapist	0.5	$4,720	Monthly	$28,320	$28,320	$0	0.0%
PT Aide	0.5	$2,903	Monthly	$17,419	$26,062	$8,643	49.6%
Occupational Therapist Aide	0.5	$2,801	Monthly	$16,808	$16,808	$0	0.0%
Rehabilitation Payroll[1]	—	—	—	**$120,654**	**$129,297**	**$8,643**	**7.2%**
Benefits		25%	of Payroll	$30,164	$32,324	$2,161	7.2%
Rehabilitation Personnel	—	—	—	**$150,818**	**$161,622**	**$10,804**	**7.2%**
Medical Supplies[2]		$525	Monthly	$6,300	$6,582	$282	4.5%
Medical Equipment[3]		$200	Monthly	$2,400	$2,400	$—	0.0%
Other Non-Personnel[4]		$64	Monthly	$768	$751	$(17)	−2.2%
Rehabilitation Non-Personnel	—	—	—	**$9,468**	**$9,733**	**$265**	**2.8%**
Total Rehabilitation	—	—	—	**$160,286**	**$171,355**	**$11,069**	**6.9%**
Rehabilitation Expense PPD	—	—	—	**$12.94**	**$13.61**	**$0.67**	**5.2%**

[1] A 3% pay increase for all Rehabilitation Department staff is approved for FY 2004.

[2] A 10% budget increase for medical supplies is approved for FY 2004.

[3] A $1,000 budget reduction in non-capital medical equipment (from a $2,500 to $1,500 limit) is approved for FY 2004.

No increases or reduction are approved or required for office supplies and subscriptions for FY 2004.

of the budget tables in this chapter contain three sections. The first section presents the past year's (in this case FY 2002) budget and actual figures, variances, and percent variances. The second section presents the FY 2003 budget and the actual 9-month figures annualized for 12 months, accompanied by variances and percent variances. The third section presents the FY 2004 budget with variances and percent variances comparing the line items to the FY 2003 budget. Explanatory notes are included at the bottom of the worksheet as needed to report administrative guidelines, assumptions, or other information relevant in reviewing the worksheet.

The summarized budget report for FY 2002 is presented in the first section of Table 6-2. The actual patient volume is very close to budgeted over the fiscal year. There is a large unfavorable personnel expense variance for the PT aide of 49.6% that is the result of 344 hours of unscheduled overtime paid at 50% over the hourly wage of $16.75. The Rehabilitation Department director was able to justify an increase in PT aide personnel from 0.5 FTE to 1.0 FTE for FY 2003. The non-personnel line items are also reported for FY 2002.

The second section of Table 6-2 reports the FY 2003 budget and actual variances. Patient days are 2.9% greater than budgeted, and both the PT and PT aide personnel expenses are the same as budgeted. The occupational therapist worked 316 hours of overtime paid at 50% over the hourly wage of $28.07, resulting in the occupational therapist expense 45.6% over budget. The occupational therapist aide (OTA) worked 254.5 hours of overtime paid at 50% over the hourly wage of $16.66, resulting in the OTA expense 36.7% over

	FY 2003 Variance							FY 2004 Incremental Budget				
FTE	Amount	Type	Budget	Annualized Actual	Variance	% Var.	FTE	Amount	Type	Budget 2004	Variance FY 2003–2004	% Var. FY 2003–2004
—	—	—	12,874	13,252	378	2.9%	—	—	—	13,657	783	6.1%
1.0	$4,992	Monthly	$59,904	$59,904	$0	0.0%	1.0	$5,142	Monthly	$61,701	$1,797	3.0%
0.5	$4,866	Monthly	$29,196	$42,503	$13,307	45.6%	0.75	$3,759	Monthly	$45,108	$15,912	54.5%
1.0	$2,993	Monthly	$35,916	$35,916	$0	0.0%	1.0	$3,083	Monthly	$36,993	$1,077	3.0%
0.5	$2,888	Monthly	$17,328	$23,689	$6,361	36.7%	0.75	$2,231	Monthly	$26,772	$9,444	54.5%
			$142,344	$162,011	$19,667	13.8%				$170,574	$28,230	19.8%
	25%	of Payroll	$35,586	$40,503	$4,917	13.8%		25%	of Payroll	$42,644	$7,058	19.8%
—	—	—	$177,930	$202,514	$24,584	13.8%	—	—	—	$213,218	$35,288	19.8%
	$585	Monthly	$7,020	$7,245	$225	3.2%	$	644	Monthly	$7,722	$702	10.0%
	$193	Monthly	$2,316	$2,316	$0	0.0%	$	198	Monthly	$1,488	$(828)	35.8%
	$78	Monthly	$936	$ 863	$(73)	−7.8%	$	78	Monthly	$936	$–	0.0%
—	—	—	$10,272	$10,424	$152	1.5%	—	—	—	$10,146	$(126)	−1.2%
—	—	—	$188,202	$212,938	$24,736	13.1%	—	—	—	$223,364	$35,162	18.7%
—	—	—	$14.62	$16.07	$1.45	9.9%	—	—	—	$16.36	$1.74	11.9%

budget. The hourly wages for the occupational therapist and OTA are not reported in Table 6-2 but are calculated by dividing the total budgeted salary by the total budgeted FTE hours. For example, the total budgeted salary for the occupational therapist is $29,196, divided by 1,040 hours in 0.5 FTE to obtain $28.07 per hour wage. The unfavorable variances in occupational therapy personnel expenses are of considerable concern when the budget is reviewed.

For FY 2004, a 3% pay increase is approved for all Rehabilitation Department staff, as shown in the FY 2004 incremental budget variances in the third section of Table 6-2 for the PT/director and the PT aide. The occupational therapist and OTA FY 2004 line items are 54.5% greater than for FY 2003. This variance is the result of the department director's decision to request an incremental increase from 0.5 to 0.75 FTE for both the occupational therapist and OTA for FY 2004, plus the 3% wage increase. The Rehabilitation Department director assumes that the direct hours required of the occupational therapist will continue to increase over FY 2004, and that by increasing occupational therapist hours it is possible to keep both the occupational therapist and OTA expenses within budget. This incremental increase is not specified in the administrative guidelines for the FY 2004 budget, so it will require justification (discussed further in the section on zero-base budgeting).

In reviewing the non-personnel expense items for the Rehabilitation Department in Table 6-2, the FY 2003 actual expenses for medical supplies are 3.2% over budget. However, a 10% increase in medical supplies for all patient care departments at Freeston ElderCare is approved for FY 2004 and is budgeted accordingly. A $1,000 budget reduction for non-capital equipment expenses is required for all patient care departments for FY 2004 (reducing the limit from $2,500 to $1,500). The FY 2004 equipment budget is $1,488. Administrative guidelines specify no change in the budget for office supplies and subscriptions (which represent the other non-personnel line item). Even though the Rehabilitation Department is well under budget for other non-personnel expenses, the budget remains the same as for FY 2003.

The advantage of incremental budgeting is that it is relatively simple and supported by administrative policy. Incremental budget decisions are largely centralized and controlled at the top administrative levels, although in some settings department directors or other staff responsible for budgets may provide input. Any budget request outside the administrative guidelines must be justified, as in the request to increase the occupational therapist and OTA FTEs from 0.5 to 0.75.

One problem with incremental budgeting is that there is a tendency to increase the budget by the maximum amount allowed without always fully analyzing the actual need for an increase. For example, a 10% increase in the medical supplies budget might be greater than actually required for the Rehabilitation Department (see Table 6-2). Incremental overbudgeting is inefficient, as more resources are budgeted than actually required.

Incremental reductions (budget cuts) may also occur without a complete analysis of their need or consequences. The actual budget requirements may vary from one department to another, so an incremental budget reduction might be excessive for one department, while other departments could manage with the same or greater budget reduction, or require a budget increase to operate most efficiently and profitably. It is difficult to know from Table 6-2 whether the budget reductions, increases, or continuations are accurate, efficient, and necessary. Because incremental budgeting relies on administrative guidelines, there may be little analysis or justification of any items in this budget other than the change in the occupational therapy personnel positions. Other budget preparation approaches, discussed in the following sections, help overcome the limitations of incremental budgeting.

Forecasting

Forecasting is a more formal process for budget preparation than incremental budgeting, using systematic methods to estimate future volume, revenues, and expenses as accurately and reliably as possible. **Qualitative forecasting** methods rely on experts or leaders basing their predictions on subjective experience. **Quantitative forecasting** methods involve the collection and mathematical analysis of measures such as patient days and dollar amounts. Many forecasting methods require knowledge of advanced research and mathematical modeling techniques that are beyond the scope of this text. Large health systems such as Kaiser Permanente have departments with experts assigned to make their forecasts.

Forecasting methods differ regarding their time perspective. **Retrospective forecasting** methods assume that future events are largely a result of past events, so retrospective forecasts are based on historical data and trends. For example, the Research Department at XYZ Health Corporation keeps records of the volume and utilization (LOS, diagnosis, and bed type) for their facilities for the last 10 years and uses these historical data to make predictions about volume for future fiscal years. **Prospective forecasting** methods assume that current information enables the prediction of future events, so prospective forecasts are based on information such as regulations and policies that are implemented. The Research Department compiles legislative reports, updates from health plans, and other current changes in reimbursement rates and policies to help forecast revenues for future fiscal years.

A combination of retrospective and prospective methods is often advisable. For example, the long-term care facility revenue forecasts made by the XYZ Health Corporation Research Department are based both on retrospective forecasts using analyses of past utilization patterns and on prospective forecasts using analyses of changes in payor policies that will be implemented over the coming fiscal year.

At Freeston ElderCare, forecasts of volume and revenue are routinely prepared by the XYZ Health Corporation Research Department. Freeston ElderCare administrators and department directors use these forecasts to prepare the statistics, revenue, and cash flow budgets. Expense budgets at Freeston ElderCare are prepared using incremental budgeting, unless there are unusual budget variances or budget requests outside of the incremental guidelines (as shown in Table 6-2) or a new program budget is proposed.

The accuracy of a forecast is expected to decrease as the time frame increases. In other words, a forecast made in FY 2003 for FY 2004 is likely to be more accurate than a forecast made in FY 2003 for FY 2010. Although the past is a relatively accurate predictor of the future, change occurs over time. As a result, uncertainty (in other words, the probability of forecasting error) increases the further the projection extends into the future. Even short-term forecasts are rarely precisely accurate, so the estimated error is typically reported, or an estimated range is presented instead of a single forecasted value. Freeston ElderCare's strategic plan is for 4 years, FY 2004–2007, and the operating and cash flow budgets are estimated from year to year.

It is important to be clear about the time frame over which the forecast is made and the assumptions involved in making forecasts. Potential sources of error should also be reported, so the reviewer understands the limitations of the forecast. Once reported, forecasts should be monitored for accuracy. Based on the extent to which the forecast fits actual experience, the forecasting method may be retained, revised, or replaced, as could the time frame and the assumptions used in making the forecast.

Figure 6-2 presents an example of forecasting that might be reported from a financial department with the skills and resources to use advanced forecasting methods. This method uses a **trend line** (a line created by a

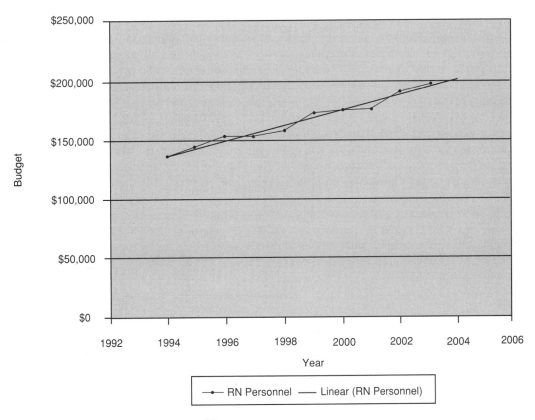

FIGURE 6.2 ■ Forecasting using trend lines.

mathematical equation that estimates the movement of an economic variable over time). In this example, Nursing Services RN personnel expense budgets (including benefits and budgeted overtime) are reported from 1994 to 2003 for Freeston ElderCare's SNF and intermediate care units. The trend line presents an estimated straight line mathematically plotted through the data points, with a forecasted personnel expense budget of $200,000 for FY 2004. This is a quantitative forecast, as the data are budget dollars, and is also a retrospective forecast that bases the FY 2004 estimate on data from FY 1994 to 2003.

⊙ **TABLE 6-3**

Patient Volume Estimates for 2004 by SNF Administrators, 2003

| | Range of Responses Method | |
| | Low Prediction | High Prediction |
Estimates		
Administrator A	2.5%	5.0%
Administrator B	4.0%	6.0%
Administrator C	7.0%	8.5%
Patient volume forecast	**4.5%**	**6.5%**

An example of a qualitative forecasting method using a range of estimates is shown in Table 6-3. This method involves recording the estimates or predictions of leaders or experts and averaging their responses. In this example, three nursing home administrators are asked to provide low and high estimates for change in patient volume from FY 2003 to 2004. The estimates are then averaged, resulting in a forecast ranging from 4.5% to 6.5%. Reporting a range of estimates helps account for forecasting error, as there are many factors that influence patient volume.

Many health care settings do not possess the expertise and resources required to make forecasts using advanced mathematical techniques or qualitative surveys. Despite its limitations, incremental budgeting is often sufficient for budget preparation. Other approaches discussed in the following sections may also help in obtaining reasonably accurate estimates for budget preparation. Box 6-2 summarizes concepts applicable to forecasting for budget preparation.

Variance Analysis and Budget Preparation

Variance analysis focusing on volume, price, or quantity is helpful in budget preparation. Table 6-4 provides examples of the application of variance analysis in preparing the FY 2004 Freeston ElderCare Ancillary Department non-personnel expense budget. The first section reports the budget and actual figures and variances for FY 2002 for comparison.

For FY 2003, the pharmaceuticals line item shows an unfavorable variance: the actual expense for pharmaceuticals for FY 2003 is $10,745, or 6.9% over budget. Investigation found that the source of this unfavorable variance is price variance (price increases) that cannot be controlled. Further investigation of price variance indicates that pharmaceutical expense for FY 2004 will be an estimated 10% above the FY 2003 budget, adjusting for volume.

The laboratory line item for FY 2003 shown in Table 6-4 represents a different result based on variance analysis. As discussed in Chapter 5, the investigation of unfavorable laboratory expense variance early in FY 2003 revealed that the source was controllable quantity variance (waste related to poor technique). Improved staff training and supervision brought this quantity variance under control by the end of FY 2003, so that the 4% increase in the laboratory expense for FY 2004 reflects the estimated increase in volume. Neither the per patient day (PPD) price nor the PPD quantity of laboratory services is expected to increase for FY 2004.

Table 6-4 reports that the FY 2003 line item for medical equipment shows an unfavorable fixed cost variance, as the purchase price for the equipment increased by $35 per month beginning in February. Although

---

B O X   6 - 2

Concepts of Forecasting

1. Forecasting requires effort, expense, and expertise.
   a. Many forecasting methods are highly advanced and not readily available to managers in health care settings.
   b. Incremental approaches often achieve similar results as forecasting, at less cost.
   c. Focus forecasting on categories of most concern that can be reasonably accurately forecasted—use incremental methods for other categories and when forecasting is not effective or realistic.
2. A combination of retrospective and prospective methods is often advisable.
   a. Retrospective methods: Assume that future events substantially result from past events, so forecasts are based on historical data and trends.
   b. Prospective methods: Assume that current information enables prediction of future events, so forecasts are based on information such as regulations and policies that will be implemented.
3. Forecasting accuracy decreases as the time frame increases.
   a. Uncertainty increases the further events are projected into the future.
   b. Short-range forecasts are usually more accurate than long-range forecasts.
4. Forecasts are rarely precisely accurate.
   a. Allowances should be made for error, or a reasonable range offered instead of a single forecasted value.
   b. Forecasts should be specific regarding the time frame of the forecast and any assumptions involved in making the forecast.
   c. Forecasts should be monitored for accuracy, and then retain, revise, or replace the methods, time frame, and assumptions based on accuracy.

---

the source of this variance could not be controlled, it will not affect the FY 2004 line item budget as no medical equipment is requested by the ancillary department for FY 2004.

The FY 2003 line item for IV supplies and solutions also shows an unfavorable variance. Over FY 2003, the price for IV supplies and solutions increased by 20%, which is reflected in a 15.2% annual increase as the existing inventory was replaced over the year. However, investigation of this unfavorable variance led the director of the ancillary department to change vendors for FY 2004, so the IV supplies and solutions line item for FY 2004 reflects a price increase of only 5% over the FY 2003 budget.

Fixed and Flexible Non-Personnel Expenses

Fixed non-personnel expenses may be estimated monthly and totaled for the year, or estimated on an annual basis and then divided into monthly budget amounts. For fixed line items, changes in price or quantity are factored into the coming fiscal year's estimate, and it is assumed that changes in volume over the coming fiscal year will not affect the fixed non-personnel expense. For example, IV supplies and solutions are a fixed budget line item for the ancillary department, as shown in Table 6-4. The IV supplies and solutions expenses are estimated for FY 2004 at $12,512, which is divided into 12 monthly budget amounts of $1,043.

Flexibly budgeted non-personnel line items must be estimated based on price, quantity, and anticipated changes in volume. If seasonal or other factors are predicted to change volume over the fiscal year, adjustments are made to the amount of flexibly budgeted line items, such as medical supplies. For example,

TABLE 6-4

Freeston Eldercare Ancillary Department Non-Personnel Expense Budget Worksheet

Line #	7400 Expense Items	Amount	Type	Budget	Actual	Variance	% Var.
				FY 2002 Variance			
	SNF & Intermediate Care Patient Days	—	—	**37,680**	**38,433**	**753**	**2.0%**
240	Pharmaceuticals[1]	$3.82	PPD	$143,968	$151,039	$7,071	4.9%
250	Laboratory[2]	$0.53	PPD	$19,940	$19,786	$(154)	−0.8%
260	Radiology	$0.16	PPD	$6,213	$6,447	$234	3.8%
230	Medical Equipment[3]	$180	Monthly	$2,160	$2,160	$0	0.0%
245	IV Supplies & Solutions[4]	$894	Monthly	$10,724	$11,868	$1,144	10.7%
246	Enteral Supplies & Formula	$1,511	Monthly	$18,128	$19,295	$1,167	6.4%
270	Oxygen & Oxygen Supplies	$653	Monthly	$7,836	$7,749	$(87)	−1.1%
300	**Ancillary Non-Personnel**	—	—	**$208,970**	**$218,344**	**$9,374**	**4.5%**
	Ancillary Non-Personnel PPD	—	—	**$5.55**	**$5.68**	**$0.14**	**2.4%**

[1] Pharmaceutical prices increasing by an estimated 10% for FY 2004.

[2] Laboratory expenses controlled, flexible budget (volume based) increase for FY 2004.

[3] No medical equipment budgeted for FY 2004.

[4] New vendor for IV supplies & solutions; price increase 5% for FY 2004.

Table 6-4 shows a budget for pharmaceuticals of $178,154 for FY 2004, a 14.4% increase over the FY 2003 budget. This budget increase partly reflects an estimated 10% increase in price but also reflects an estimated 4% increase in volume.

Fixed and Flexible Personnel Expenses

Budgeting for **fixed staff** (employees who must be available regardless of patient volume or acuity) is relatively simple to estimate for the coming fiscal year. For example, most institutions, departments, and work units require fixed management or administrative staff, such as one nurse manager per unit, one department director per department, and a specified number of administrative support staff. These fixed staff are budgeted by dividing the annual salary by the 12 months of the fiscal year to obtain a monthly fixed personnel expense, and adding benefits to the total personnel expense as required.

However, a flexible budget in which hourly staff are scheduled is more complicated, involving the elements of volume, quantity (direct care hours), and price (hourly wage). One concern in estimating flexible budget hourly personnel expenses is the anticipated workload or total number of hours of direct care required. For 24-hour, direct patient care services such as SNF or hospital nursing care, the first step in calculating the anticipated workload is obtaining estimates or forecasts of patient volume. Patient volume may be difficult to forecast because it is based on a number of external and uncontrollable factors. If forecasts are not provided by the financial department, then a volume variance analysis may be useful in estimating volume for the coming fiscal year. At Freeston ElderCare, forecasts of patient volume are provided by its parent company, XYZ Health Corporation. Table 6-5 shows that for the SNF unit, the budgeted FY 2003 volume is 12,874 patient days, with 13,657 patient days forecasted for FY 2004. Table 6-5 does not include FY 2002 figures, as it focuses solely on direct care hours, FTE, and wage changes between FY 2003 and FY 2004.

		FY 2003 Variance						FY 2004		
Amount	Type	Budget	Annualized Actual	Variance	% Var.	Amount	Type	Budget	FY 2003–2004 Variance	% Var.
—	—	39,128	40,348	1,220	3.1%	—	—	40,693	1,565	4.0%
$3.98	PPD	$155,729	$166,475	$10,745	6.9%	$4.38	PPD	$178,154	$22,425	14.4%
$0.54	PPD	$21,129	$22,883	$1,754	8.3%	$0.54	PPD	$21,974	$845	4.0%
$0.17	PPD	$6,652	$6,943	$291	4.4%	$0.17	PPD	$6,918	$266	4.0%
$150	Monthly	$1,800	$2,185	$385	21.4%	$0	Monthly	$0	$(1,800)	−100.0%
$993	Monthly	$11,916	$13,727	$1,811	15.2%	$1,043	Monthly	$12,512	$596	5.0%
$1,642	Monthly	$19,704	$18,617	$(1,087)	−5.5%	$1,642	Monthly	$19,704	$0	0.0%
$674	Monthly	$8,088	$8,025	$(63)	−0.8%	$674	Monthly	$8,088	$0	0.0%
—	—	$225,018	$238,855	$13,837	6.1%	—	—	$247,350	$22,331	9.9%
—	—	$5.75	$5.92	$0.17	2.9%	—	—	$6.08	$0.33	5.7%

The second step in calculating the anticipated workload is to estimate the direct care hours required by each type of staff (such as RN, LPN, and CNA). Direct care hours are then multiplied by patient volume to estimate the total workload. Flexibly budgeted staff are also referred to as **variable staff**, because a change in volume or direct care hours changes the amount of staff required. Concepts used in estimating direct care hours are discussed in the following section.

Estimating Direct Care Hours

Direct care hours may be estimating using staffing standards established by administrative, regulatory, or accreditation requirements. At Freeston ElderCare, the FY 2003 staffing standards assigned 0.2 direct hours PPD for RNs, 1.0 direct hours PPD for LPNs, and 2.4 direct hours PPD for CNAs, as shown in Table 6-5. For FY 2004, new requirements increase RN direct care hours to 0.4 hours PPD.

Another factor in calculating direct care hours is the **acuity** (estimated severity of various disorders), frequently measured by the various hours of direct care required by each acuity classification per patient day. In acute care settings this is often referred to as the case mix or patient acuity mix. The case mix represents the various levels or amounts of care (typically measured by hours of direct care required per day) that various types of patients need (see Chap. 4). Case mix in acute care settings is a complex calculation based on multiple measures, including staff observations and judgment as well as the patient census. Many hospitals employ computerized patient acuity classification systems to record the average care hours provided per patient on each hospital unit and shift to help estimate and predict the case mix. At Freeston ElderCare, the required direct care hours differ between the SNF and the intermediate care units, but there is no case mix estimate within each of these units.

Staffing (determining the number and mix of staff and staff time) is required for nearly all health care settings. Scheduling for 24-hour care every day of the year makes staffing a complex process in which accurate prediction of staffing needs and resources becomes difficult. Health care management texts discuss staffing and scheduling in more detail. The reason it is important to consider staffing in budget preparation is that it directly affects the personnel expense budget, which is frequently the largest budget amount that is prepared, monitored, and controlled in health care settings.

TABLE 6-5

Freeston EdlerCare SNF Nursing Personnel Direct Care & FTE Budget Worksheet, FY 2004

Nursing Staff Positions	FY 2003 Budget								FY 2004 Budget							
	Patient Days	ADC	Hours PPD	Total Hours	Hourly Wage	Total Expense	FTE	Adj. FTE	Patient Days	ADC	Hours PPD[1]	Total Hours	Hourly Wage[2]	Total Expense	FTE	Adj. FTE
RN	12,874	35.3	0.2	2,575	$29.32	$75,493	1.24	1.90	13,657	37.4	0.4	5,463	$30.49	$166,576	2.6	4.0
LPN	12,874	35.3	1.0	12,874	$18.40	$236,882	6.19	9.49	13,657	37.4	1.0	13,657	$19.14	$261,340	6.6	10.1
CNA	12,874	35.3	2.4	30,898	$10.72	$331,222	14.85	22.78	13,657	37.4	2.4	32,777	$11.15	$365,422	15.8	24.2
Total SNF Direct Care Wages	—	—	—	—	—	$643,597	—	—	—	—	—	—	—	$793,338	—	—

[1] RN direct hours increased to 0.4 hours PPD per staffing standards for FY 2004.

[2] Hourly wage increase of 4% for all nursing staff for FY 2004.

One consideration in staffing is determining the **staff mix** (the various types or skill levels of staff required to provide care). It is not unusual for a variety of licensed and non-licensed health care personnel to be employed for a given health care unit, department, or program. For example, Freeston ElderCare nursing staff include RNs, LPNs, and CNAs, each with standards for hours of direct care.

Another element in staffing is determining the FTEs. As discussed in Chapter 5, many health care settings, including most 24-hour acute care facilities, measure staffing using FTEs rather than job positions, to enable hiring and scheduling hourly part-time personnel to fill full-time hourly positions. An FTE represents 40 hours of work per week multiplied by 52 weeks for a year, resulting in 2,080 work hours per year, or 260 work days per year (2,080 work hours per year ÷ 8 work hours per day).

However, there are two additional issues in determining staff FTEs. The first issue is nonproductive time. Employees typically require sick leave, holidays, vacations, and some weekends off, so in actual practice the same employee cannot be scheduled for a full 2,080 work hours per year. The second issue is that settings that must staff for 24 hours 7 days a week must plan for sufficient FTEs to cover the entire schedule. These issues require calculating an **adjusted FTE** that accounts for productive time (direct care), nonproductive time (vacation, sick leave, holidays), and, if applicable, 24-hour and weekend scheduling.

For example, Donna, Director of Nursing at Freeston ElderCare, knows that 1.0 FTE equals 260 work days. Freeston ElderCare nursing staff have 9 paid holidays, 3 paid sick days, and 10 paid vacation days allowed (22 nonproductive days), so 1.0 FTE staff actually is scheduled for 238 productive days (260 work days − 22 nonproductive days). Full coverage of the SNF unit including weekends requires 365 days per year of staffing. Donna therefore calculates the following adjusted FTE:

$$\text{Adjusted FTE} = \text{Total Staffed Days} \div \text{Total Productive Days per FTE}$$

$$\text{Adjusted FTE} = 365 \text{ Days} \div 238 \text{ Days}$$

$$\text{Adjusted FTE} = 1.53 \text{ FTEs}$$

In other words, to staff for nonproductive time and for 7 days a week, Donna must budget 1.5 nursing staff FTEs for every 1 FTE of direct care. Table 6-5 shows that for the SNF RNs in FY 2003, there are 2,575 direct care hours (12,874 patient days × 0.2 hours PPD), resulting in 1.2 RN FTEs (2,575 direct care hours ÷ 2,080 hours per FTE). The adjusted FTE is 1.9, calculated as follows:

$$\text{SNF RN Adjusted FTE} = \text{FTE} \times \text{Adjusted FTE}$$

$$1.9 \text{ RN Adjusted FTE} = 1.24 \text{ FTE} \times 1.53 \text{ Adjusted FTE}$$

Donna must budget 1.9 RN FTEs to cover the 1.24 FTEs of direct care required for FY 2003.

The budgeted FTEs and adjusted FTEs increase for RNs for FY 2004 to 2.6 FTEs and 4.0 FTEs, respectively (see Table 6-5). Part of the increase is the result of volume variance, as the patient days increase from FY 2003 to FY 2004. Another reason for this increase is quantity variance, as new regulations require 0.4 RN direct care hours PPD. The dollar amount FY 2004 budget increase is also partly related to price variance, resulting from a 4% hourly wage increase.

The FTE and budgeted FTE calculations presented in Table 6-5 do not show how staff may be scheduled for each 8-hour shift. This budget worksheet simply totals the direct hours, FTEs, and related hourly direct care expenses for the entire fiscal year. Hourly wages are averaged for simplicity.

Box 6-3 summarizes concepts in preparing a flexible budget for hourly personnel.

Flexible Personnel Budget for Nursing Services

Budget preparation requires focusing on the greatest level of budget detail: the line items and groups of line items making up the budget. Donna closely monitors the RN overtime expense over FY 2003, not only to

☐ **BOX 6·3**

Flexible Budgeting for Hourly Personnel

1. Workload estimate = patient volume × total direct hours
2. Direct hours estimate:
   a. Staffing standards
   b. Patient acuity (case mix)
3. Staffing
   a. Staff mix
   b. Scheduling requirements
   c. Adjusted FTE = total staffed days ÷ total productive days
      i. Adjusts for 24-hour, 7-days-per-week staffing
      ii. Adjusts for nonproductive time

investigate and control this expense but also to gather information for preparing the FY 2004 Nursing Services budget.

Table 6-6 presents a budget worksheet for the Nursing Services SNF unit RN total personnel expenses. Some details were not provided in the earlier Nursing Services personnel budgets reported in previous chapters. For simplicity, the Nursing Services personnel budgets reported in the earlier chapters reported a 4% overtime expense calculated for all nursing staff within the SNF or intermediate care unit rather than by staff type. This overtime estimate was added to the total direct hours expense for all nursing staff within the SNF or intermediate care unit as part of the calculation of total nursing personnel expenses.

○ **TABLE 6·6**

Freeston Eldercare SNF Unit RN Personnel Total Budget Worksheet

Line #	7210 SNF Personnel	Amount	Type	FY 2002 Variance			
				Budget	Actual	Variance	% Var.
SNF Patient Days		—	—	**12,791**	**12,992**	**201**	**1.6%**
RN Direct Hours Target		0.2	Direct Care Hours PPD	**2,558**	**2,598**	**40**	**1.6%**
RN Scheduled Hours		—	—	2,456	2,619	61	2.4%
001	RN Expense	$29.32	Wage	$75,006	$76,789	$1,783	2.4%
RN Overtime		4%	of Direct Care Hours	102	98	(5)	−4.7%
101	RN Overtime Expense	150%	of Wage	$4,500	$4,288	$(212)	−4.7%
120	Benefits	25%	of Wages	$18,752	$19,197	$446	2.4%
RN Registry Services		—	—	0	0	0	—
145	RN Registry Expense	—	—	$0	$0	$0	—
Total RN Direct Hours		—	—	**2,558**	**2,717**	**$158**	**6.2%**
130	**Total SNF RN Personnel**	—	—	**$98,258**	**$100,274**	**$2,016**	**2.1%**
Average SNF RN PPD		—	—	**$7.68**	**$7.72**	**$0.04**	**0.5%**

Table 6-6 provides more detail and accuracy in budgeting and reporting direct care hours and expenses. This additional detail is helpful in preparing flexible budgets. Following the patient days line, there is a line showing the target hours for RN direct care. These target hours are calculated by multiplying the target hours PPD by the volume. Therefore, the budgeted target RN direct care hours for FY 2002 are 2,558 (0.2 × 12,791) and the actual target RN direct care hours are 2,598 (0.2 × 12,992). For this line item, the actual hours represent the target amount based on the actual volume, not the amount of hours actually worked by RNs.

The following line in Table 6-6 is identified as hours actually scheduled for RN direct care. The budgeted scheduled hours are 2,456 because the 102 budgeted overtime hours are considered to be included in the scheduling. The 2,456 RN budgeted scheduled hours represent the target direct care hours less the budgeted overtime hours (2,558 − 102). In other words, RNs are budgeted to work up to 4% of the targeted direct hours as overtime as a replacement for regularly scheduled staff. The budgeted personnel expense for RNs scheduled at the base hourly wage of $29.32 is $75,006 ($29.32 × 2,456). The budgeted overtime expense for RNs for FY 2002 is $4,500 (102 overtime hours $29.32 base wage × 1.5 overtime wage increase), which reflects the overtime wage at 50% above the base wage.

The actual RN scheduled hours in Table 6-6 shows the number of hours RNs worked at the regularly scheduled hourly wage. The actual RN overtime hours shows the actual number of overtime hours worked. As a result, the actual RN expense for scheduled hours is $76,789 ($29.32 × 2,619). The actual RN expense for overtime is $4,288 (98 overtime hours × $29.32 base wage ×1.5 overtime wage increase).

For simplicity, benefits in Table 6-6 are calculated as 25% of scheduled direct care hours, although benefits are also added to overtime hours at specified rates in most health care settings. For FY 2002, no registry RN services are budgeted. To review and compare total RN direct care hours with the target hours, a line is included for total RN direct hours. For FY 2002, this represents the sum of scheduled and overtime

| | | FY 2003 Variance | | | | FY 2004 | | | | |
Amount	Type	Budget	Annualized Actual	Variance	% Var.	Amount	Type	Budget FY 2004	Variance FY 2003–2004	% Var. FY 2003–2004
—	—	12,874	13,252	378	2.9%	—	—	13,657	783	6.1%
0.2	Direct Care Hours PPD	2,575	2,650	76	2.9%	0.4	Direct Care Hours PPD	5,463	2,888	112.2%
—	—	2,472	2,426	(148)	−5.8%	—	—	4,204	1,732	70.1%
$29.32	Wage	$72,473	$71,142	$(1,331)	−1.8%	$30.49	Wage	$128,201	$55,727	76.9%
4%	of Direct Care Hours	103	255	152	147.6%	4%	of Direct Care Hours	219	116	112.2%
150%	of Wage	$4,530	$11,215	$6,685	147.6%	150%	of Wage	$9,995	$5,465	120.7%
25%	of Wages	$18,118	$17,786	$(333)	−1.8%	25%	of Wages	$32,050	$13,932	76.9%
—	—	0	0	0	—	—	—	1,040	1,040	—
—	—	$0	$0	$0	—	$35	Hourly Fee	$36,400	$36,400	—
—	—	2,575	2,681	107	4.1%	—	—	5,463	2,888	112.2%
—	—	$95,121	$100,142	$5,021	5.3%	—	—	$206,645	$111,524	117.2%
—	—	$7.39	$7.56	$0.17	2.3%	—	—	$15.13	$7.74	104.8%

hours. The budgeted total hours match the budgeted target hours of 2,558. The actual total RN direct hours are 2,717, or 6.2% above budget.

The first section of Table 6-6 summarizes the FY 2002 budget performance, showing that actual performance was close to budget. The second section of the budget worksheet shows a large unfavorable variance in hours and expenses for RN overtime, as annualized based on the first 9 months of FY 2003. Investigation of this variance finds that staffing shortages are an uncontrolled source of variance contributing to the overtime expense increases. Scheduling problems are also a source of unfavorable RN personnel expense in that there are 2,681 actual total direct hours reported as worked for FY 2003, more than the 2,650 actual target direct hours. In other words, RNs are working more hours in FY 2003 than the staffing target requires, adjusted for patient volume.

The third section of Table 6-6 presents the proposed FY 2004 budget. The total targeted direct hours reflect the new guidelines requiring 0.4 hours of RN direct care PPD, as was reported in Table 6-5. Even with staffing shortages, Donna budgets overtime at no more than 4% because, in her experience at Freeston ElderCare, staff satisfaction and retention are adversely affected when overtime exceeds 4% of total direct care hours (this assumption may differ in other settings). The line for RN registry expense is discussed in the following section on adding new budget lines.

Revenue Budgeting and Budget Balancers

The preparation of the revenue budget is only briefly discussed because it is typically based on expert forecasts of both volume and reimbursement from financial departments. The concepts of revenue budgeting are similar to budgeting for expenses. Volume, price (reimbursement), and quantity (intensity of services) are all relevant factors in preparing the revenue budget. A pro forma P&L statement allows for estimating profits or losses by calculating the difference between projected revenues and projected expenses for the coming fiscal year. The following section discusses approaches to adjusting projected revenues as well as volume and expenses to balance a budget under preparation.

Estimating and Using Budget Balancers. Budget balancers represent management strategies for generating additional volume or operating revenues, or reducing operating expenses to achieve desired profit levels. Budget balancers are used so that the budget under preparation will address the volume and revenue that must be generated, and the limits to expenses that can be incurred to meet profitability targets. Chapter 8 discusses the use of break-even analysis as a method to estimate the amount of profit or loss, useful in developing budget balancers.

Table 6-7 shows a budget worksheet for Accurate Labs. The first section presents an approach using the volume of a given laboratory procedure as the budget balancer. In FY 2003, the estimated volume of the procedure was 1,600, generating $2,720 in expenses, $3,200 in revenues, and $480 in profit, $80 more than the profitability target (based on $0.25 of profit per procedure). However, the actual volume of this procedure fell below budget estimates to 1,523, and the profits were below the targeted amount. In FY 2004, the costs of the procedure are expected to rise, with total expenses estimated at $3,100; to maintain a competitive price, the laboratory director may not raise the revenue (price) per procedure above $2. Therefore, the laboratory director focuses on strategies to increase volume, establishing additional contracts with local clinics to increase the volume estimated for FY 2004 to 1,800. Despite increased costs and no increase in price, the laboratory is expected to meet and exceed its profitability target for FY 2004.

Another way to use budget balancers is to focus on revenues. Continuing the Accurate Labs example, the second section of Table 6-7 shows the laboratory director's budget worksheet using revenue as a budget balancer. In this example, volume is estimated to remain the same from FY 2003 to FY 2004, and expenses for the laboratory procedure are estimated to increase from $2,720 to $3,000. The laboratory director proposes

Accurate Labs Budget Balancer Worksheet, FY 2004

Item	Volume as Budget Balancer			Revenue as Budget Balancer			Expense as Budget Balancer		
	Budget 2003	Actual 2003	Budget 2004	Budget 2003	Actual 2003	Budget 2004	Budget 2003	Actual 2003	Budget 2004
Volume	**1,600**	**1,523**	**1,800**	**1,600**	**1,523**	**1,600**	**1,600**	**1,585**	**1,600**
Total expenses	**$2,720**	**$2,693**	**$3,100**	**$2,720**	**$2,693**	**$3,000**	**$2,720**	**$2,919**	**$2,734**
Revenue per procedure	$2.00	$2.00	$2.00	$2.00	$2.00	$2.15	$2.00	$2.00	$2.00
Total revenues	**$3,200**	**$3,046**	**$3,600**	**$3,200**	**$3,046**	**$3,440**	**$3,200**	**$3,170**	**$3,200**
Pro forma P&L	$480	$353	$500	$480	$353	$440	$480	$251	$466
Profitability target	$400	$381	$450	$400	$381	$400	$400	$396	$400

and negotiates an increase in the revenue per unit (price) for the procedure from $2.00 to $2.15, which exceeds the profitability target for FY 2004.

One other way to use budget balancers is to find ways to reduce fixed or flexible budgeted costs to achieve the desired profit levels. Returning to the Accurate Labs example, the third section of Table 6-7 presents a worksheet prepared by the laboratory director using expenses for a given procedure as the budget balancer. As in the first example using the laboratory procedure, the revenue per procedure (price) is set at $2. The laboratory director does not anticipate any increase in volume, and actual expenses put the profit below the profitability target for FY 2003. By monitoring and controlling expenses related to this procedure (see Chap. 5), it is possible to keep FY 2004 estimated expenses at $2,734, close to the budget for FY 2003, thus meeting the profitability target of $0.25 per procedure.

Budgeting for New Line Items

It is important to consider and anticipate new line items for the next fiscal year in both personnel and non-personnel categories. These new line items are included in the budgets of continuing programs and departments, representing previously unbudgeted sources of revenue or expense that are new for the next fiscal year. Budgeted amounts for the new line item revenue or expense are obtained by forecasting or by making the best available estimate.

One example of budgeting for a new line item is shown in Table 6-6. Donna, the Director of Nursing at Freeston ElderCare, plans to add a line item for RN registry services to the Nursing Services SNF unit RN personnel expense budget. In reviewing the FY 2004 proposed budget, it is reported that, even with 219 hours of overtime, the scheduled direct hours fall below budget by 1,040 hours (4,204 = 5,463 − 219 − 1,040). Donna decides to budget these 1,040 hours as a nursing registry expense, as with nursing shortages she does not think she can recruit an RN for 0.5 FTE to fill these hours. Therefore, a new budget line for RN registry is added for FY 2004, and Donna will be required to justify this request.

Preparing the Capital Budget

Capital budgets present estimates of expenses for high-cost and long-term items such as equipment, major maintenance and repair, renovation, and construction. Recall that capital budgets are typically linked to the long-term strategic plan. Capital budgets usually require written justification and are reviewed and approved by the top administrators of the organization. Chapters 8 and 9 provide financial analysis techniques that are useful in preparing estimates of cost and profitability for capital budgets, and Chapter 12 discusses the preparation of a business plan, which is often prepared as a justification for large capital expenses.

Preparing the Cash Flow Budget

Chapter 4 discusses the importance of carefully tracking cash flow to ensure that obligations such as payment of salaries and bills are met, and to maintain the day-to-day financial health of the program, department, or organization. Settings in which cash flow is monitored require the preparation of cash flow budgets. The preparation of the cash flow budget is more complicated than preparing operating expense and capital budgets and is often done by or with the assistance of financial departments.

Considerations in preparing the cash flow budget include anticipating the amount of revenue likely to be received over specified time periods from each revenue source. Refer to Freeston ElderCare's FY 2003 collections worksheet in the "Supplemental Tables and Documents" section of the Back-of-Book CD-ROM for an example of these estimates. Estimates of uncollectible revenue are then presented in a worksheet. A cash

TABLE 6-8

Freeston Eldercare Nursing Services Hourly Wages "What-If" Worksheet, FY 2004

7200 Nursing Services Item	FY 2003			FY 2004 Scenario A			FY 2004 Scenario B		
	Hourly Wage	Benefits	Total	Hourly Wage	Benefits	Total	Hourly Wage	Benefits	Total
RN	$29.32	25%	**$36.65**	$30.64	25%	**$38.30**	$30.49	27%	**$38.73**
LPN	$18.40	25%	**$23.00**	$19.23	25%	**$24.04**	$19.14	27%	**$24.30**
CNA	$10.72	25%	**$13.40**	$11.20	25%	**$14.00**	$11.15	27%	**$14.16**

Scenario A: increase all wages by 4.5%, no increase in benefits.

Scenario B: increase wages by 4%, benefits increased to 27% of hourly wages.

flow worksheet is then prepared that includes monthly estimates of the revenue amounts expected to be collected over specified time frames, as well as operating and capital expenses estimated from the operating and capital budgets. These estimates are used to prepare the cash flow budget, as presented in the Back-of-Book CD-ROM.

Additional Budget Preparation Concepts

This section presents some concepts useful for budget preparation in various settings or situations. This section also briefly discusses the situation of closing or ending a program or service. Budgeting is a complex function that may require the application of approaches other than those presented so far in this chapter. Additional approaches may be used in other settings or learned with experience.

"What-If" Calculations

"What-if" calculations are one or more sets of estimates based on different assumptions, forecasts, scenarios, approaches, or other management strategies to compare and select among alternative budget decisions. "What-if" calculations are useful in budget preparation as well as in making other financial estimates. Computer spreadsheets are well suited to making "what-if" calculations, as the following example illustrates. Calculating various "what-if" estimates allows for the review of potential alternative outcomes.

Table 6-8 shows "what-if" calculations comparing possible changes in Freeston ElderCare Nursing Services hourly staff wages and benefits. The first section shows the average hourly wages and benefit rates for FY 2003, with the total hourly wages and benefits. The second section shows Scenario A, in which wages increase by 4.5% but benefits remain the same. The third section shows Scenario B, in which wages increase by only 4% but benefits increase to 27%. For example, under Scenario A total RN wages and benefits are $38.30 hourly, and under Scenario B total RN wages and benefits are $38.73 hourly. Entering these data into a spreadsheet as "what-if" calculations allows for a quick comparison of alternative choices.

Step-Fixed FTEs and Budgeting

Step-fixed staff remain at a constant FTE amount until the volume reaches a certain point, then increase (or decrease) by a given step. Table 6-9 gives an example of step-fixed staffing and budgeting using Wellness, Inc., a non-profit health care agency. Wellness, Inc. employs health educators, who are assigned a caseload of up to 35 clients each. When the caseload for the first health educator exceeds 35 clients, a second health educator is hired. When the second health educator's caseload exceeds 35 clients, a third health educator is hired. This approach is more responsive to changes in volume than fixed budgeting but not as sensitive to changes in volume as flexible budgeting. Step-fixed budgeting may be applied to non-personnel line items as well as to personnel line items that are applicable to changes occurring in measurable steps.

TABLE 6-9

Wellness, Inc. Step-Fixed Health Educator Personnel Budget Worksheet, FY 2004

Total Clients	FTE	Expense
1 to 35	1.0	$38,272
36 to 70	2.0	$76,544
71 to 105	3.0	$114,816

Zero-Base Budgeting

Zero-base budgeting is an approach that treats a continuing budget as if it were for a new program or service requiring approval. This approach was developed to address potential problems with the incremental expense budgeting approach, thus improving accuracy, efficiency, and control. In some situations, incremental changes are made to expense budgets without thoroughly analyzing or justifying whether these increases or reductions represent the most accurate estimates and the most efficient use of resources.

Zero-base budgeting requires preparation of the next year's budget as if it were a new, not continuing budget. In other words, the budget begins at zero, requiring justification of every line item and dollar amount. The budget justification is more detailed than for an incremental budget, as each line item must be justified, as well as the total budget. Benefits of zero-base budgeting include increased efficiency, cost savings, better allocation of resources, and generation of improved performance strategies.

Although zero-base budgeting has the advantage of increasing efficiency, this approach is complex, requiring considerable time and effort, and is burdensome to require of all budgets each year. A frequent alternative approach is to require zero-base budgets for selected programs or line items, particularly when there are concerns about budget accuracy and control.

Marie, administrator at Freeston ElderCare, uses zero-base budgeting to address concerns about the Rehabilitation Department's budget. Frank Mitchell, PT and Director of the Rehabilitation Department, prepared the incremental budget worksheet reviewed in Table 6-2. The occupational therapist worked about 6.6 hours of overtime each week (316 overtime hours ÷ 48 work weeks), and the OTA worked about 5.3 hours of overtime each week (254.5 overtime hours ÷ 48 work weeks). Rather than implementing strategies to investigate and control this unfavorable variance, Frank requests an incremental budget increase in the occupational therapist and OTA FTE for FY 2004, justifying this request on the basis of the reported overtime. Marie does not believe this approach is efficient or feasible and is concerned about the increasing personnel costs.

Table 6-10 presents a zero-base budget for the occupational therapy personnel line items for the Rehabilitation Department. Marie develops this budget using the following assumptions:

1. The FTE hours for both the occupational therapist and OTA are for the most part directly related to patient care and thus can be budgeted as a flexible budget.
2. The direct care provided by occupational therapy personnel is for SNF patients, so SNF volume figures are used in budgeting.
3. Using historical data and industry statistics, the occupational therapist is expected to perform evaluations on about 30% of the SNF admissions, requiring about 2 hours per evaluation.
4. Using historical data and industry statistics, the occupational therapist is expected to perform about 3.5 therapeutic procedures on each evaluated patient, requiring about 1.5 hours per procedure.

○ **TABLE 6-10**

Freeston ElderCare Rehabilitation Department, Zero-Base Budget Worksheet for Occupational Therapy Personnel, FY 2004

Items	Budget 2003	Budget 2004	Variance	% Var.
SNF Patient Days	**12,874**	**13,657**	**783**	**6.1%**
SNF Admissions	382	396	14	3.7%
Occupational Therapist				
Evaluation Procedures	115	119	4	3.7%
Evaluation Direct Hours	229	238	8	3.7%
Therapeutic Treatment Procedures	401	416	15	3.7%
Therapeutic Treatment Direct Hours	602	624	22	3.7%
Total Occupational Therapist Direct Hours	**831**	**861**	**30**	**3.7%**
Occupational Therapist Direct FTE	0.4	0.4	0	3.7%
Occupational Therapist Indirect FTE	0.1	0.1	0	0.0%
Total Occupational Therapist FTE	**0.50**	**0.5**	**0**	**2.9%**
Occupational Therapist Aide				
Therapeutic Treatment Procedures	516	535	19	3.7%
Therapeutic Treatment Direct Hours	516	535	19	3.7%
Other Direct Assistance Hours	500	500	0	0.0%
Total OTA Direct Hours	**1,016**	**1,035**	**19**	**1.9%**
Total OTA FTE	**0.5**	**0.5**	**0**	**1.9%**

5. The Rehabilitation Department budgets 0.1 indirect FTE for the occupational therapist for tasks such as record keeping and supervision of the OTA.
6. Using historical data and industry statistics, the OTA is expected to perform about 4.5 therapeutic procedures on each evaluated patient, requiring about 1 hour per procedure.
7. The OTA is budgeted 500 hours of other direct assistance, such as transferring and transporting patients, and preparing for occupational therapy procedures.

Table 6-10 indicates that, based on the above assumptions, the budgeted 0.5 FTE for the occupational therapist and the OTA should be sufficient for the required direct care hours. Further investigation indicates that scheduling and patient transport problems led to delays and considerable wasted time for occupational therapy personnel. Marie expects Frank to exercise closer monitoring and control of the occupational therapy personnel budget for FY 2004.

Closing a Program

In some situations, a product, service, or program is found to be unprofitable or to no longer fit with the objectives of the department or organization. In such a case, it may be necessary to discontinue the program. For example, there might be a decision to contract for laundry services with an outside vendor and close the internal laundry unit at Freeston ElderCare. In such a case, the personnel and non-personnel line items are removed from the departmental budget.

Typically, the major concern in closing a program is not the budget adjustment, but the issues of human resources. If the employees working in the unit that is closed are retained, they require reassignment to other

---

BOX 6-4

Factors in Budget Preparation

- The budget cycle
- Preparation of the strategic plan
- Assumptions, priorities, goals, objectives, and performance targets for the next fiscal year
- Incremental budgeting basing the next year's budget on administrative guidelines
- Forecasts of volume, revenues, and expenses for the next fiscal year
- Variance analysis applied to estimating next fiscal year's budget
- Budgeting for new line items anticipated for next year
- Budget balancers to meet profitability targets
- "What-if" calculations to determine alternative budget decision outcomes
- Step-fixed budgets
- Zero-base budgeting to control incremental increases and increase budget accuracy
- Closing a program
- New products, programs, or services

---

departments or work, and possibly retraining. If employees are to be released, they require termination benefits and possibly job counseling and other services. Budget planning must therefore include these requirements in decisions around making the closure.

Conclusion

This chapter presents approaches and concepts for budget preparation in health care settings. Box 6-4 summarizes the factors to consider in budget preparation discussed throughout this chapter. Box 6-5 presents Internet resources for additional information on health care budgeting.

BOX 6-5

On-line Sources for Information on Budgeting

Academy for Health Services Research and Health Policy—Glossary of Terms:
http://www.academyhealth.org/publications/glossary-healthcare.htm
BetterManagement.com—Resource Planning General Concepts: www.bettermanagement.com
Edward Lowe's Peerspectives—Acquiring and Managing Finances—Budgeting:
http://peerspectives.org/
Evaluating the Impact of Value-Based Purchasing—A Guide for Purchasers:
http://www.ahrq.gov/about/cods/valuebased/
Free, On-Line Nonprofit Organization and Management Development Program—Module 8:
http://www.managementhelp.org
Health Care Financing Review on-line: http://www.hcfa.gov/pubforms/ordpub.htm
July 1998 Special Issue of Provider On-Line—Analyzing and Tracking Long-Term Care Costs:
http://www.ahca.org/news/provider/pv-archive.htm

■ CRITICAL THINKING EXERCISES

1. If possible, bring budgets from your health care setting that include budgeted and actual figures, concealing the setting's identity as appropriate. Prepare budget estimates for the next fiscal year for at least 3 months. Explain how you derive your assumptions, forecasts, and estimates.
2. If outside budgets are not available, use information from the Freeston ElderCare operating budget and prepare a budget for the next fiscal year for at least 3 months, explaining your assumptions and estimates.

■ REFERENCES

Baker, J. J., & Baker, R. W. (2000). *Health Care Finance: Basic Tools for Nonfinancial Managers*. Gaithersburg, MD: Aspen.

Cleverley, W. O., & Cameron, A. E. (2002). *Essentials of Health Care Finance*, 5th ed. Gaithersburg, MD: Aspen.

Eichenberger, J. (1998). Project Management, Part III: Budgets for Projects. *AAOHN Journal, 46*(5), 268–270.

Finkler, S. A., & Kovner, C. T. (2000). *Financial Management for Nurse Managers and Executives*, 2nd ed. Philadelphia: W. B. Saunders.

Gapenski, L. C. (2002). *Healthcare Finance: An Introduction to Accounting and Financial Management*, 2nd ed. Chicago: Health Administration Press.

Herkimer, A. G. (1988). *Understanding Health Care Budgeting*. Gaithersburg, MD: Aspen.

McGuffin, J. (1999). *The Nurse's Guide to Successful Management: A Desk Reference*. St. Louis, MO: Mosby.

Neumann, B. R., Suber, J. D., & Zelman, W. N. (1988). *Financial Management: Concepts and Applications for Health Care Providers*, 2nd ed. Owings Mills, MD: National Health Publishing.

Nowicki, M. (2001). *The Financial Management of Hospitals and Healthcare Organizations*. Chicago: Health Administration Press.

Shim, J. K., & Siegel, J. G. (1988). *Handbook of Financial Analysis, Forecasting & Modeling*. Englewood Cliffs, NJ: Prentice-Hall, Inc.

CHAPTER 7

Cost Allocation and Cost-Finding

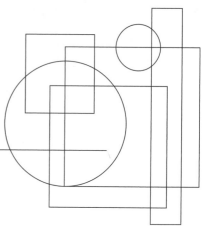

▢ Learning Objectives

1. Differentiate between direct and indirect costs, explaining the importance of identifying sources of both direct and indirect costs in health care settings.
2. Demonstrate the application of at least one approach to cost allocation and cost-finding.
3. Define and explain the application of DRGs, CPT®, HCPCS codes, RBRVS, and RVUs.

◯ Key Terms

Activity-based costing
Cost allocation
Cost center
Cost driver
Cost-finding
Cost pool
Current Procedural Terminology (CPT®) code
Direct distribution
Healthcare Common Procedure Coding System (HCPCS)

Non-revenue cost center
Product line
Profit center
Reciprocal distribution
Relative Value Unit (RVU)
Resource-Based Relative Value Scale (RBRVS)
Revenue cost center
Step-down distribution
Support service
Surcharge

Chapter 4 discusses the difference between direct costs, which are costs generated in the provision of health care goods and services, and indirect costs, which are costs generated by the operation of an organization as a whole, or indirectly generated in the provision of health care goods and services. For example, costs for nursing services represent direct costs, while costs for administration and housekeeping represent indirect costs. Chapters 4, 5,

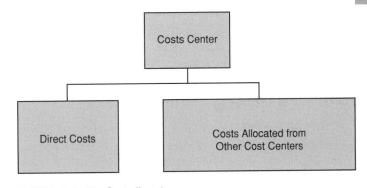

FIGURE 7.1 ■ Cost allocation.

and 6 focus largely on departmental budgets and whether these departments provide direct or indirect services. This chapter discusses ways to budget indirect costs that are generated by departments that provide direct services. Many health care settings must budget and report indirect costs in their operating expense budgets and identify the direct and indirect costs per service unit, so it is helpful to have an overview focused on the allocation of indirect costs. The term "overhead" is used in this textbook to identify a specified amount or rate of indirect costs included in an operating expense budget line; often the terms "indirect costs," "administrative costs," and "overhead" are used interchangeably.

The text defines **cost allocation** as determining the total direct and indirect costs of **cost centers** (work units that generate and report operating expenses), using accepted methods for identifying and assigning costs from other cost centers. Figure 7-1 illustrates that cost allocation identifies a cost center's direct costs, and assigns costs from other cost centers. For examples, Nursing Services is a cost center that generates costs for dietary services. Therefore, a portion of the dietary department's costs are assigned to Nursing Services when using a cost allocation approach.

In this text, **cost-finding** refers to determining the total direct and indirect costs of a service unit such as a patient day using accepted methods for identifying and assigning costs. Cost-finding is frequently completed after costs are allocated to cost centers. Figure 7-2 illustrates that cost-finding identifies the direct and indirect costs for a service unit. For example, the total cost of an SNF unit patient day would include direct costs such as nursing care, and indirect costs such as dietary services. The terms and definitions of cost-finding and cost allocation are frequently used interchangeably in health care settings, but the text differentiates the two terms to make the related concepts clearer to the reader. As in other areas of financial practice, it is important to learn the terms and definitions used in one's own work setting.

Cost Centers and Cost Drivers

The types and definitions of cost centers vary among work settings. A **non-revenue cost center** is a cost center that generates expenses but not revenues, and typically provides indirect services. A **revenue cost center** or **profit center** is a cost center that generates both expenses and revenues, and typically provides direct services. Although this text distinguishes between revenue and non-revenue cost centers, in many settings the term "cost center" applies to all types of cost centers.

The group or selection of costs that are allocated to a cost center make up the **cost pool**. For example, the costs of the Dietary Department at Freeston ElderCare might be considered a cost pool. The following examples designate cost pools by department, using their total operating expense budgets. Revenue cost centers are identified as departments that report an operating revenue budget (thus indicating the generation

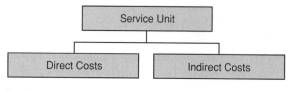

FIGURE 7.2 ■ Cost-finding.

of revenues). For simplicity, these examples assume that Assisted Living and Nursing Services are the only revenue cost centers for Freeston ElderCare, ignoring the revenues generated by Ancillary Services. Nursing Services is a cost pool that combines the operating expenses for Nursing Administration, the SNF unit, and intermediate care.

The following section provides a detailed explanation and example of cost allocation and cost-finding based on the departments at Freeston ElderCare. Other approaches to cost-finding and cost allocation are discussed later in this section. The calculation of many of these methods and approaches is beyond the scope of the text. Frequently finance staff must prepare the cost reports, but an overall understanding of the concepts involved is helpful in reviewing and monitoring these reports and in attempting to control indirect costs. The purpose of this review of cost allocation methods is to facilitate reviewing and monitoring these reports rather than preparing them. Calculations are explained to show how selected cost allocations and cost-finding are developed.

Cost Drivers

Cost drivers are measures or specifications for the allocation of costs from a cost pool. In allocating costs from the Dietary Department cost pool, cost drivers might be the costs per patient day (PPD), the costs per meal, or the costs by types of meals provided. It is important to develop cost drivers that allow for the most acceptable allocation of costs among cost centers. First of all, cost drivers must be measurable, and in relevant units of measurement. For example, costs PPD are frequently used in inpatient settings, and costs per patient visit in outpatient settings. In some settings, it is more relevant to measure costs per procedure rather than costs per patient, or to find other measures that fit the services provided and associated resources used.

Second, the cost drivers should be "fair," or related to the actual amount of indirect resources used by the cost center. For example, assume that the Freeston ElderCare Assisted Living residents consume a greater quantity and demand a higher variety of meals, thus incurring more dietary costs than the patients in Nursing Services. Rather than allocating the same per diem costs to all units, the Dietary Department costs might be better allocated by determining the dietary costs for Assisted Living and for Nursing Services. Allocating the per-pound cost of laundry and the per-square-foot cost of housekeeping might be better measures to differentiate among units in term of actual resource use than costs per patient visit or PPD.

Third, cost drivers ideally allow for cost control by the cost center to which the costs are allocated. In many cases it is difficult or impossible for a department director to control indirect costs, such as expenses for security or landscaping. However, it might be possible to control some indirect costs by preventing waste, damage, or theft. For example, if laboratory tests are allocated as an indirect cost to a nursing unit, supervision in the use of correct collection procedures could reduce costs related to waste. Criteria for cost drivers are summarized in Box 7-1.

Direct Distribution Cost Allocation and Cost-Finding

This section discusses approaches for allocating costs to cost centers in order to help in understanding concepts of cost allocation. These examples are simplified, but cost allocation approaches and decisions can be quite complex. The allocation of indirect costs is therefore often the responsibility of executive management and financial staff. Department directors may be required to monitor and control costs allocated to their work units and may also participate in decisions about how to allocate costs.

The **direct distribution** method allocates indirect costs (costs generated by non-revenue cost centers or cost pools) to revenue cost centers. Non-revenue cost centers or cost pools that contribute costs to revenue

---

☐ BOX 7 · 1

Cost Driver Criteria

- ■ Measurable in units relevant to the cost center
- ■ "Fair"—related to the actual amount of indirect resource use by the cost center
- ■ Allows for cost control by the cost center

---

cost centers or cost pools are also frequently referred to as **support services**. Two approaches to direct distribution for cost allocation are discussed in the following sections, using examples from Freeston ElderCare.

Overhead Rate Method of Direct Distribution

One of the simplest methods of allocating indirect costs is to calculate an overall overhead rate for direct distribution. This method averages all indirect costs by the number of service units such as patient days or patient visits. Chapter 8 gives an example of a per-visit overhead rate added to the costs for each patient visit to cardiac rehabilitation.

Overhead Rate Cost-Finding

Unlike the other methods of cost allocation discussed in this chapter, the overhead rate method begins with cost-finding, or calculating indirect costs per service unit. Table 7-1 shows the calculation of an overhead rate for Freeston ElderCare. In this example, the Administration, Rehabilitation, Ancillary, Dietary, and Plant Operations departments, as well as the line items for property expenses, are assumed to be non-revenue cost centers. The costs for each of these departments are estimated using the total FY 2003 operating expense budgets. Total overhead is $4,256,086, and the overhead rate is calculated as follows:

$$\text{Overhead Rate} = \text{Total Overhead} \div \text{Total Service Units}$$

$$\$77.34 = \$4,256,086 \div 55,034 \text{ patient days}$$

The rate of overhead that will be applied to the revenue cost centers at Freeston ElderCare is $77.34 PPD. The second column of Table 7-1 shows the percent contributed by each non-revenue cost center to total overhead.

Overhead Rate Cost Allocation

Table 7-2 shows how the overhead rate calculated in Table 7-1 is used to allocate costs to the Freeston ElderCare departments designated as revenue cost centers. With 15,906 patient days budgeted for FY 2003, the Assisted Living department is allocated $1,230,100 in overhead costs ($77.34 × 15,906). Nursing Services (which includes the SNF and intermediate care units as well as Nursing Administration) is allocated

◯ TABLE 7 · 1

Freeston ElderCare Overhead Rate Worksheet, FY 2003

	Overhead FY 2003	% Overhead
Total Patient Days	**55,034**	—
Administration	$178,281	4.2%
Rehabilitation	$188,202	4.4%
Ancillary	$265,676	6.2%
Dietary	$871,370	20.5%
Plant Operations	$715,654	16.8%
Property Expense	$2,036,904	47.9%
Total Overhead	**$4,256,086**	**100%**
Overhead PPD (Overhead Rate)	**$77.34**	—

TABLE 7·2

Freeston ElderCare Overhead Distribution Worksheet, Budget FY 2003

	Overhead	Assisted Living	Nursing Services	Total Costs
Total Patient Days	55,034	15,906	39,128	—
Direct Costs	—	$100,434	$3,058,616	—
Direct Cost PPD	—	$6.31	$78.17	—
Total Overhead	$4,256,086	$1,230,100	$3,025,987	
Monthly Overhead	$354,674	$102,508	$252,166	—
Total Costs	4,256,086	1,330,534	6,084,603	7,415,137
Total Cost PPD	$77.34	$83.65	$155.51	—

$3,025,987 in overhead costs. These overhead costs are budgeted monthly at $102,508 for Assisted Living and $252,166 for Nursing Services.

Total costs are calculated in Table 7-2 by adding the revenue cost center's direct costs (total operating expenses) to its overhead costs. The final step in cost-finding is to calculate the total costs per service unit. In this example, total costs PPD are calculated by adding the direct costs PPD and the indirect costs PPD. For Assisted Living, the direct costs PPD are $6.31 and the indirect costs PPD are $77.34, for a total cost PPD of $83.65. Note that the direct costs for Assisted Living are much lower than the indirect costs. This is related to the relatively low need for these clients for direct care, compared to their high use of supportive services such as room and board (plant and dietary services), laundry, and housekeeping.

The last column of Table 7-2 adds the total costs for Assisted Living ($1,330,534) and Nursing Services ($6,084,603), which results in $7,415,137. This calculation serves as a check in that $7,415,137 represents the total operating expenses for Freeston ElderCare in FY 2003 (see the Freeston ElderCare operating expense budget in the "Supplemental Tables and Documents" section of the Back-of-Book CD-ROM).

The overall overhead rate is relatively simple to calculate as it represents the average indirect cost per service unit. An average overhead rate is applicable to cost pools such as landscaping or the lease, for which the amount of resource use would not be expected to differ across revenue cost centers. However, other types of resource use may differ substantially among revenue cost centers and their service units. For example, the amount of laundry and housekeeping required per patient for Nursing Services might be substantially greater than for Assisted Living. Although in some settings or for some indirect costs the overhead rate is an acceptable cost driver, in other situations more refined methods are required.

Cost Pool Method of Direct Distribution

The cost pool method of direct distribution is an approach to cost allocation that attempts to overcome the limitations of the overhead rate method. The first steps, identifying direct costs for each cost center and differentiating between revenue and non-revenue cost centers, are the same as for calculating an overhead rate. The difference in the cost pool method is that instead of combining all indirect costs and averaging them over all service units, cost drivers are developed that reflect the estimated resource use by the respective revenue cost centers. Costs are then allocated from the cost pools to revenue cost centers using the cost drivers. Box 7-2 summarizes direct distribution methods of cost allocation.

Cost Pool Cost Allocation

Table 7-3 presents an example using the cost pool method of direct distribution to allocate costs from support services at Freeston ElderCare to revenue cost centers. The first column indicates the total budgeted patient days

☐ **B O X   7 - 2**

Direct Distribution Method of Cost Allocation

1. Identify all direct costs for each cost center (operating expense budget)
2. Classify cost centers
   a. Revenue or profit centers (operating revenue budget)
   b. Non-revenue cost centers
3. Determine cost drivers using accepted criteria
4. Allocate costs using the overhead rate
   a. Overhead Rate = Total Overhead ÷ Total Service Units
   b. Simple, but resource use may differ among cost centers and service units
5. Allocate costs using cost pools
   a. Cost pool is a group of costs to allocate from non-revenue cost centers
   b. Allocate costs from cost pools using associated cost drivers
   c. Relatively simple, but ignores indirect costs generated by non-revenue cost centers

and the patient days budgeted to be generated by Assisted Living and Nursing Services. Percents are also calculated, indicating that Assisted Living is budgeted to generate 29% of the patient days for FY 2003 and Nursing Services 71% of the patient days. The cost pools, designated as departments providing support services, are indicated in Table 7-3 in the section for non-revenue cost centers, with a separate section for revenue cost centers. The direct costs for each department is in the first row, using the operating expense budget for FY 2003.

Costs are then allocated between Assisted Living and Nursing Services using cost drivers for each cost pool. Costs for administration and property expenses are allocated at 29% to Assisted Living and 71% to Nursing Services. This cost driver approximates the overhead rate PPD, based on the rationale that administrative costs and expenses such as utilities and the lease should be averaged out or equally spread over all service units. The cost drivers for ancillary services, rehabilitation, and plant operations allocate fewer costs to Assisted Living compared to Nursing Services, based on the rationale that Assisted Living makes less use of these resources compared to Nursing Services. The selection of 5% for Rehabilitation, 15% for Ancillary, and 20% for Plant Operations cost drivers are based on assumptions about indirect costs generated by the revenue cost centers for each of these support services. The allocation for Dietary is 40% for Assisted Living, assuming that the per patient costs for Assisted Living meals are somewhat greater compared to Nursing Services. Under different assumptions, the cost drivers would differ from these examples.

The cost allocations per cost pool are reported in Table 7-3 as negative numbers because they represent deductions from the total costs generated by each support service. The total amount of indirect costs allocated to Assisted Living is $1,181,176, with a total of $3,074,910 allocated to Nursing Services. These amounts are added to the direct costs for each revenue cost center to obtain the total cost of $1,281,610 for Assisted Living and $6,133,527 for Nursing Services. The sum of the total costs for Assisted Living and Nursing Services is calculated in the last column of Table 7-3 as a check. This amount is $7,415,374, which equals the total operating expense budget for Freeston ElderCare in FY 2003.

Cost Pool Cost-Finding

Table 7-3 shows that the direct costs PPD for Assisted Living are $6.31 and for Nursing Services $78.17. The indirect costs PPD for Assisted Living are $74.26 (or $1,181,176 ÷ 15,906) and for Nursing Services $78.59. Total costs for each revenue cost center PPD are calculated by dividing the total costs by the number of patient days. For Assisted Living the total costs PPD are $80.58 and for Nursing Services the total costs PPD are $156.76.

TABLE 7-3

Freeston ElderCare Direct Distribution Worksheet, Budget FY 2003

	Patient Days	Administration	Rehabilitation	Non-Revenue Cost Centers				Revenue Cost Centers		Total Costs
				Ancillary	Dietary	Plant Operations	Property Expense	Assisted Living	Nursing Services	
Direct Costs	55,034	$178,281	$188,202	$265,676	$871,370	$715,654	$2,036,904	$100,434	$3,058,616	7,415,137
Direct Cost PPD	—	—	—	—	—	—	—	$6.31	$78.17	—
% Assisted Living	29%	29%	5%	15%	40%	20%	29%	—	—	—
Assisted Living	15,906	$(51,527)	$(9,410)	(39,851)	(348,548)	(143,131)	(588,709)	$1,181,176	—	—
Assisted Living PPD	—	—	—	—	—	—	—	$74.26	—	—
% Nursing Services	71%	71%	95%	85%	60%	80%	71%	—	—	—
Nursing Services	39,128	$(126,754)	$(178,792)	$(225,824)	(522,822)	(572,523)	(1,448,195)	—	3,074,910	—
Nursing Services PPD	—	—	—	—	—	—	—	—	$78.59	—
Total %	100%	100%	100%	100%	100%	100%	100%	—	—	—
Total Costs	—	$0	$0	$0	$0	$0	$0	$1,281,690	$6,133,683	$7,415,374
Total Cost PPD	—	—	—	—	—	—	—	$80.58	$156.76	—

[1] Ancillary assumed to not generate revenues for simplicity.

[2] Nursing Administration costs included in Nursing Services as direct costs.

The identification of cost pools and the development of cost drivers are expected to vary among work settings. For example, rather than using the total operating expenses for a department as a cost pool, costs might be pooled that represent specific services. For example, rather than using the entire Plant Operations expense budget as a cost pool, the costs for central supply, laundry, and housekeeping might be used instead. In some settings, revenue cost centers are charged by departments providing support services, so cost drivers represent specific amounts charged for laundry, dietary, and other indirect costs rather than a percent of costs assigned to the revenue cost center.

In cost allocation, it is helpful to separate the costs of individual programs. For simplicity, the text does not differentiate between non-personnel expenses for the SNF, Intermediate Care, and Nursing Administration units in the Freeston ElderCare Nursing Services operating expense budget. Increasing the detail of the Nursing Services budget would make it possible to separate the SNF and intermediate care units as revenue cost centers and to assign the costs for nursing administration as indirect costs. The added detail in budget reporting would increase the complexity of the budget but would refine the cost allocation process by more specifically assigning costs to each of the Nursing Services units.

Increasing the detail and complexity of non-revenue cost centers at Freeston ElderCare would also refine cost allocation. For example, it might be advisable to report laundry and housekeeping as separate cost pools so that each of these costs would be allocated in a more accurate way to the revenue cost centers. These examples assumed that ancillary services did not generate revenues, though revenues are reported in the operating revenue budget (see the "Supplemental Tables and Documents" section of the Back-of-Book CD-ROM). It should be apparent that cost allocation methods and reporting are frequently complex and involve input from executive administrators, department directors, and financial officers.

Other Cost Allocation Methods

One limitation of the direct distribution method of cost allocation is that it overlooks indirect costs generated by non-revenue cost centers. For example, the Dietary Department at Freeston ElderCare requires housekeeping services and uses space included in the lease.

The **reciprocal distribution** method allocates costs for support services to all cost centers, not just to revenue cost centers. This is a more complex process than the direct method but is also more accurate as it takes all sources of costs into account rather than only focusing on costs generated by revenue cost centers. The preparation of a reciprocal distribution cost report requires mathematical calculations beyond the scope of this text. Such reports would be prepared by finance departments.

Step-Down Distribution Method

The **step-down distribution** method, mandated by Medicare for cost reports, addresses the limitations and difficulties of direct and reciprocal distribution methods. Costs are allocated among non-revenue as well as revenue cost centers. However, as all the costs from a cost center are allocated, the cost center is removed from further cost allocation procedures. Cost centers are entered into the allocation process in sequential order. This method improves the accuracy of cost allocation by assigning costs generated from one support service to another, such as the use of housekeeping by a dietary department, yet is simpler to calculate than the more complex reciprocal distribution method. This is one of the most common methods of cost allocation because it must be used in Medicare cost reports.

Table 7-4 presents an example of step-down distribution that allocates costs for Freeston ElderCare. Costs are first allocated from the Property Expenses cost pool, with 5% or $101,845 in property expenses allocated to Administration, 15% or $305,536 to Plant Operations, and to the remaining cost centers until 100% of property expenses are allocated to other non-revenue and revenue cost centers. The allocations are entered as negative numbers because these costs are transferred from the property expense cost pool until its total costs after step-down distribution is $0.

TABLE 7-4

Freeston ElderCare Step-Down Distribution Worksheet, Budget FY 2003

Cost Allocations	Non-Revenue Cost Centers						Revenue Cost Centers		Total Costs
	Property Expense	Administration	Plant Operations	Dietary	Ancillary	Rehabilitation	Assisted Living	Nursing Services	
Total Costs	**$2,036,904**	**$280,126**	**$1,029,593**	**$1,345,351**	**$493,354**	**$434,743**	**$1,426,988**	**$6,030,959**	**7,415,137**
Direct Costs	**$2,036,904**	$178,281	$715,654	$871,370	$265,676	$188,202	$100,434	$3,058,616	7,415,137
Direct Cost PPD	—	—	—	—	—	—	$6.31	$78.17	—
Property Expense									—
% Property Expense									—
Administration	$(101,845)	**$101,845**							—
% Administration	5%								—
Plant Operations	$(305,536)	$(8,404)	**$313,939**						—
% Plant Operations	15%	3%							—
Dietary	$(305,536)	$(14,006)	$(154,439)	**$473,981**					—
% Dietary	15%	5%	15%						—
Ancillary	$(142,583)	$(33,615)	$(51,480)	$0	**$227,678**				—
% Ancillary	7%	12%	5%	0%					—
Rehabilitation	$(61,107)	$(42,019)	$(51,480)	$(67,268)	$(24,668)	**$246,541**			—
% Rehabilitation	3%	15%	5%	5%	5%				—
Assisted Living	$(448,119)	$(56,025)	$(205,919)	$(538,140)	$(74,003)	$(4,347)	**$1,326,554**		—
% Assisted Living	22%	20%	20%	40%	15%	1%			—
Assisted Living PPD							**$83.40**		—
Nursing Services	$(672,178)	$(126,057)	$(566,276)	$(739,943)	$(394,683)	$(430,396)	$(42,810)	**$2,972,342**	—
% Nursing Services	33%	45%	55%	55%	80%	99%	3%		—
Nursing Services PPD								**$75.96**	—
Total Step-Down Costs	**$0**	**$0**	**$0**	**$0**	**$0**	**$0**	**$1,384,178**	**$6,030,959**	**$7,415,137**
Total % Allocated	**100%**	**100%**	**100%**	**100%**	**100%**	**100%**	**3%**	**0%**	—
Total Step-Down Cost PPD	—	—	—	—	—	—	**$87.02**	**$154.13**	—

The next cost pool allocated using the step-down method shown in Table 7-4 is administration. The total costs for administration are $280,126. This figure represents the sum of $178,281 in direct costs plus $101,845 in indirect costs allocated from the property expense cost pools. Administration costs are allocated at 3% or $8,404 to Plant Operations, 5% or $14,006 to Dietary, and to the remaining cost centers until 100% of administration costs are allocated, with total step-down costs at $0. The property expense cost pool is removed from the procedure as all its costs have been allocated.

Table 7-4 shows the step-down distribution continuing for all of the non-revenue cost centers, with each cost center removed as its costs are completely allocated. When revenue cost centers are allocated, Assisted Living only allocated 3% or $42,810 of its total costs to Nursing Services, leaving a balance of $1,384,178 ($1,426,988 − $42,810) in total step-down cost allocation. Nursing Services' step-down cost allocation is $6,030,959. As in previous examples, the final column of Table 7-4 sums the total costs for Assisted Living and Nursing Services, resulting in $7,415,137, which equals the total operating expense budget for Freeston ElderCare for FY 2003.

Cost-finding is shown in Table 7-4 in the lines for direct costs, which report $6.31 for Assisted Living and $78.17 for Nursing Services. Patient days used to calculate costs PPD are not shown in Table 7-4 but are the same as in Table 7-3. Indirect costs PPD for Assisted Living are $83.40 ($1,326,554 ÷ 15,906) and $75.96 for Nursing Services. The total costs PPD for Assisted Living are $89.71, of which $6.31 are direct costs and $83.40 are indirect costs. The total costs PPD for Nursing Services are $154.13.

In reviewing Table 7-4 and the process of step-down distribution, note that the sequence in which cost centers are entered into cost allocation affects their indirect and total costs. At either extreme, using the example in Table 7-4, the cost pool for property expenses is not allocated any costs from other cost centers, while Nursing Services could not allocate any of its costs to other cost centers. The rationale used in selecting the sequence in this example is based on the assumption that property expenses such as utilities and the lease should be shared by all cost centers, administrative costs shared by all remaining cost centers, and plant operations by most of the cost centers. Next, the costs of support services of dietary, ancillary, and rehabilitation are allocated based on the assumption that their services largely support the revenue centers to a greater extent than the non-revenue centers. Finally, there was an assumption that Assisted Living provides some support services to Nursing Services. If different assumptions were made about allocation, the order of entry into the step-down distribution would differ from this example, which would change the total costs allocated the departments.

Although the step-down distribution method better accounts for support services among non-revenue cost centers, the sequence of entry into cost allocation is also a limitation. For example, there might be housekeeping or dietary costs generated by administration that are not allocated in the example shown in Table 7-4. Nursing Services may provide some support services to other cost centers that are not recognized in this example. It is important to carefully consider the sequencing of cost centers in step-down distribution as well as the cost drivers employed to allocate costs. Box 7-3 summarizes the procedure for step-down distribution.

Activity-Based Costing

Activity-based costing (ABC) is a cost allocation method that focuses on the indirect and direct costs of specific activities performed within cost centers, with the cost of these activities used as the cost drivers for cost allocation and cost-finding. Figure 7-3 illustrates that the sources of costs for specified activities involved in the services provided by a given cost center are based on the direct costs for each activity and the costs of relevant activities provided by each support service. For example, Nursing Services provides direct nursing care as an activity, but Plant Operations provides housekeeping as a support service activity for Nursing Services.

☐ **B O X   7 · 3**

Step-Down Method of Cost Allocation

1. Identify all direct costs for each cost center (operating expense budget)
2. Classify cost centers as non-revenue or revenue cost centers
3. Determine cost drivers using accepted criteria
4. Select the order of entering cost centers into the step-down process, beginning with non-revenue cost centers
5. Remove cost centers from step-down procedures when all their costs are allocated
6. Calculate total indirect costs and total costs allocated to each revenue cost center

---

Table 7-5 provides a simplified example of ABC from Freeston ElderCare's Assisted Living unit. The column at the left lists several selected activities involved in providing Assisted Living services. Admission procedures are the first activity, which is a support service activity of administration, with an estimated cost of $50 per admission. Budgeted indirect costs for admission procedures are therefore $18,100 ($50 × 362) for FY 2003. The intake assessment performed on admission is estimated at $200 per admission and is a direct cost for the Assisted Living unit. Indirect costs are allocated from dietary and plant operations (for housekeeping) based on costs PPD, and direct costs allocated for home health services. The total indirect costs for Assisted Living services based on its activities are $256,690 and total direct costs are $98,560.

Cost-finding using the ABC method is shown in Table 7-5 as $16.14 PPD for indirect costs and $6.20 PPD for direct costs, with total costs PPD of $38.47. These figures, particularly for indirect and total costs, are much lower for Assisted Living than in previous examples because property expenses and other activities provided by support services such as laundry and maintenance are ignored for simplification.

The types and level of detail of activities selected for ABC are important in costing various services. For example, direct nursing care could be aggregated over a given number of patient days or hours per patient day, or could be listed in much greater detail, such as by the number of IVs started and other nursing procedures done PPD. It is necessary to think about what activities are most relevant to the service provided, and which activities can and should be reported and monitored for direct and indirect costs.

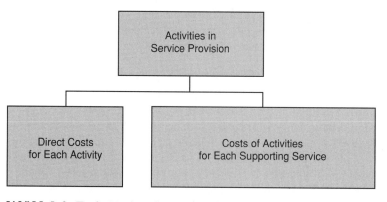

FIGURE 7.3 ■ Activity-based costing (ABC).

ABC is more useful in settings providing services that involve direct and indirect activities that can be measured or reported in terms of costs. For example, it might be feasible to track specific procedures (activities) performed in an emergency room setting as direct costs, and support services such as laboratory tests, radiology procedures, and time spent by security services as indirect costs.

TABLE 7·5

Freeston ElderCare Activity-Based Costing for Assisted Living, FY 2003

Activity	Cost Driver	Unit Cost	Support Services			Assisted Living
			Administration	Dietary	Plant Operations	Total Direct & Indirect Costs
Patient Days	—	—	—	—	—	15,906
Patient Admissions	—	—	—	—	—	362
ADC	—	—	—	—	—	43.6
Indirect Costs						
Admission procedures	per admission	$50	$18,100	—	—	$18,100
Dietary Services	PPD	$10	—	$159,060	—	$159,060
Housekeeping	PPD	$5	—	—	$79,530	$79,530
Total Indirect Costs	—	—	—	—	—	**$256,690**
Total Indirect Cost PPD	—	—	—	—	—	**$16.14**
Direct Costs						
Intake Assessment	per admission	$200	—	—	—	$72,400
Home Health Services	25% of ADC/month	$100	—	—	—	$26,160
Total Direct Costs	—	—	—	—	—	**$98,560**
Total Direct Cost PPD	—	—	—	—	—	**$6.20**
Total Costs	—	—	$18,100	$159,060	$79,530	**$611,956**
Total Cost PPD	—	—	—	—	—	**$38.47**

ABC might also be useful in determining the cost of care for various diagnoses or types of patients, when the activities associated with patient care are measurable and can be assigned costs.

Classification and Weighted Approaches to Costing Services

Besides direct distribution, step-down, and ABC approaches to costing health care services and service units, approaches using various classifications or grouping of patients or procedures may be employed. This section provides an introduction to some of these approaches that are commonly seen in health care settings.

Product Line Costing

A **product line** is a group of patients with a common characteristic that allows for grouping by classification, such as a common diagnosis or procedure. For example, product lines at Freeston ElderCare include SNF patients, Intermediate Care patients, and Assisted Living patients. There are several methods for product line costing. One of the most common methods is calculating the average cost per service unit. Examples have been provided throughout this chapter calculating costs PPD (also known as per diem costs). Costs PPD are averages because the total cost is divided by the number of patient days, resulting in an average cost PPD. Other calculations of average cost per service unit include costs per patient visit, per procedure, or per episode.

Another approach to product line costing is the calculation of total direct care hours for each product line, discussed in Chapter 6. Costs are then assigned by the amount of total direct care hours required per product line, using the hourly rate (wage) of various levels of staff providing care. For example, if product line costing for the Rehabilitation Department at Freeston ElderCare were applied to patients grouped as having total hip replacement surgery, the number and cost of direct hours of physical therapist time as well as physical therapist assistant time would be calculated. These direct hours are then multiplied by the hourly wage for each staff level and totaled to obtain the product line cost for physical therapy staff.

MDC and DRG Classifications

As discussed in Chapter 2, in the 1980s the prospective payment system of Medicare reimbursement established diagnostic related groups (DRGs) based on major diagnostic category (MDC) classifications of illness and standardized expected length of inpatient care. The diagnostic categories for a patient's principal admitting diagnosis are based on the "International Classification of Diseases, 9th Revision, Clinical Modification" (IDC-9-CM). Besides their utility in prospective payment systems (which are now being extended beyond acute care to home health and long-term care settings), MDCs and DRGs enable the identification of average patient resource consumption by diagnosis.

Table 7-6 presents a few examples of DRGs based on the MDC 04, respiratory disorders and diseases. A brief description is included for each DRG, followed by the number and percentage of hospital discharges for the DRG as a primary admitting diagnosis for the United States for the year 2000. The average charge and LOS for the DRG are then reported. Information about mortality, gender, and age makes up the remainder of Table 7-6. These data could be compared to utilization, costs, mortality rates, and demographic characteristics for the same DRGs in hospital settings across the United States.

CPT® and HCPCS Codes

The Physicians' **Current Procedural Terminology (CPT®) code** is a coding system developed by the American Medical Association that identifies specific medical services and procedures used to classify outpatient services and costs. Inpatient cost centers may also use CPT® codes to group costs, as in radiology departments or other work units performing procedures that fit the coding system. The **Healthcare Common Procedure Coding System (HCPCS)** is a coding system that incorporates and expands CPT® codes to classify services and products not included in the CPT® codes. HCPCS codes were also developed to reduce the use of miscellaneous or non-classified codes for programs, products, and services. Table 7-7 shows CPT® and HCPCS codes for a few selected physical and occupational therapy services and procedures.

RBRVS and RVUs

The Medicare **Resource-Based Relative Value Scale (RBRVS)** was developed in 1992 to quantify physician services for reimbursement purposes. The cost assigned to each **Relative Value Unit (RVU)** developed under the RBRVS corresponds to a CPT® or HCPCS code and includes three components. Approximately 55% of the cost assigned to the RVU is the value of the physician's work. The second component of the RVU, approximately 42% of the cost of the physician services, is the practice expense. Malpractice liability insurance expense is the third component assigned as the remaining portion of the RVU.

The approach in developing RVUs is similar to the ABC approach in that the specific service (activity) is analyzed for its direct and indirect resource use. This is also referred to as a weighted procedure because the various components of the RVU are assigned different amounts. The type of procedure (medical or surgical), type of setting (facility representing inpatient and non-facility representing outpatient), and level of malpractice risk are weighted and combined differently for each RVU, as shown in Table 7-7.

For example, for the CPT® code 97001, a medical procedure for physical therapy evaluation, the RVUs for physician work, non-facility practice expense, and malpractice insurance costs are provided, with a recommended level for Medicare reimbursement. The calculations of RVUs are not in the scope of this text but are included in Table 7-7 to show how they may be reported. Direct, indirect, and total costs for procedures in a given setting could be compared with the standard Medicare reimbursement and RVUs.

U.S. Hospital Stays, Selected DRGs from Medical Diagnosis Category (MDC) 04, Respiratory Disorders and Diseases, Healthcare Cost and Utilization Project (HCUP), Nationwide Inpatient Sample (NIS), 2000

MDC		DRG	Number of Discharges	% of Discharges	Mean Charges (dollars)	Mean Length of Stay (days)	% Died	% Male	Mean Age
04	SURG 75	Major chest procedures	101,219	0.3%	$36,025	9.2	4.2%	56.6%	58
04	SURG 76	Other resp system O.R. procedures w CC[1]	72,553	0.2%	$34,043	10.7	7.9%	52.3%	65
04	SURG 77	Other resp system O.R. procedures w/o CC	8,106	0.0%	$16,133	4.6	n/a[2]	50.0%	53
04	MED 78	Pulmonary embolism	72,746	0.2%	$15,412	6.3	4.3%	40.9%	63
04	MED 79	Respiratory infections & inflammations age >17 w CC	239,308	0.7%	$19,819	8.5	14.4%	54.3%	75
04	MED 80	Respiratory infections & inflammations age >17 w/o CC	16,726	0.0%	$13,072	6.6	4.9%	55.7%	65

Source: Adapted from HCUPnet, Healthcare Cost and Utilization Project. Agency for Healthcare Research and Quality, Rockville, MD. 2000 National Statistics Results. http://www.ahrq.gov/data/hcup/hcupnet.htm Accessed Dec. 30, 2002.

[1] CC defined as complications and/or comorbidities.

[2] Values based on 70 or fewer unweighted cases are not reliable and have been suppressed.

◯ TABLE 7-7

Selected CPT/HCPCS Codes and Associated RVUs, 2002

CPT/HCPCS		Description	2002 Physician Work RVUs	2002 Fully Implemented Non-facility Practice Expense RVUs	2002 Malpractice RVUs	Benchmark Reimbursement[1]
97001	Medical	PT Evaluation	1.2	0.56	0.1	$55.85
97002	Medical	PT Re-evaluation	0.6	0.35	0.04	$21.87
97003	Medical	OT Evaluation	1.2	0.69	0.05	—
97004	Medical	OT Re-evaluation	0.6	0.69	0.02	—
97010	Medical	Hot or cold packs therapy	0.06	0.04	0.01	—
97012	Medical	Mechanical traction therapy	0.25	0.11	0.01	—

Source: American Physical Therapy Association (APTA). 2002 Relative Value Units. http://www.apta.org/Govt_Affairs/regulatory/privatepractice/feeschedule/RVU2002 Accessed Dec. 30, 2002.

[1] Source: INTELLIMED International. MyHealthScore.com Physician Procedures. http://www.myhealthscore.com Accessed Dec. 30, 2002.

Other Cost-Finding Methods

As discussed earlier in the text, average resource use per service unit (such as PPD or per patient visit) is a frequently used approach to cost-finding. This calculation is relatively simple once direct and indirect costs are identified, but it treats all patients, patient visits, or other service units as if they consume the same amount of resources. Two other methods may be applicable in settings in which the average per service unit is not a satisfactory cost-finding measure.

Hourly Rate

In settings in which costs per hour or minute of care are relevant and can be tracked and reported, the hourly rate or rate per minute is a useful approach to cost-finding. Settings such as surgery or rehabilitation, with procedures that can be tracked by costs per hour or per minute, are highly suitable for this method. The hourly rate may be a measure used in the ABC and the product line approach, focusing on the time spent per activity or per patient classification. This is similar to the calculation of direct care hours discussed in the section on product line costing but is calculated as the amount of time per procedure rather than PPD.

The hourly rate approach is not useful for services or activities that are difficult to assign costs for each hour or minute involved. It is also possible to overlook the amount of personnel and non-personnel resources for each given procedure per time period. For example, a procedure taking an hour for one patient may require twice the personnel and supplies as an hour-long procedure for another patient. Classification by patient and procedure type may help refine the applicability of the hourly rate so that an hour for a more complex procedure or a more acutely ill patient reflects higher costs per hour than for a less complex procedure or less ill patient.

Surcharge

A **surcharge** involves adding a percent of the inventory value to items such as supplies or pharmaceuticals to allocate costs for storage and processing. For example, a hospital's inventory of 5,000 units of an IV solution might be valued at $150,000, or $30 per unit. However, the storage and processing costs might be estimated at 5%, so that a 5% surcharge is added to each unit of the IV solution, making the charge $31.50 ($30 × 1.05).

□ B O X 7 - 4

Approaches to Cost Allocation and Cost-Finding

1. Cost allocation methods
   a. Direct distribution
   b. Reciprocal
   c. Step-down (mandated by Medicare)
2. Activity-based costing
3. Classification and weighted approaches
   a. Product line costing
   b. MDCs and DRGs
   c. CPT® and HCPCS codes
   d. RBRVS and RVUs
4. Cost-finding methods
   a. Average cost per service unit
   b. Hourly rate
   c. Surcharge

Basing surcharges on the inventory value overlooks situations in which a higher-cost inventory generates relatively few costs for storage and processing, and a lower-cost inventory requires high costs for storage and processing. It may also be difficult to assign a different surcharge to each type of item that may be inventoried. In such cases a standard minimum surcharge might be applied, or the surcharge based on past reports of associated indirect costs.

Box 7-4 summarizes the approaches to cost allocation and cost-finding discussed in this chapter.

Monitoring and Preparing Cost Reports

Concepts in Chapter 5 may be applied in monitoring cost reports, particularly controllable costs. For example, if the laundry costs are above the allocation, investigation might find excessive use, and staff training and supervision might help bring the costs into better control. When cost allocations are prepared for the coming fiscal year, department directors often have input regarding the use of indirect resources to improve the cost allocation estimates.

□ B O X 7 - 5

On-Line Sources for Information on Cost Allocation and Cost-Finding

Centers for Medicare and Medicaid Services (CMS). Activities Based Costing Training.
http://cms.hhs.gov/contractors/abc/abc2.asp
Department of Health and Human Services (HHS) Health Care Financing Administration (HCFA).
(May 2000). Medicare Provider Reimbursement Manual Part 1.
http://cms.hhs.gov/manuals/pm_trans/R414PRM.pdf Transmittal 414.
Healthcare Financial Management Association (HFMA). http://www.hfma.org

Conclusion

This chapter presents concepts and approaches to cost allocation and cost-finding in health care settings. Box 7-5 provides Internet resources for further information about allocation and cost-finding.

■ CRITICAL THINKING EXERCISES

1. If available, obtain cost allocation or cost-finding reports from your own health care setting, concealing the setting's identity as appropriate. Review and interpret these reports, applying the concepts covered in this chapter. Does the method used for cost allocation or cost-finding appear to be accurate and fair? Discuss.

2. Use information from the operating expense budget for Freeston ElderCare in the Chapter 4 Appendix to practice cost allocation and cost-finding, using at least one approach discussed in this chapter. Evaluate the results based on accuracy and fairness. Discuss.

■ REFERENCES

American Physical Therapy Association (APTA). 2002 Relative Value Units. http://www.apta.org/Govt_Affairs/regulatory/privatepractice/feeschedule/RVU2002 Accessed Dec. 30, 2002.

Baker, J. J., & Baker, R. W. (2000). *Health Care Finance: Basic Tools for Nonfinancial Managers.* Gaithersburg, MD: Aspen.

Centers for Medicare & Medicaid Services (CMS). Activities-Based Costing Training. http://cms.hhs.gov/contractors/abc/abc2.asp Accessed Dec. 30, 2002.

Claritas Inc. (1999). Diagnosis Related Group Codes. *http://www.connect.claritas.com/doc/dbh_hdrg.htm* Accessed Dec. 30, 2002.

Cleverley, W. O., & Cameron, A. E. (2002). *Essentials of Health Care Finance*, 5th ed. Gaithersburg, MD: Aspen.

Finkler, S. A., & Kovner, C. T. (2000). *Financial Management for Nurse Managers and Executives*, 2nd ed. Philadelphia: W. B. Saunders.

Gapenski, L. C. (2002). *Healthcare Finance: An Introduction to Accounting and Financial Management*, 2nd ed. Chicago: Health Administration Press.

HCUPnet, Healthcare Cost and Utilization Project. Agency for Healthcare Research and Quality, Rockville, MD. 2000 National Statistics Results. http://www.ahrq.gov/data/hcup/hcupnet.htm Accessed Dec. 30, 2002.

INTELLIMED International. MyHealthScore.com Physician Procedures. *http://www.myhealthscore.com* Accessed Dec. 30, 2002.

Johnson, S. E., & Newton, W. P. (March 2002). Resource-based Relative Value Units: A primer for academic family physicians. *Family Medicine, 34*(3), 172–176.

Medicare Provider Analysis and Review (MEDPAR). Medicare Provider Analysis and Review (MEDPAR) of Short-Stay Hospitals List of Diagnosis Related Groups (DRGs) FY 2000. http://cms.hhs.gov/statistics/medpar/Drg00dsc.pdf Accessed Dec. 30, 2002.

CHAPTER 8

Break-Even Analysis

▢ Learning Objectives

1. Differentiate between fixed and variable costs.
2. Apply concepts of volume, cost, and revenue to calculate a break-even equation with and without profit.
3. Apply concepts of volume, cost, revenue, and profit to calculate a contribution margin with a specified level of profit.

◯ Key Terms

Break-even analysis
Contribution margin (CM)
Contribution margin per unit (CMU)
Fixed cost (FC)
Payor mix
Product mix
Revenue per unit (RU)

Total cost (TC)
Total fixed cost (TFC)
Total fixed cost per unit
Total revenue (TR)
Total variable costs (TVC)
Variable costs
Variable costs per unit (VCU)

How do managers figure out how many goods or services they must deliver, and how much they must charge to cover their budgets and generate profits? This chapter discusses the concept of **break-even analysis**–calculating how much one must charge (setting a price) or how much volume (numbers of clients or units of service) one must generate to cover the costs of business, then make a profit (the amount of revenue exceeding expenses). The first section discusses factors in break-even, then break-even analysis is presented for covering costs without profit. Next discussed is break-even analysis when profit is an added factor, then some complicating factors in break-even analysis and break-even under capitation financing are introduced. The calculation and application of the **contribution margin** and the importance of including indirect costs (some of which are accounted for as overhead) into a break-even analyses for profitability are additional concepts covered in this chapter.

Break-even analysis has many applications and uses. This technique helps the manager in profit planning by identifying how profitable it may be to purchase new equipment or expand a program, and by targeting projects that are unprofitable and may need to be terminated or downsized. Managers can demonstrate the impact of changes in price or volume on profitability and can determine the optimal price or volume by using this analysis. Moreover, break-even analysis is a way to evaluate productivity and management efficiency. Break-even analysis is also a tool in estimating profit and loss for developing budget balancers, or management strategies used when preparing a budget to generate additional revenues or reduce expenses to achieve desired profit levels (discussed in Chap. 6).

Break-Even Without Profit

The first formulas presented will calculate break-even without considering profit. This is the most simplistic approach to a break-even analysis: simply calculating the amount of volume (clients or units of goods or services) or revenue (income or reimbursement) required to cover the costs of operation. It is assumed that any volume or revenue that is actually generated beyond this calculation will generate profits. In many cases, managers may want to factor in a specified target for profit; therefore, after reviewing break-even analyses in their simplest form, profit will be entered into the break-even formula.

The fundamental principle of break-even analysis is that profits change with changes that occur in costs, revenue, and volume. It is essential to understand, identify, and estimate costs, volume, and revenue (reimbursement or price) to undertake a break-even analysis in its simplest form before including a specified profit target.

Volume

Volume (designated as Q, or the quantity of a relevant unit of volume) is the number of the relevant units of goods, services, or clients. In identifying volume, it is critical to clearly define the relevant unit of measurement. For example, in identifying volume for an outpatient clinic or service, the number of patients likely do not represent volume; rather, the number of patient visits represents volume. In other words, one patient may make many visits for outpatient services, with each service representing costs and revenues and affecting the volume.

Frequently, one can only estimate an expected volume over the coming year. To ensure the accuracy of the break-even analysis, it is critical to estimate volume as accurately as possible. On the other hand, in this ever-changing health care climate, accurate volume estimations may be difficult. When reporting a break-even analysis in which any estimations, whether cost, volume, or revenue may be subject to unexpected change, this limitation should be reported.

This chapter uses the example of ABC Hospital, which runs an inpatient cardiac rehabilitation unit. Its administrators are considering opening an outpatient cardiac rehabilitation unit as well. To consider whether this new venture would be feasible and profitable, Joe, the exercise physiologist who manages the inpatient unit, is assigned to gather data and do a financial analysis. Here are some initial assumptions that guide Joe's estimates and calculations:

1. Estimated fixed costs (equipment, staff) for the unit budget over the projected budget year are $250,000.
2. The unit operates only on business days, 250 days over the projected budget year.
3. Reimbursement for patient visits is at or above the Medicare rate of $60 per visit.
4. Calculations are made on a per-day basis so Joe can estimate the volume as well as revenue (on average) needed each day to cover costs.

Joe decides to estimate various possible levels of daily patient volume (visits to the cardiac rehabilitation unit) in increments of 5 from the low, worst-case scenario of 15 visits to a high of 35 visits (Table 8-1).

Costs

Costs represent any and all resources involved in providing a service or producing a good (see Chapter 1). One way to identify costs is to use an expense budget focused on the service or good of interest. For example, Joe prepares an expense budget to start the outpatient cardiac rehabilitation unit, from which he obtains data regarding fixed and variable costs.

In relating costs to volume, it is important to identify and estimate **fixed costs** and **variable costs**. Fixed costs are costs one assumes will not vary (at least over the budget year) regardless of changes in volume. For example, the costs of permanent staff, capital equipment, and, in some cases, rent are generally assumed to remain unchanged, at least over the time of an annual budget. Whether the cardiac rehabilitation unit serves 5 patients or 50 on a given day, the cost of the equipment purchased for the unit will not change. Of course, if in the coming year one estimates that additional equipment must be purchased to accommodate an increasing or larger-than-expected volume of patient visits, the fixed cost budget must be adjusted accordingly. However, for the current year in which the unit equipment is budgeted, costs typically do not change based on change in volume. One assumption for the cardiac rehabilitation unit is that it will cost about $250,000 in budgeted fixed costs to purchase equipment and staff the unit (see Table 8-1).

There is one other important point in calculating fixed costs for programs, units, or departments contained within a larger organization. Frequently, it is necessary to add a specified amount of overhead to a program

TABLE 8-1

ABC Hospital, Outpatient Cardiac Rehabilitation Unit, Break-Even Analysis without Profit, 2001

Volume	FC per Day*	FC per Visit	Overhead per Day	Overhead per Visit	TFC per Day	TVC per Visit	TC per Day	TC per Visit	TR per Visit**	Break Even
15	$1,000	$67	$225	$15	$1,225	$5	$1,300	$87	$60	($400)
20	$1,000	$50	$300	$15	$1,300	$5	$1,400	$70	$60	($200)
25	$1,000	$40	$375	$15	$1,375	$5	$1,500	$60	$60	$0
30	$1,000	$33	$450	$15	$1,450	$5	$1,600	$53	$60	$200
35	$1,000	$29	$525	$15	$1,525	$5	$1,700	$49	$60	$400

* Estimate $250,000 annual unit budgeted FC and 250 days of operation.

** Medicare reimbursement; assume non-Medicare clients' reimbursement at or above Medicare reimbursement level.

budget to account for the indirect costs borne by one unit or department on behalf of another. For example, opening the outpatient cardiac rehabilitation unit will add to the workload and costs for the outpatient admissions office, housekeeping, security, and other departments. As discussed in Chapter 7, organizational policy generally determines whether and to what amount overhead costs are to be included as budgeted fixed costs.

Therefore, **total fixed costs (TFC)** include all fixed costs in the budget, plus any specified overhead costs. The CFO at ABC Hospital instructs Joe to estimate $15 overhead per visit, adjusting the TFC per visit and per day accordingly (see Table 8-1). The formula for calculating total fixed costs (TFC) is:

$$\text{Fixed Costs (budgeted)} + \text{Overhead (if required)} = \text{Total Fixed Costs}$$

$$\text{FC} + \text{Overhead} = \text{TFC}$$

In some cases, managers want to know what their TFC amount to per patient, per patient visit, or per other unit of goods or services provided—the **total fixed costs per unit**. The formula to calculate TFC per unit is as follows:

$$\text{Total Fixed Costs} \div \text{Volume} = \text{Total Fixed Costs per Unit}$$

$$\text{TFC} \div \text{Q} = \text{TFC per unit}$$

Table 8-1 shows that the fixed costs per day are $1,000 regardless of the volume of patient visits. The amount of overhead increases with increases in patient volume, so for 25 patient visits it is $375 per day. Therefore, the calculations for TFC and TFC per unit are as follows:

$$\text{TFC} = \$1,000 + \$375$$

$$\text{TFC} = \$1,375$$

$$\text{TFC per Unit} = \$1,375 \div 25$$

$$\text{TFC per Unit} = \$55$$

Variable costs are always directly tied to changes in volume. For example, in a cardiac rehabilitation unit, each patient uses a set of disposable ECG contact pads during the visit. Any supplies directly tied to individual clients or client visits represent sources of variable costs. In addition, temporary staff who must be obtained when volume surpasses estimates for which permanent staff have been hired may represent variable costs. Review the section in Chapter 4 regarding flexible budgeting based on volume, which reflects adjustments in staffing (largely treated as a variable cost) based on changes in volume.

While one may simply estimate and sum up all of the fixed costs for a given good or service to identify TFC, estimating **total variable costs (TVC)** is a little more difficult. First, one must estimate the variable costs associated with each individual client, client visit, or other relevant transaction, commonly referred to as the **variable costs per unit (VCU)**. For example, to identify the VCU identified with a cardiac rehabilitation unit, any supplies used on a per-visit basis must be taken into account. For cardiac rehabilitation, there are typically very few variable costs, and their calculation is quite simple (see Table 8-1). In some settings, as in a wound clinic, where the individual costs of dressing changes may vary considerably, one might average the costs of a dressing change, or set a financial target for typical dressing change costs. Remember, the more accurate the cost estimate, the more accurate and reliable the resulting break-even analysis.

The next step in estimating TVC is to multiply the VCU by the estimated volume (Q). The formula for calculating TVC costs is:

$$\text{Total Variable Costs} = \text{Variable Costs Per Unit} \times \text{Volume}$$

$$\text{TVC} = \text{VCU} \times \text{Q}$$

One must include both a total of the fixed costs involved in producing a given good or service and a total of the estimated variable costs to calculate the **total costs (TC)** for producing a given good or service over a budget year. Therefore, the basic formula for total costs is:

$$\text{Total Costs} = \text{Total Fixed Costs} + \text{Total Variable Costs, or}$$

$$\text{TC} = \text{TFC} + \text{TVC}$$

A more expanded formula for TC is:

$$\text{Total Costs} = \text{Total Fixed Costs} + (\text{Variable Costs Per Unit} \times \text{Volume}), \text{or}$$

$$\text{TC} = \text{TFC} + (\text{VCU} \times \text{Q})$$

While the second, expanded formula for TC appears a bit more complicated, it enables one to more clearly identify and factor in both the VCU and the estimated volume in calculating total costs. Table 8-1 shows the variable and total costs for the outpatient cardiac rehabilitation unit.

Revenue

Revenue, also referred to as **revenue per unit**, is the income derived from the reimbursement provided or the price set for goods or services. **Total revenue (TR)** is the revenue per unit multiplied by the volume of clients, visits, or other transactions, such as laboratory tests. The revenue per unit of goods or services must be identified or estimated, then multiplied by the estimated volume of clients, visits, examinations, or other relevant units of volume measurement. The revenue per visit for the outpatient cardiac rehabilitation unit is at or above the $60 Joe assumes is allowed by Medicare (see Table 8-1). Therefore, the formula for estimating total revenue is very similar to the formula for TVC, as shown below:

$$\text{Total Revenue} = \text{Revenue per Unit} \times \text{Volume, or}$$

$$\text{TR} = \text{RU} \times \text{Q}$$

Estimates of costs, revenue, and volume are needed to compute a break-even formula. The next section completes the formula for the break-even analysis.

The Break-Even Principle and Formula

As stated at the beginning of this chapter, the fundamental principle of break-even analysis is that revenues and costs change with changes in volume. "Breaking even" means that the revenue from selling goods or services equals the total costs of producing goods or services; in other words, one's revenues covers one's costs. This principle is represented by the following formula:

$$\text{Total Costs} = \text{Total Revenue, or}$$

$$\text{TC} = \text{TR}$$

An expanded formula for break-even analysis is:

$$\text{Total Fixed Costs} + (\text{Variable Costs Per Unit} \times \text{Volume}) = \text{Revenue per Unit} \times \text{Volume, or}$$

$$\text{TFC} + (\text{VCU} \times \text{Q}) = \text{RU} \times \text{Q}$$

Although the second, more expanded formula may seem a bit confusing, remember that it allows for the direct identification of revenues per unit, estimated volume, fixed costs, and variable costs per unit to enter

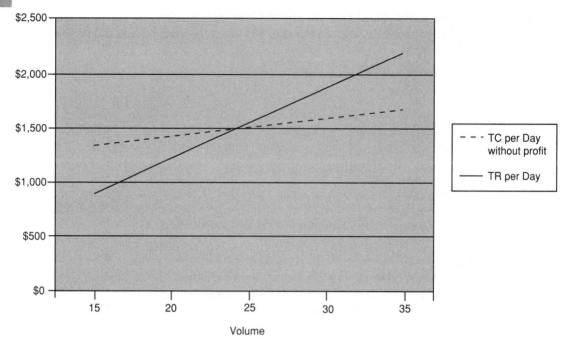

FIGURE 8.1 ■ ABC Hospital Outpatient Cardiac Rehabilitation Unit, break-even without profit, 2001.

into the formula. Figure 8-1 graphs the break-even point for Joe's cardiac rehabilitation unit without factoring in profit (in other words, the point at which just enough revenues are generated to cover the costs of operation). The break-even point is the point at which the total costs (TC) and total revenues (TR) lines intersect.

Now it is possible to apply the break-even formula to begin to answer some practical questions useful in health care management. Continue to refer to Table 8-1 as the source of data in the following formulas.

Keeping Costs Within Budget

Earlier chapters in this text discussed budgeting, and the importance of adhering to a budget was emphasized. Break-even analysis can be applied using the basic formula TC = TR to identify how well a manager adheres to a budget and to monitor both volume and sources of costs. Obviously, if the overall costs of providing a good or service exceed the revenues, there are problems in management efficiency that must be addressed.

The extent to which total revenue exceeds total costs determines the profitability of the goods or services provided. If a particular profit target is not specified, it is still possible to calculate profit according to the following formula:

$$\text{Profit} = \text{Total Revenue} - \text{Total Costs, or}$$

$$P = TR - TC$$

Note Joe's calculations in Table 8-1. Given the estimated total costs and total revenues, the break-even point (when profit is not factored into the break-even formula) is reached at a volume of 25 patient visits per day. Any additional patient visits per day generate a certain proportion of profit; from Table 8-1, 30 patient visits generate $200 of profit per day, and 35 patient visits generate $400 in profit. Figure 8-1 graphs the profit increase beyond the break-even point as volume increases.

When Reimbursement Is Set

In many cases, the revenue or reimbursement for health care goods or services is set by the payor. For example, one cannot negotiate with state or federal authorities to make changes in Medicaid or Medicare reimbursements. Increasingly, insurance plans may also negotiate a preset, often discounted reimbursement for some goods or services provided. In such a situation, it would not make sense to focus on estimating how to price a given good or service to break even; remember, the price or reimbursement has already been decided. However, a break-even formula could be useful to determine the volume of goods or services, given the fixed reimbursement, that would be required to cover costs. The formula for calculating a break-even analysis to determine volume is as follows:

$$\text{Break-Even Volume} = \text{Total Fixed Costs} \div (\text{Revenue per Unit} - \text{Variable Costs per Unit}), \text{ or}$$

$$Q = TFC \div (RU - VCU)$$

For example, assume Joe has not made the volume estimates indicated in Table 8-1 but has estimated a total fixed cost (TFC) per day of $1,375 and knows the revenue per unit (RU) is $60 and the variable cost per visit (VCU) is $5. Entering the data into the break-even formula for volume, Joe finds the outpatient cardiac rehabilitation unit must attract 25 patient visits per day to break even (without generating profit).

$$Q = \$1,375 \div (\$60 - \$5)$$

$$Q = \$1,375 \div \$55$$

$$Q = 25$$

Using Break-Even Analysis to Set the Price

There are cases in which it is important to know what price must be set or what units of revenue are required to cover the costs of operation (in other words, break even). In this case, the focus is on the revenue generated per unit of a given good or service provided (RU), and the volume of goods or services is estimated. The formula for the break-even price (RU) is as follows:

$$\text{Break-Even Price} = \text{Total Costs} \div \text{Volume}, \text{ or}$$

$$RU = TC \div Q$$

The expanded formula is:

$$\text{Break-Even Price} = (\text{Total Fixed Costs} + [\text{Variable Costs Per Unit} \times \text{Volume}]) \div \text{Volume}, \text{ or}$$

$$RU = (TFC + [VCU \times Q]) \div Q$$

For example, assume Joe does not have a Medicare rate to use to make the revenue estimates. Entering the data into the break-even formula for price, and assuming there are 25 patient visits per day (see Table 8-1), Joe finds the outpatient cardiac rehabilitation unit must charge $60 per visit to break even (without generating profit).

$$RU = (\$1,375 + [\$5 \times 25]) \div 25$$

$$RU = \$1,500 \div 25$$

$$RU = \$60$$

Break-Even With Profit

Profit is an additional and very important factor to consider in break-even analysis. Some financial experts refer to break-even analysis as "cost-volume-profit (CVP) analysis," which directly describes the relationships involved. For-profit enterprises need to generate profit, but nonprofit enterprises must also generate profit to be able to grow and maintain the quality of their goods and services. For this reason, profit may also be referred to as "operating income." Some people make a mistake of thinking of their own salaries as profit. When budgeting and calculating a break-even analysis for starting up one's own business, one's salary should be calculated into the personnel budget, not the profit target. People are expected to earn a salary, regardless of the profitability of the enterprise.

The principle of calculating break-even with profit is that the revenues or volume generated must cover both costs and profit. The amount of profit is specifically targeted in this analysis and entered into the formula, as shown in the following formula:

$$\text{Total Revenue} = \text{Total Costs} + \text{Profit, or}$$

$$TR = TC + P$$

An expanded formula for break-even analysis with profit is:

$$\text{Revenue per Unit} \times \text{Volume} = \text{Total Fixed Costs} + (\text{Variable Costs Per Unit} \times \text{Volume}) + \text{Profit, or}$$

$$RU \times Q = TFC + (VCU \times Q) + P$$

Figure 8-2 graphs the break-even point with a \$200-per-day profit target for Joe's outpatient cardiac rehabilitation unit. As in Figure 8-1, the lines for total costs (TC) and total revenue (TR) intersect at the break-even point.

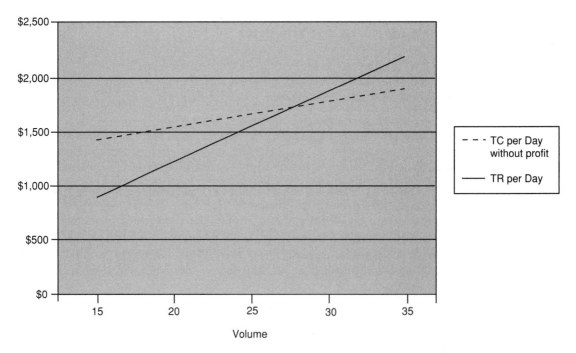

FIGURE 8.2 ■ ABC Hospital Outpatient Cardiac Rehabilitation Unit, break-even with profit, 2001.

TABLE 8-2

ABC Hospital, Outpatient Cardiac Rehabilitation Unit, Break-Even Analysis with Profit, 2001

Volume	FC per Day*	Overhead per Day	Overhead per Visit	TFC per Day	TVC per Day	TVC per Visit	Profit per Day	TC per Day	TR per Visit**	Break-Even
15	$1,000	$225	$15	$1,225	$75	$5	$200	$1,500	$60	($600)
20	$1,000	$300	$15	$1,300	$100	$5	$200	$1,600	$60	($400)
25	$1,000	$375	$15	$1,375	$125	$5	$200	$1,700	$60	($200)
30	$1,000	$450	$15	$1,450	$150	$5	$200	$1,800	$60	$0
35	$1,000	$525	$15	$1,525	$175	$5	$200	$1,900	$60	$200

* Estimate $250,000 annual unit budgeted FC and 250 days of operation.

** Medicare reimbursement; assume non-Medicare clients' reimbursement at or above Medicare reimbursement level.

Table 8-2 presents Joe's data for calculating break-even analyses with a profitability target of at least $200 per day. Refer to Table 8-2 for data to use in formulas presented throughout this section.

Break-Even Volume to Generate a Profit Target

To calculate a break-even analysis with profit that determines the volume of goods or services necessary to provide under a fixed reimbursement, the formula is:

$$\text{Break-Even Volume with Profit} = (\text{Total Fixed Costs} + \text{Profit}) \div (\text{Revenue per Unit} - \text{Variable Costs per Unit}), \text{ or}$$

$$Q = (TFC + P) \div (RU - VCU)$$

For example, assume Joe has not made the volume estimates indicated in Table 8-2 but has estimated a total fixed cost (TFC) per day of $1,450 with a profit target of $200, so the TFC per day with profit is $1,650. Joe also knows the revenue per unit (RU) is $60 and the variable cost per visit (VCU) is $5. Entering the data into the break-even formula for volume, Joe finds the outpatient cardiac rehabilitation unit must attract 30 patient visits per day to break even (without generating profit).

$$Q = (\$1,450 + 200) \div (\$60 - \$5)$$

$$Q = \$1,650 \div \$55$$

$$Q = 30$$

Break-Even Price to Generate a Profit Target

To calculate a break-even analysis with profit that determines the price of goods or services necessary to provide under an estimated volume, the formula is as follows:

$$\text{Break-Even Price with Profit} = (\text{Total Costs} + \text{Profit}) \div \text{Volume, or}$$

$$RU = (TC + P) \div Q$$

The expanded formula is:

$$\text{Break-Even Price with Profit} = ([\text{Total Fixed Costs} + \text{Profit}] + [\text{Variable Costs} \\ \text{Per Unit} \times \text{Volume}] + \text{Profit}) \div \text{Volume, or}$$

$$RU = ([TFC + P] + [VCU \times Q]) \div Q$$

For example, assume Joe does not have a Medicare rate to use to make the revenue estimates. The break-even formula for price includes a $200-per-day profit target (see Table 8-2). Joe assumes there are 30 patient visits per day, and finds the outpatient cardiac rehabilitation unit must charge $60 per visit to break even and generate the profit target of $200 per day.

$$RU = (\$1,450 + \$200) + [\$5 \times 30]) \div 30$$

$$RU = (\$1,650 + \$150) \div 30$$

$$RU = \$1,800 \div 30$$

$$RU = \$60$$

Guidelines for Breaking Even

Guidelines to remember in breaking even are fairly simple and obvious after working through a few of these formulas. One guideline is that to whatever extent the revenue per unit (selling price) of the goods or services provided can be increased, the more the break-even volume may decrease while covering costs, with or without profit. For example, if Medicare and other insurance rates for outpatient cardiac rehabilitation increases to $65 per visit, the volume needed to break even decreases accordingly. Table 8-3 presents revised break-even calculations with and without the $200 per day profit target, based on a $65 revenue per visit.

The actual break-even volumes with and without profit shown in Table 8-3 fall somewhere between 20 and 25 visits (without profit) and somewhere between 25 and 30 visits (with profit). Joe would need to do some additional calculation for break-even volume to determine the exact break-even points under this new scenario. However, a lower volume than under the $60 reimbursement scenario would be required to break even, whether the profit target of $200 a day is specified or the revenues merely cover the costs.

If, instead, the volume of goods and services generated can be increased, the corresponding revenue per unit (selling price) can be reduced—another guideline for breaking even. This principle is demonstrated when customers are attracted by sales: the seller reduces the price, thereby increasing volume by attracting more customers to purchase their goods or services. For example, Joe develops a strategy in which referrals to outpatient cardiac rehabilitation from cardiologists and cardiac surgeons in ABC Hospital's catchment area increase by two thirds, increasing actual patient visits per day by 50%. Table 8-4 shows the effect of increased volume on break-even and shows how revenues could be reduced to $58 per visit with break-even points at just under 27 visits per day without profit, and 32 visits per day with the profit target of $200 per day.

When it is possible to reduce fixed or variable costs (or both), either break-even volume or break-even revenue (or both) can also decrease and costs (with or without profit) will still be covered. These are also guidelines in breaking even. For example, the more Joe can control and reduce fixed and variable costs, the lower the volume or revenue per unit needed for the cardiac rehabilitation center to break even.

Of course, all of these guidelines hold true in the reverse. If fixed or variable costs increase, break-even volume or revenue (or to some extent, both) must increase for costs (with or without profit) to be covered.

ABC Hospital, Outpatient Cardiac Rehabilitation Unit, Break-Even Analysis at $65 per Visit, 2001

Volume	FC per Day*	Overhead per Day	Overhead per Visit	TFC per Day without Profit	TFC per Day with Profit	TVC per Visit	Profit per Day	TC per Day without Profit	TC per Day with profit	Revenue per Visit**	Break Even without Profit	Break-Even with Profit
15	$1,000	$225	$15	$1,225	$1,425	$5	$200	$1,300	$1,500	$65	($325)	($525)
20	$1,000	$300	$15	$1,300	$1,500	$5	$200	$1,400	$1,600	$65	($100)	($300)
25	$1,000	$375	$15	$1,375	$1,575	$5	$200	$1,500	$1,700	$65	$125	($75)
30	$1,000	$450	$15	$1,450	$1,650	$5	$200	$1,600	$1,800	$65	$350	$150
35	$1,000	$525	$15	$1,525	$1,725	$5	$200	$1,700	$1,900	$65	$575	$375

* Estimate $250,000 annual unit budgeted FC and 250 days of operation.

** Hypothetical new Medicare and other insurance reimbursement increased from $60.

● TABLE 8 - 4

ABC Hospital, Outpatient Cardiac Rehabilitation Unit, Break-Even Analysis at 50% Projected Increase in Volume, 2001

Volume***	FC per Day*	Overhead per Visit	TFC per Day without Profit	TFC per Day with Profit	TVC per Visit	Profit per Day	TC per Day without Profit	TC per Day with profit	Revenue per Visit**	Break Even without Profit	Break-Even with Profit
22	$1,000	$15	$1,330	$1,530	$5	$200	$1,440	$1,640	$58	($175)	($375)
27	$1,000	$15	$1,405	$1,605	$5	$200	$1,540	$1,740	$58	$13	($188)
32	$1,000	$15	$1,480	$1,680	$5	$200	$1,640	$1,840	$58	$200	$0
37	$1,000	$15	$1,555	$1,755	$5	$200	$1,740	$1,940	$58	$388	$188
42	$1,000	$15	$1,630	$1,830	$5	$200	$1,840	$2,040	$58	$575	$375

* Estimate $250,000 annual unit budgeted FC and 250 days of operation.

** Reduction in charges below assumed Medicare rate of $60 per visit.

*** Rounded downward for a conservative volume estimate.

Joe must anticipate increased costs of purchasing and replacing equipment, salary increases, increased overhead costs, more ambitious profit targets, cuts in reimbursement from Medicare and other insurers, and possible drops in volume.

Table 8-5 illustrates the guidelines for breaking even by showing the relationships between all the factors in a break-even analysis. The interaction between volume, costs, revenue, and profit demonstrates how a change in one factor affects the other factors in a break-even equation, given an increase in each factor. A decrease in any of these factors would reverse the direction of the relationship.

Contribution Margin

The contribution margin (CM) represents the dollar amount available to first cover fixed costs (including overhead), then contribute to profits. Total revenues minus total variable costs result in the contribution margin:

$$\text{Total Revenue} - \text{Total Variable Costs} = \text{Contribution Margin, or}$$

$$TR - TVC = CM$$

When total fixed costs are subtracted from the contribution margin, the resulting amount represents profit:

$$\text{Contribution Margin} - \text{Total Fixed Costs} = \text{Profit, or}$$

$$CM - TFC = P$$

The contribution margin makes it possible to calculate a break-even analysis from yet another perspective. When the contribution margin equals the total fixed costs, the break-even point is reached. The following formula illustrates this concept:

$$\text{Break-even Contribution Margin} = \text{Break-even Total Fixed Costs}$$

$$CM = TFC$$

Expanding the formula should more clearly illustrate this concept. Remember that the classic break-even formula is represented as:

$$\text{Total Revenues} = \text{Total Costs, when expanded:}$$

$$\text{Total Revenues} = \text{Total Fixed Costs} + \text{Total Variable Costs, so that}$$

$$\text{Total Revenues} - \text{Total Variable Costs} = \text{Total Fixed Costs, so that}$$

$$\text{Contribution Margin} = \text{Total Fixed Costs, or}$$

$$TR = TFC + TVC$$

$$TR - TVC = TFC$$

$$CM = TFC$$

When calculating a break-even including profit using the contribution margin, the formula is adjusted as follows:

$$\text{Total Revenues} = \text{Total Costs} + \text{Profit, so that}$$

$$\text{Total Revenues} = (\text{Total Fixed Costs} + \text{Total Variable Costs} + \text{Profit}), \text{so that}$$

TABLE 8-5

Relationships Between Factors in Break-Even, Assuming Increase in Value of Factors

Given changes in volume, costs, overhead, or profit, the effects on volume, costs, revenue, and profit are displayed.

Interaction Given Increase	Volume Increases	FC per Day Increases	Fixed Cost per Visit Increases	Overhead per Day Increases	Overhead per Visit Increases	TVC per Day Increases	TVC per Visit Increases	Profit Target per Day Increases	Profit Target per Visit Increases	TR per Day Increases	Revenue per Visit Increases
Volume	—	NC	NC	NC	NC	NC	NC	NC	NC	NC	NC
FC per Day	NC	—	increase	NC	NC	NC	NC	NC	NC	NC	NC
Fixed Cost per Visit	decrease	increase	—	NC	NC	NC	NC	NC	NC	NC	NC
Overhead per Day	increase	NC	NC	—	increase	NC	NC	NC	NC	NC	NC
Overhead per Visit	NC	NC	NC	increase	—	NC	NC	NC	NC	NC	NC
TFC per Day without Profit	increase	increase	increase	increase	increase	NC	NC	NC	NC	NC	NC
TFC per Visit without Profit	decrease	increase	increase	increase	increase	NC	NC	NC	NC	NC	NC
TFC per Day with Profit	increase	increase	increase	increase	increase	NC	NC	increase	increase	NC	NC
TFC per Visit with Profit	decrease	increase	increase	increase	increase	NC	NC	increase	increase	NC	NC
TVC per Day	increase	NC	NC	NC	NC	—	increase	NC	NC	NC	NC
TVC per Visit	NC	NC	NC	NC	NC	increase	—	NC	NC	NC	NC
Profit Target per Day	NC	NC	NC	NC	NC	NC	NC	—	increase	NC	NC

Metric										
Profit Target per Visit	decrease	NC	NC	NC	NC	NC	increase	—	NC	NC
Profit per Day	increase	decrease	decrease	decrease	decrease	decrease	NC	NC	increase	increase
Profit per Visit	increase	decrease	decrease	decrease	decrease	decrease	NC	NC	increase	increase
TC per Day without Profit	increase	increase	increase	increase	increase	increase	NC	NC	NC	NC
TC per Visit without Profit	decrease	increase	increase	increase	increase	increase	NC	NC	NC	NC
TC per Day with Profit	increase	increase	increase	increase	increase	increase	increase	increase	NC	NC
TC per Visit with Profit	decrease	increase	increase	increase	increase	increase	increase	increase	NC	NC
TR per Day	increase	NC	NC	NC	NC	NC	NC	NC	increase	increase
Revenue per Visit	NC	NC	NC	NC	NC	NC	NC	NC	increase	—
CM	increase	increase	NC	NC	NC	decrease	NC	NC	increase	increase
Break Even without Profit	increase	decrease	decrease	decrease	decrease	decrease	NC	NC	increase	increase
Break-Even with Profit	increase	decrease	decrease	decrease	decrease	decrease	decrease	decrease	increase	increase

$$\text{Total Revenues} - \text{Total Variable Costs} = \text{Total Fixed Costs} + \text{Profit, so that}$$

$$\text{Contribution Margin} = \text{Total Fixed Costs} + \text{Profit, so that}$$

$$\text{Profit} = \text{Contribution Margin} - \text{Total Fixed Costs, or}$$

$$TR - TVC = TFC + P$$

$$CM = TFC + P$$

$$P = CM - TFC$$

Table 8-6 presents Joe's data used to calculate the contribution margin under each patient volume scenario.

Unit Contribution Margin

The **contribution margin per unit (CMU)** may be calculated by subtracting the variable costs per unit from the revenues per unit:

$$\text{Contribution Margin per Unit} = \text{Revenue per Unit} - \text{Variable Cost per Unit, or}$$

$$CMU = RU - VCU$$

It is then possible to calculate the total contribution margin by multiplying the contribution margin per unit by the total volume:

$$\text{Total Contribution Margin} = \text{Contribution Margin per Unit} \times \text{Volume, or}$$

$$CM = CMU \times Q$$

In a previous section of this chapter, the following formula was to calculate a break-even analysis to determine the volume required:

$$\text{Break-Even Volume} = \text{Total Fixed Costs} \div (\text{Revenue per Unit} - \text{Variable Costs per Unit}), \text{ or}$$

$$Q = (TFC \div [RU - VCU])$$

Because the contribution margin per unit equals the revenue per unit less the variable costs per unit, the break-even analysis for volume can be calculated using the contribution margin:

$$\text{Break-Even Volume} = \text{Total Fixed Costs} \div \text{Contribution Margin per Unit, or}$$

$$Q = TFC \div CMU$$

Table 8-6 shows the variable costs, revenue, and contribution margins per visit (i.e., per unit) for Joe's outpatient cardiac rehabilitation unit given changes in volume.

Contribution Margin and Pro Forma P&L Statements

Break-even analysis may be used as a tool to develop pro forma P&L statements (forecasted estimates of profit or loss) when preparing or reviewing budgets, as discussed in previous chapters. The results of the pro forma P&L would indicate profitable operations or the need to employ control mechanisms or to develop budget balancers. In using financial data to develop a pro forma P&L statement, the volume, revenue per unit (price), and costs are assumed or estimated and used to calculate the estimated amount of profit or loss.

ABC Hospital, Outpatient Cardiac Rehabilitation Unit, Break-Even Contribution Margins, 2001

Volume	FC per Day*	Overhead per Day	TFC per Day without Profit	TFC per Day with Profit	TVC per Day	TVC per Visit	Profit per Day	TR per Day	Revenue per Visit**	CM	CM per Visit	Break Even CM without Profit	Break-Even CM with Profit
15	$1,000	$225	$1,225	$1,425	$75	$5	$200	$900	$60	$825	$55	($400)	($600)
20	$1,000	$300	$1,300	$1,500	$100	$5	$200	$1,200	$60	$1,100	$55	($200)	($400)
25	$1,000	$375	$1,375	$1,575	$125	$5	$200	$1,500	$60	$1,375	$55	$0	($200)
30	$1,000	$450	$1,450	$1,650	$150	$5	$200	$1,800	$60	$1,650	$55	$200	$0
35	$1,000	$525	$1,525	$1,725	$175	$5	$200	$2,100	$60	$1,925	$55	$400	$200

* Estimate $250,000 annual unit budgeted FC and 250 days of operation.

** Medicare reimbursement; assume non-Medicare clients' reimbursement at or above Medicare level.

◯ TABLE 8-7

ABC Hospital, Outpatient Cardiac Rehabilitation Unit, Pro Forma P&L Based on Volume, 2001[1]

Volume	15	20	25	30	35
Total Revenues[2]	$225,000	$300,000	$375,000	$450,000	$525,000
Total Variable Costs	$18,750	$25,000	$31,250	$37,500	$43,750
Total Contribution Margin	$206,250	$275,000	$343,750	$412,500	$481,250
Total Fixed Costs	$250,000	$250,000	$250,000	$250,000	$250,000
Pro forma P&L	($43,750)	$25,000	$93,750	$162,500	$231,250

[1] Estimate $250,000 annual unit budgeted FC and 250 days of operation per year.

[2] Assume Medicare rate of $60 per visit.

The first step is to calculate the contribution margin. Table 8-7 annualizes the volume, revenue, and cost data that Joe uses for the cardiac rehabilitation unit. Total revenue for 2001 is estimated as $60 per visit multiplied by the estimated daily volume, then multiplied by the 250 days the unit is expected to operate per year. For an estimated volume of 15 patient visits per day, estimated revenues for 2001 are $225,000. Variable costs per unit are estimated at $5 per day, so for an estimated volume of 15 visits per day and 250 days of operation, the total variable costs for 2001 are estimated at $18,750. The contribution margin equals total revenues less total variable costs, which is $206,250 for an estimated 15 visits per day for 2001.

The next step, shown in Table 8-7, is to subtract total fixed costs from the contribution margin to calculate the estimated amount of profit or loss. For a volume of 15 patient visits per day, the estimated total fixed costs of $250,000 per year are subtracted from the contribution margin of $206,250 for an estimated loss of $43,750 for 2001. The cardiac rehabilitation unit shows a profit at an increased estimated volume of 20 visits per day, and continues to increase in profitability as the volume increases. This is another way to analyze and report volume, revenue, and cost data from the perspective of generating profit or loss.

Complicating Factors in Breaking Even

The above formulas represent the simplest forms of the break-even analysis without and with profit. Many factors greatly complicate the calculation of break-even. This text does not cover these complicating factors in detail, but a few of them are mentioned below to provide an idea of how quickly break-even can become complex. A few complicating factors include:

- Taxes (where would taxes be entered in the break-even formula?)
- **Product mix** (producing various goods and services with various combinations of costs, volume, and prices)
- **Payor mix** (various sources of reimbursement with various rates of reimbursement for the same goods and services)
- Case mix (clients requesting or requiring different combinations of goods or services)
- Volume forecasting (the extent of accuracy possible in forecasting volume)
- Changes in prices and costs

Preparing break-even analyses in these more complex scenarios is beyond the scope of this text; a more advanced text and course in financial analysis is recommended for those who want to incorporate these and other complicating factors into their calculations. However, one further scenario, capitation financing, is worth discussing in the light of the concepts covered in examining the break-even analysis.

Break-Even in Capitation

Think about the fundamental principles of capitation financing: a fixed payment, per health plan enrollee, paid to the provider or provider system for a defined set of services over a prescribed period of time. Given that under capitation the total revenue is fixed by the payor, think about what the break-even point would be. Clearly, under capitation, the enterprise breaks even when the total costs for covering the population of health plan enrollees equal the total fixed capitation payment. The enterprise generates a profit is it is able to keep the health plan costs under the capitation payment, and loses money if costs exceed the capitation payment.

Conclusion

This chapter presents the use of break-even analysis and the contribution margin to better understand and apply the relationships between volume, cost, and revenue in determining whether a program or service is profitable. Box 8-1 presents Internet resources for further exploration of the calculation and use of break-even analysis.

■ C R I T I C A L   T H I N K I N G   E X E R C I S E S

1. Compile or estimate program or project data from your work setting or a health care setting of interest. Identify the following:
   a. Volume
   b. Price, charges, or reimbursement
   c. Fixed costs
   d. Overhead
   e. Variable costs
   f. Profit or profit target

2. Prepare a break-even analysis to determine:
   a. Volume required to cover costs with and without a specified profit target
   b. Price, charges, or reimbursement to cover costs with and without a specified profit target
   c. Contribution margin that equals total fixed costs (breaks even)
3. Consider the relationship of costs to changes in volume and profitability. Using concepts from this chapter, give at least two reasons for the current emphasis of health care managers on cost control and cost reduction.

■ REFERENCES

Baker, J. J., & Baker, R. W. (2000). *Health Care Finance: Basic Tools for Nonfinancial Managers*. Gaithersburg, MD: Aspen.

Finkler, S. A., & Kovner, C. T. (2000). *Financial Management for Nurse Managers and Executives*, 2nd ed. Philadelphia: W. B. Saunders.

Gapenski, L. C. (2002). *Healthcare Finance: An Introduction to Accounting and Financial Management*, 2nd ed. Chicago: Health Administration Press.

Neumann, B. R., Suber, J. D., & Zelman, W. N. (1988). *Financial Management: Concepts and Applications for Health Care Providers*, 2nd ed. Owings Mills, MD: National Health Publishing.

CHAPTER 9

Cost-Benefit Analysis and Cost-Effectiveness Analysis

☐ Learning Objectives

1. Compare and contrast the application of cost-benefit analysis and cost-effectiveness analysis in the financial analysis of health care programs and services.
2. Explain the procedures for conducting a cost-benefit analysis.
3. Explain the procedures for conducting a cost-effectiveness analysis.

◯ Key Terms

Benefit
Benefit-cost ratio (B/C ratio)
Compounded
Cost-benefit analysis (CBA)
Cost-effectiveness analysis
  (CEA)
Default
Discount rate
Discounting
Externality
Human capital
Intangible

Net benefits
Net contribution
Objective function
Present value
Primary benefit
Program evaluation
Quality-adjusted life year
  (QALY)
Rule of Seventy
Secondary benefit
Tangible
Willingness to pay

Chapters 4, 5, and 6 discussed the use of budgeting, and Chapter 8 discussed the use of break-even analysis in understanding financial performance and making financial decisions. This chapter presents two additional analysis techniques useful to health care professionals. **Cost-benefit analysis (CBA)** is a method of evaluating the benefits produced by resources (inputs) used within a given project, program, or other intervention. **Cost-effectiveness analysis (CEA)** is a method of evaluating and comparing the benefits and resources used between two or more alternative interventions. This chapter first discusses basic concepts of CBA, then basic concepts of CEA. Sample reports (see Appendices A and B) illustrate the application of each of these methods.

Cost-Benefit Analysis

CBA has several applications that are useful to health care professionals. It is a technique that can help guide decision-making by determining the benefits achieved by a specific intervention. CBA helps identify the optimal size for projects or programs and can provide a framework for program evaluation or the financial analysis in a business plan (see Chap. 12). CBA requires that resources and benefits be expressed as **tangibles** (inputs or outputs that are or can be converted to monetary units such as dollars).

For example, a nurse case management program for pregnant diabetic women might measure the number and cost of physician visits and hospital days as tangible resources, and reduction in physician visits and hospital days resulting from complications of pregnancy or diabetes as tangible benefits. The findings from the CBA analysis of the case management program are used in making decisions about the program, including its optimal size and overall evaluation.

CBA is less useful when the analysis involves **intangibles** (inputs or outputs that cannot be quantified as monetary units). For example, the pregnant diabetic women might experience reduced fear and worry because they are monitored by the nurse case managers. Unless a way is found to quantify the dollar value of patient fear and worry, these intangibles cannot be included in the CBA.

The usefulness of CBA is also limited when **externalities** (events beyond the control of the intervention) increase risk or uncertainty about outcomes. Risk represents a calculated or estimated probability of an external event or outcome. For example, if there is a 30% chance of rain predicted for the day of an outdoor community health fair, the event may be canceled regardless of the CBA.

Uncertainty represents a completely unknown probability of an external event or outcome. In health care, the use of accepted practice guidelines, procedures, and clinical pathways helps reduce uncertainty, as practice is linked to patient outcomes. In the nurse case management program, the use of accepted guidelines, procedures, and pathways would reduce uncertainty about the outcomes for pregnant diabetic women and would more clearly establish that the resources used by the program did (or did not) result in tangible benefits.

CBA Procedures

The first step in conducting a CBA is to identify the **objective function** or functions (what the intervention is intended to achieve). The objective functions must be tangible and measurable. For example, the nurse case management program for pregnant diabetic women is expected to reduce complications related to pregnancy and diabetes. The rate of complications for the case-managed group of women is an example of an objective function.

Costs are resources required as inputs in producing the objective function of health care goods or services. Costs must be measurable, and in monetary units or in a form that can be converted to monetary units. For example, intangible costs, such as discomfort, must be quantified and converted to dollars to be entered in the analysis. Opportunity costs are the dollar value of an alternative benefit that could result during the same time period or with the same amount of resources as invested in the current activity. For example, if it is possible to convert the value of the time a client spends waiting for health care services, it may be entered into the CBA as an opportunity cost.

Costs may be direct costs, or resources used as inputs in the production of an objective function. For example, the wages and benefits paid for nursing services in the nurse case management program are a direct cost. Indirect costs are resources used that are not direct inputs in the production of an objective function. Expenses paid for the staff of the nurse case management program to attend conferences is an example of an indirect cost (Chaps. 4 and 7 discuss direct and indirect costs).

Benefits are the outputs or contributions produced by the objective function, including cost savings achieved by the intervention. Benefits, like costs, must either be in monetary units or in a form that can be converted to monetary units. For example, a reduction in hospital days achieved by reducing complications of pregnancy and diabetes with nurse case management results in a tangible cost savings that can be measured using inpatient charges. Intangible benefits, such as patient satisfaction with the monitoring provided by the nurse case management program, must be quantified and converted to monetary units if entered into the analysis.

Benefits may be classified as **primary benefits**, which result directly from the objective function. For example, the reduction in hospital costs for the pregnant diabetic women is a primary benefit of the nurse case management program. **Secondary benefits** represent indirect contributions that result from the objective function. For example, improved school performance of the children born to the participants of the nurse case management program is a secondary benefit.

Once the objective functions, costs, and benefits are identified and the costs and benefits converted to monetary units, the **net benefit** (also referred to as **net contribution**) is calculated. The dollar values of all of the costs are subtracted from the dollar values of all the benefits to determine the net benefits. If benefits exceed costs, the intervention generates more benefits than costs and may be recommended or supported on that basis. In many cases, benefits represent cost savings generated by the objective function. If costs exceed benefits, the intervention generates more costs than benefits and may be considered too costly or inefficient.

For example, the nurse case management program reports that its annual cost, including direct and indirect costs, is $250,000, with benefits over the same year of $375,000. The "benefits" largely represent reductions in hospital and physician visit costs by reducing the rate of complications of diabetes and pregnancy among the clients. Net benefits are calculated as follows:

$$\text{Net Benefits} = \text{Total Benefits} - \text{Total Costs}$$

$$\$125,000 \text{ Net Benefits} = \$375,000 - \$250,000$$

In other words, the nurse case management program generated $125,000 in net benefits (cost savings) over the year of operation (or made a net contribution of $125,000), so its evaluation is highly satisfactory.

Another calculation used in CBA is the **benefit-cost ratio (B/C ratio)**, calculating by dividing the total benefits by the total costs. This calculation allows for comparisons across similar interventions that may vary in size. Interventions with B/C ratios greater than 1 generate more benefits than costs; if the B/C ratio is less than 1, the costs exceed benefits. A B/C ratio of 2.0 means that for every dollar of cost, the intervention generates $2 in benefits. By contrast, a B/C ratio of 0.5 indicates that for every dollar of cost, the intervention only generates $0.50 in benefits.

For example, the nurse case management program generates $250,000 in costs and $375,000 in benefits over the same year. The B/C ratio is calculated as follows:

$$\text{B/C Ratio} = \text{Total Benefits} \div \text{Total Costs}$$

$$1.5 \text{ B/C Ratio} = \$375,000 \div \$250,000$$

In other words, the nurse case management program generates $1.50 in benefits for every $1.00 in cost. The sample CBA presented in Appendix A presents both the net benefits and the B/C ratios for an adult asthma education program evaluation.

Discounting, Discount Rate, and Present Value

Discounting (converting the future value of a monetary unit to its present value) is discussed briefly and only in general terms in this text. The goal of this chapter is to enable the reader to conduct a simpler, short-term CBA for which discounting is not needed, and discounting is not included in the sample CBA or in the exercises at the end of the chapter. More information on discounting is available in advanced health care finance texts.

Discounting enables the calculation and analysis of costs and benefits for specified numbers of years into the future. Discounting is required when very costly, long-term projects such as a major renovation or construction is the objective function. Calculation of discount rates is usually not required for smaller, short-term projects of only 1 year.

The **discount rate** is the rate of interest used in the discounting calculation. Theoretically, the discount rate is determined by the rate at which people or institutions are willing to give up current consumption for future consumption by establishing savings. The discount rate also reflects the rate at which a borrower pays for funds, which depends to a large extent on the amount of risk, which may be real or perceived by the lender. The greater the risk of **default** (failure to repay the loan), the higher the interest rate charged to the borrower. The longer the life of the project, the higher the interest rate, as long-term projects requiring long-term debt are considered to carry more risk than short-term projects carrying short-term debt.

Discounting is calculated by finding the **present value** (monetary value of an investment) and its discount (interest) rate for a specified number of years into the future. The calculation of the present value requires estimates of the interest rate (discount rate), time period of the investment, and future value of the investment. It is assumed that the interest is **compounded** (the interest earned in each time period earns interest in future time periods). If the cost of the investment equals or exceeds the present value, then the project may not be worth the investment. If the cost of the investment is less than the present value, the project is likely to be profitable.

For example, if the managers of XYZ Health Corporation evaluate a business plan to borrow money to build a new long-term care facility, they will determine the interest rate and the time period of the loan. Assume for this example there is an 11% interest rate and a 20-year loan. They then estimate the present value of each of the annual cash inflows for the long-term care facility over the time period of the loan. Assume for this example that the long-term care facility is built in 2 years, so it operates for 18 years of the loan generating cash flow. The sum of the present values for the cash inflows from year 3 (when the long-term care facility begins generating revenue) through year 20 (the last year of the loan) is $6,200,000.

If the business plan proposes an investment of $6,200,000, the XYZ Health Corporation managers may reject the plan and put the money in what they feel might be a better, more profitable investment. If the investment proposed exceeds the present value of $6,200,000, the managers will almost certainly reject the proposal as unprofitable. However, if the business plan proposes an investment less than the present value of $6,200,000 (for example, showing that the long-term care facility can be built with a current investment of only $5,500,000), then the managers are likely to see this as a profitable investment and accept the plan.

Table 9-1 shows the impact of various discount rates applied over selected time periods given a future value of $100. Note that as the discount rate increases, the present value of the investment decreases. For example, a $78.35 investment is required over 5 years for a $100 future value at a 5% discount rate, but only $49.72 is required when the discount rate increases to 15% for the same time period and future value. In addition, as the time period increases, the present value of the investment decreases. For example, a $78.35 investment is required over 5 years for a $100 future value at a 5% discount rate, but only $37.69 is required when the time period increases to 20 years.

A rule of thumb used in estimating financial returns is the **Rule of Seventy**: an investment earning 7.2% compounded annually is estimated to double every 10 years. Table 9-1 shows that

○ **TABLE 9-1**

Effect of Discount Rates over Specified Time Periods for Future Value of $100

Year	5%	7.2%	10%	12.5%	15%
5	$78.35	$70.64	$62.09	$55.49	$49.72
10	$61.39	$49.89	$38.55	$30.79	$24.72
15	$48.10	$35.24	$23.94	$17.09	$12.29
20	$37.69	$24.89	$14.86	$9.48	$6.11

the Rule of Seventy also works in reverse. In other words, at a discount rate of 7.2%, the present value (investment) is about half the future value in 10 years. The present value of $49.89, located at the intersection of 7.2% discount rate and a 10-year time period, is about half of the future value of $100.

The discount rate is closely related to the time frame of the intervention and analysis. For example, if benefits are analyzed over 10 years, a 10% discount rate reduces all long-term benefits to zero. One suggestion is to calculate net benefits using the best available discount rate, then recalculate net benefits without including a discount rate to see the impact a discount rate makes on the long-term estimates. If discounting makes a substantial impact on the net benefits, then discounting should be included in the CBA.

Cost-Effectiveness Analysis and Procedures

CEA is useful in comparing alternative interventions to determine the least costly means to obtain the desired benefit. Unlike CBA, CEA does not compare benefits to costs but assumes a benefit is produced by an objective function. Therefore, CEA is highly applicable when benefits may be intangible or cannot be converted to dollar values (a situation in which CBA may be meaningless).

For example, a county public health department might assume that good prenatal care for women with high-risk pregnancies is a desired benefit, although a dollar value is not attached to this benefit. The health department might then compare the nurse case management prenatal program with other prenatal programs to see which program provides the most and best prenatal care for high-risk pregnant women at the lowest cost. The health department would then be expected to choose the least costly program (which achieves the desired benefit) for funding and support.

Although benefits need not be quantified for a CEA, it is essential to quantify and convert all costs into monetary units so the interventions may be compared to find the least costly alternative to achieve the desired benefit. Both direct and indirect costs may be included, as in performing a CBA. If the project is long term, discounting may also be applied to the total costs of each program.

For example, the nurse case management program for pregnant diabetic women costs $250,000 over a given year. The program is compared for the same year to Program A, operated at a cost of $300,000, Program B, operated at a cost of $150,000, and Program C, operated at a cost of $245,000. Assuming that all four programs achieve the same level of benefits, the director of the nurse case management program might want to examine the operation of Program B more closely and consider switching to that program, as it operates at far less cost than the other programs. A sample CEA featured in Appendix B compares alternative interventions for postsurgical pain reduction.

Box 9-1 summarizes the fundamental applications and differences between CBA and CEA.

□ B O X   9 - 1

Cost-Benefit Analysis vs. Cost-Effectiveness Analysis

CBA	**CEA**
Both benefits and costs are evaluated.	Costs are evaluated, but benefits are assumed to be of value.
Must quantify and convert both costs and benefits to monetary units.	Costs must be in monetary units, but benefits may be intangible.
Compares the costs of a project, program, or process to its benefits.	Compares the costs of two or more alternative projects, programs, or processes, assuming the same benefits.

Valuing Human Life

In some cases, it is important to consider the valuation of human life and quality of life in calculating a CBA or CEA. As with discounting, this text introduces the topic of valuing human life, but more information is available in advanced health care economics texts. An example of valuing human life is included in the sample CBA focused on adult asthma education (see Appendix A).

One method of valuing human life is the **human capital** approach, in which the present value of a person's future earnings is estimated. This approach is commonly applied in assessing legal damages for death or disability. The human capital approach may also be applied in estimating the overall loss in national output from morbidity and mortality (such as the human capital costs of HIV), or the production gains for saving and extending life (such as the human capital benefits of influenza immunizations).

Another approach in valuing human life is estimating the **willingness to pay** for risk or safety. For example, wage differentials may be established based on the amount of occupational risk in work settings such as foundries or construction sites. This approach is also used in determining the amount consumers are willing to pay for safety devices such as bike helmets or smoke detectors.

Quality-Adjusted Life Years

The calculation of **quality-adjusted life years (QALYs)** enables one to assess the proportion of the state of health experienced by an individual over a year. QALY is a method to assign dollar values to life and the benefits of health care by weighting each remaining year of life by the expected quality-of-life measure for that year. A CBA might then compare the costs of a treatment to the benefits as valued by the QALY calculation. A CEA might compare costs per QALY among different treatments to find the treatment with the lowest cost per QALY.

QALYs are calculated using quality-of-life measures from standardized instruments such as the 15-D Health-Related Quality of Life Index. For example, an adult with emphysema might have a 15-D score of 0.75 (out of a maximum score of 1.0, which represents optimal health) for a given year. Multiplying the score by 1 year results in a QALY of 0.75. In other words, the individual lost 0.25 QALY because of the emphysema.

The person with emphysema might be expected to live for 10 years, experiencing a 15-D score of 0.75 for 5 years (designated as weight) and a 15-D score of 0.5 for the remaining 5 years of life (designated as weight). The QALY calculation for these 10 years of life is as follows:

$$QALY = (QALY \text{ weight} \times \text{years of life}) + (QALY \text{ weight} \times \text{years of life})$$

$$6.25 \text{ QALY} = (0.75 \times 5) + (0.5 \times 5)$$

In other words, the person with emphysema experiences 6.25 QALYs from the 10 remaining years of life. The sample CBA calculates a dollar value based on the QALY scores and productivity.

Program Evaluation

Program evaluation is the application of analytic methods to determine whether a program is needed, utilizes its resources effectively, operates as planned, and meets its objectives. When applied to health care settings, program evaluation can be used to identify strengths and problem areas, justify a program's continued existence, and support program expansion. In applying CBA to program evaluation, the first step is to identify measurable program objectives and expected outcomes. The direct and indirect costs for resources used to meet the program objectives are calculated, as well as the dollar value of the benefits from the outcomes. Costs are then subtracted from the benefits (or vice versa) to determine if the program's benefits equal or exceed its costs. A B/C ratio is also calculated to determine the value of benefits generated per dollar of costs.

In applying CEA to program evaluation, the total costs of the program under evaluation may be compared to the total costs of other programs providing similar benefits to decide if the program under evaluation keeps its costs at or under those of the comparison programs. The CBA or CEA may be the primary method of evaluating the program, or one of multiple methods may be used in combination for program evaluation.

Limitations of CBA and CEA

The CBA and CEA have limitations. First, the analyses are only as accurate and complete as the data available. Therefore, if the data are not available or are of poor quality, the analysis may be inaccurate or limited in focus to factors that have good measures. Second, it may not be possible or feasible to measure all of the relevant costs and benefits or to convert all relevant measures to dollars, or some of the relevant costs and benefits may be overlooked. For example, externalities and opportunity costs may be important factors but are frequently overlooked or are impossible to measure or quantify. Third, health care "is about health care," not solely about saving money. In many cases a CBA or CEA is not an adequate analysis for planning or evaluation in and of itself. Other ways of determining the value of a program, project, or intervention, such as its fit with the organizational mission, expert opinion, and community support, should be considered as well.

BOX 9-2

On-line Sources for Information on Cost-Benefit Analysis and Cost-Effectiveness Analysis

CCH Business Owner's Toolkit—Major Purchases & Products:
   http://www.toolkit.cch.com/text/P06_6000.asp
Focus on Cost-Effectiveness Analysis at AHRQ:
   http://www.ahrq.gov/research/costeff.htm
Free, On-Line Nonprofit Organization and Management Development Program—Module 12, Program
   Evaluation: http://www.managementhelp.org
Performance Improvement 2002: Evaluation Activities of the U.S. Department of Health and Human
   Services: http://aspe.hhs.gov/pic/perfimp/2002/index.htm
Project HOPE Center for Health Affairs Publications—Health Care Costs and Financing:
   http://www.projecthope.org/CHA/pubs/finance.htm

Conclusion

This chapter presents concepts in developing a CBA or CEA focused on health care programs or services. A sample CBA and a sample CEA are in Appendices A and B. Note that the sample CBA is a retrospective evaluation of a program over the prior fiscal year, while the CEA is a prospective projection for use in a business plan. However, a CBA could be developed and reported prospectively, and a CEA can make retrospective comparisons as well. Box 9-2 provides some Internet resources for further information on CBA and CEA.

■ CRITICAL THINKING EXERCISES

1. Using an example from Chapter 8 and the cardiac rehabilitation unit, calculate net benefits, a B/C ratio, or CEA.
2. Think of a project or program in your work setting, or in a setting of interest, and list all of the direct and indirect costs. Quantify these costs into dollar terms. Are there any costs that cannot be quantified and converted to dollars? Discuss.
3. Think of a project or program in your work setting, or in a setting of interest, and list all of its primary and secondary benefits. Quantify these benefits into dollar terms. Are there any benefits that cannot be quantified and converted to dollars? Discuss.
4. Explain how you would evaluate a project or program in your work setting, or in a setting of interest. Discuss reasons for selecting CBA or CEA to evaluate this project or program.

■ REFERENCES

Bissinger, R., Allred, C., Arford, P., & Bellig, L. (1997). A cost-effectiveness analysis of neonatal nurse practitioners. *Nursing Economics, 15*, 92–99.

Buerhaus, P. I. (Third Quarter, 1998). Milton Weinstein's insights on the development, use, and methodologic problems in cost-effectiveness analysis. *Image, 30*(3), 223–227.

Financial Maths in Context: Teaching and Assessment (accessed 7/27/2002). The Rule of Seventy. *http://education.qld.gov.au/tal/kla/finance/ruleof.htm*

Folland, S., Goodman, A. C., & Stano, M. (1997). *The Economics of Health & Health Care*, 2nd ed. Upper Saddle River, NJ: Prentice Hall.

Gilmartin, M. J. (2001). Economic issues in health care. In J. L. Creasia & B. Parker (Eds.), *Conceptual Foundations: The Bridge to Professional Nursing Practice* (3rd ed., pp. 228–255). Philadelphia: Mosby.

Jacobs, P., & Rapoport, J. (2002). *The Economics of Health and Medical Care*, 5th ed. Gaithersburg, MD: Aspen.

Mullahy, C. (October 1998). Cost benefit analysis reports: An effective outcomes reporting tool. *Journal of Care Management, 4*(5), 32–42.

Posavac, E. J., & Carey, R. G. (1997). *Program Evaluation Methods & Case Studies*, 5th ed. Upper Saddle River, NJ: Prentice Hall.

Pruitt, R., & Jacox, A. K. (March-April 1991). Looking above the bottom line: Decisions in economic evaluation. *Nursing Economics, 9*(2), 87–91.

Santerre, R. F., & Neun, S. P. (1996). *Health Economics: Theory, Insights, and Industry Studies*. Chicago: Irwin.

Serxner, S., Miyaji, M., & Jeffords, J. (May/June 1998). Congestive heart failure disease management study: A patient education intervention. *CHF*, pp. 23–28.

Wise, L. C., Bostrom, J., Crosier, J. A., White, S., & Caldwell, R. (1966). Cost-benefit analysis of an automated medication system. *Nursing Economics, 14*(4), 224–231.

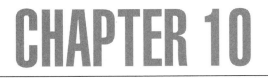

CHAPTER 10

Basics of Financial Accounting and Reporting

☐ Learning Objectives

1. Identify at least two regulatory bodies that establish financial standards for health care organizations.
2. Explain the concept of depreciation and one method for calculating depreciation.
3. Identify the components and purpose of the annual report, income statement, balance sheet, and statement of cash flows.

○ Key Terms

Accelerated depreciation
Accounts payable (A/P)
Accounts receivable (AR)
Accrual basis of accounting
Accrued expenses
Accumulated depreciation
Amortization
Annual report
Assets
Balance sheet
Board-restricted accounts
Book value
Capital
Capital in excess of par

Cash basis of accounting
Cash flow statement
Collateral
Collectibles
Common stock
Contra-asset account
Contributed capital
Current assets (CA)
Current liabilities (CL)
Current maturities of long-term
 debt
Default
Depreciation
Disclosure

continued

Key Terms (continued)

Earnings before interest and taxes (EBIT)	Net income
	Net receivables
Equity	Net surplus
Excess of revenue over expenses from operations	Net working capital
	Non-current assets (NCA)
Fair market value	Non-current liability (NCL)
Financial accounting	Operating fund
Fiscal conservatism	Operating profit
Fixed assets	Owner's equity
Functional classification	P&L statement
Fund accounting	Par
General fund	Payout ratio
Goodwill	Principal
Illiquid asset	Real assets
Income statement	Receivables
Incurred but not reported expense (IBNR)	Restricted assets
	Retained earnings
Input	Retention ratio
Intangible asset	Secured loan
Interest	Statement of cash flows
Inventory	Statement of financial operations
Just-in-time	Statement of financial position
Liability	Stockholders' equity
Liquid asset	Straight-line depreciation
Liquidation	Tangible assets
Managerial accounting	Trade credit
Marketable securities	Transaction costs
Matching principle	Unrestricted fund
Materiality principle	Unsecured loan
Natural classification	Working capital
Net assets	Written off
Net deficit	

This chapter presents some introductory concepts of financial accounting and reporting so that health care professionals can review and interpret financial statements. A brief history of financial accounting and regulation is provided, followed by an overview of relevant accounting concepts. The chapter then presents and discusses frequently encountered financial statements and their interpretation. Chapter 11 introduces concepts of analyzing financial performance using data from financial statements. Chapter 3 discusses approaches to financial reporting and analysis developed specifically for capitated and managed care plans.

Financial statements, like budgets, serve several purposes. Financial statements are assessments and indicators of the financial health of the organization. In addition, they show the decisions affecting finances made by leadership as well as the impact of those decisions. Financial statements also reflect the perspective, tax status, and priorities of organizations. Box 10-1 summarizes the purposes of financial statements.

The setting for the financial reporting examples in this chapter is SouthSide Hospital, a 24-hour acute care facility with 110 beds in service and an operating (expense) budget of approximately $566 million in FY 2003. SouthSide Hospital is a non-profit enterprise, discussed in more detail in the section addressing for-profit versus non-profit financial status and reporting. The same financial statements developed in this chapter are reviewed in Chapter 11 to further analyze the financial performance and operations of SouthSide Hospital. The terms *organization*, *enterprise*, *business*, and *company* are used interchangeably to refer to either a for-profit or non-profit health care setting that generates revenues and expenses.

☐ BOX 10·1

Purposes of Financial Statements

- ■ Assess and provide indicators of financial health
- ■ Show the owners' and managers' decisions affecting financial health and the impact of those decisions
- ■ Reflect the perspective, tax status, and priorities of the organization

History and Regulation of Financial Reporting

Financial accounting and reporting has progressed through history from using piles of stones to using spread-sheet software to measure and report exchanges of goods and services. Improvements in technology greatly increased the types and amounts of financial data that may be accumulated, analyzed, and reported. Today, managers frequently have computer capabilities that allow fairly sophisticated financial recording, reporting, and analysis. However, the age-old difficulty of translating resources, economic activities, and intangibles into financial (monetary) units persists. For example, what is the best way to place a value on SouthSide Hospital? Its price on the market? The cost of its physical plant and inventories? The qualifications of its medical, nursing, and allied health staff? What about the value of its reputation in the community?

Financial regulations in the United States were prompted by the economic upheaval and disorder brought about by the Great Depression in the late 1920s and 1930s. Health care organizations are generally required to implement accepted financial practices and periodic audits to ensure financial accountability. Examples of regulatory bodies and organizations that establish financial standards relevant to health care organizations are presented in Table 10-1.

○ TABLE 10·1

Regulatory Bodies and Organizations Establishing Financial Standards for Health Care Settings

Acronym	Name	Purpose
SEC	Securities & Exchange Commission	U.S. government regulatory agency that specifies & enforces the form & content of financial statements. Noncompliant businesses are prohibited from selling securities to the public.
FASB	Financial Accounting Standards Board	A private organization the SEC delegates to establish standards
GASB	Government Accounting Standards Board	Similar to FASB, but established for public businesses
GAAP	Generally accepted accounting principles	A set of objectives, conventions & principles established as guidelines issued from the FASB & other regulatory organizations that continue to develop over time.
AICPA	American Institute of Certified Public Accountants	Professional association of public financial accountants, with similar authority as the AMA exerts over physicians
HFMA	Healthcare Financial Management Association	An organization that participates in setting specific standards for health care finance

Measuring and Recording Financial Activities

Chapters 4 and 5 discussed the level of detail for both the time period and the line items in reviewing and monitoring budgets. These chapters also discuss measuring in terms of volume (the number of units of goods, services, or clients), dollars (revenue, expense, profit, or loss), and percents (percent variance and collection rates). Financial accounting and reporting also involves measuring and entering financial activities, usually within a revenue-generating enterprise or organization such as SouthSide Hospital rather than a smaller department or work unit.

Financial accounting includes activities involved in collecting, reporting, and analyzing organization-level data to present in financial statements. This chapter and Chapter 11 present concepts relevant to financial accounting. By contrast, **managerial accounting** involves activities often focused at the level of departments or work units, such as budgeting and planning. Chapters 4, 5, and 6 focused on managerial accounting related to budgeting and budget reports.

Time Periods

As in budgeting and budget analysis, it is important to consider the time period for recording financial activities. The time periods are usually reported as months, quarters, or the fiscal year (a 12-month period for financial reporting that may or may not represent a calendar year). One fiscal year may also be compared to another to report and analyze financial performance over the longer term.

Basis of Accounting

The way in which revenues and payments are perceived and recorded by the financial manager may vary. There are two approaches to recording financial activities relevant to health care organizations. The main difference between these two approaches is the timing of the reporting of financial events.

The first approach is the **cash basis of accounting**, in which revenue represents and is recorded at the time of receipt of payment, and expenses represent and are recorded at the time of expenditures or monetary disbursements. In cash accounting, revenues are reported within the same accounting time period as when the payment is received, typically at or very close to the time the goods or services are provided, and expenses are reported when payments are made for **inputs** (items such as personnel, supplies, and equipment that generate costs in providing goods and services). The following example illustrates cash accounting.

At Central City Clinic, Mr. Jones visits a nurse practitioner, who cleans and dresses a wound from a rusty nail and gives him a tetanus booster vaccination. Mr. Jones pays the nurse practitioner $30 cash. The revenue and payment are recorded within the same accounting time period as the service is provided. In other words, in cash accounting, the financial event is recorded and reported at the time cash is exchanged. Cash accounting is the system most of us use to balance our checkbooks and manage our personal finances. Most people acknowledge revenues (income) when they receive a paycheck or fee, and acknowledge expenses when they pay bills or make cash disbursements for goods or services. This is a simple and intuitive approach to recording financial activities.

Cash accounting is useful to health care organizations in managing their cash flow, as the discussion of the cash budget in Chapters 4 and 6 and the discussion of reporting cash flows will demonstrate later in this chapter. The cash flow budget reflects a cash accounting perspective. It is important to be able to cover day-to-day expenses and to meet financial obligations, such as payment of salaries and wages, on time. Therefore, cash accounting is used for an organization's cash management.

However, as Chapter 4 points out, in most health care organizations there is often a lag, sometimes of considerable duration, between the time goods or services are provided and payment is made. In these situations, it makes more sense to use the **accrual basis of accounting**, in which revenues are recorded when earned, representing an obligation for payment, and expenses are recorded when financial obligations are created, such as when inputs are employed, used, or consumed. The following example illustrates accrual accounting:

On March 5, during the first quarter of the fiscal year, the nurse practitioner treats Mr. Jones' wound and gives him a tetanus booster vaccination. Mr. Jones pays the $5 co-pay in cash, and the nurse practitioner bills Mr. Jones' insurance company for the remaining $25 for his care. The entire $30 is recorded as revenue at the time of service, although the $25 is not actually paid by the insurance company to the Central City Clinic until May 21, the second quarter of the fiscal year.

In accrual accounting, revenue is reported in the same accounting time period as the goods or services are provided, generating an obligation to pay, which may not be fulfilled until a future accounting time period. In other words, the recording of revenue does not represent the receipt of payment, but the implied promise of payment. Frequently, services are provided under the provisions of an existing contract for payment.

In accrual accounting, expenses represent the utilization of personnel, supplies, or equipment, such as the hours of direct nursing care scheduled or the amount of supplies used over a given time period, not the financial expenditures or cash disbursements made over another time period to pay for these inputs. Frequently, disbursements for accrued expenses are made in compliance with contract terms and conditions. For example, employees typically expect to be paid semi-monthly or monthly, not at the end of each workday. Although somewhat more complicated and less intuitive than cash accounting, accrual accounting is a standard accounting method that is more applicable to health care financial activities and payment systems.

The operating revenue and expense budgets are prepared using an accrual accounting approach. For example, at Freeston ElderCare (See "Supplemental Tables and Documents" on the Back-of-Book CD-ROM), the per diem bed revenues are recorded according to the monthly census (in other words, as services are provided), not when the payment is received. Expenses, such as for hourly staff, are recorded within the time periods in which they are used. Capital and operating budgets both forecast and record financial activity over specified time periods. Accrual accounting records and reports these financial activities over a comparable time period.

One advantage of using accrual accounting is that it more realistically and accurately portrays the financial activities of most health care organizations. The operating revenue and expense budgets reflect the application of accrual accounting. For example, Paul Jackson, Director of Central Supply at SouthSide Hospital, approves the purchase of 300,000 pairs of sterile latex gloves for patient care. The order is prepaid in February 2001, received in March 2001, and used within the second quarter (April through June) 2001. Paul budgets and records this expense for the second quarter 2001, not February 2001, as that is the time period within which these inputs are used.

Another advantage of using accrual accounting is that it helps guard against financial manipulation. Cash accounting reports result only when money is exchanged, not when goods and services are actually provided or inputs are actually utilized. A manager could therefore make costs appear lower by delaying payment on bills due at the end of the fiscal year. Accrual accounting uses the **matching principle**, in which revenue is matched to the time revenue is earned and, to the greatest extent possible, revenue is matched with the expenses used to generate that revenue.

Consistency and Conservatism

Consistency is an important factor in measuring and recording financial activities. Financial accountants not only use accepted accounting rules and practices to maintain consistency, but apply the same rules from year to year to allow meaningful comparisons of financial status and performance. Regulatory and industry bodies such as the FASB determine standards as new accounting issues evolve, such as capitation and risk pools.

Another accounting practice employed in measuring and recording financial activities is **fiscal conservatism**, in which probable losses to a business are recorded if they may be reasonably estimated, while gains are not recorded until they are actually realized. In other words, if SouthSide Hospital's financial officers have strong reason to suspect that diagnostic equipment will become obsolete, they may write it off as a loss; however, even after negotiating a profitable managed care contract, the revenues are not reported until they are generated.

Another example of fiscal conservatism is that many physician group practices distribute their income on a cash basis rather than on an accrual basis. This is the more conservative approach, as if their charges are not paid, the physicians are not attempting to distribute money they do not possess.

Materiality

Another factor in measuring and recording financial activities is the **materiality principle**, in which separate categories of financial entries are recorded only if they are relevant to the financial condition of the enterprise or organization, or to understand the financial statements. In addition, figures are frequently rounded rather than exact, as long as the reviewer obtains a fairly stated view of the entity's financial condition. Some of the financial statements used as examples in this chapter round SouthSide Hospital's financial figures to the nearest thousand. Chapter 4 discusses the level of detail for revenue and expense line items in reviewing and monitoring budgets: in some cases managers require a high level of detail, and in other cases an overall summary is of greater use. Financial statements also include detail or summarize entries for the same reason.

Disclosure

The final accounting principle, **disclosure**, is closely related to the principle of materiality. It is important to report with reasonable accuracy on all aspects of financial transactions: "how much, what, and when." Accountants also use footnotes, notes, attachments, and explanations of assumptions to provide a fair view of financial activities, condition, and performance. Disclosure is important because it is possible that information could be omitted from the financial statements which would make the financial situation appear better than it actually is.

Periodic (frequently annual) financial audits performed by qualified, objective, and independent accounting firms require full disclosure and review of the financial accounting practices of health care organizations. The use of financial audits increases confidence in the organization's financial reporting. An example of a financial audit report is presented as part of SouthSide Hospital's annual report in the "Supplemental Tables and Documents" section of the Back-of-Book CD-Rom.

Box 10-2 summarizes the factors involved in measuring and recording financial activities discussed in this section.

Financial Statements

The following sections discuss four financial statements commonly encountered in health care organizations. Related financial concepts are discussed in the context of these statements. The **annual report** is an overall summary of an organization's financial performance, prepared largely for the review of persons outside the organization. The **income statement** discloses the profitability of an organization and the use of any profits; the income statement section explains concepts of for-profit versus non-profit status. The **balance sheet** provides information about the organization's resources (**assets**) and how they are acquired. The **statement of cash flows** provides details about the sources of cash and how cash is used.

Frequently, the form of financial statements used is determined by the finance committee or the board of directors. Therefore, while the text follows standard organization and layout, financial statements may vary

---

□ B O X   1 0 - 2

Factors in Measuring and Recording Financial Activities

- Time period: months, quarters, or the fiscal year (FY)
- Basis of accounting
  - –Cash accounting (report revenue when payment is received) vs.
  - –Accrual accounting (report revenue when goods or services are provided, generating an obligation to pay)
- The matching principle
  - –Match revenue with the accounting period in which it is generated
  - –Match expenses with related revenues if possible
- Consistency
  - –Use accepted accounting rules and practices
  - –Apply the same rules from year to year to allow meaningful comparison
- Fiscal conservatism
  - –Record probable losses if they may be reasonably estimated
  - –Do not record gains until they are actually realized
- Materiality
  - –Create categories only for entries related to financial performance
  - –Figures reported may be rounded or estimated, not exact, as long as they provide a fair view of financial activities, condition, and performance
- Disclosure
  - –Related to the principle of materiality
  - –Report how much, what, and when for financial transactions
  - –Use footnotes, notes, attachments, and explanations of assumptions to provide a fair view of financial activities, condition, and performance

---

among different health care organizations, so it is important to learn the conventions and layout used in one's own work setting.

The Annual Report

The annual report is the financial statement with which most people, including health care professionals, are familiar. Serving as an overall summary of an organization's financial position, the annual report is generally the most important financial statement released to the general public and others outside the organization. The annual report is the financial statement that is also typically more widely available and widely distributed within health care organizations.

The annual report consists of three major parts. First is the text, usually in the form of a letter from the chief executive officer (CEO) or head of the organization. This section presents the current status of the organization (in the most positive perspective possible) and goals and plans for the future. The next section presents an overall summarized income statement, balance sheet, and statement of cash flows, often comparing the current year to the prior year. Financial statements prepared for the annual report frequently provide far less detail than standard financial statements. The final section of the annual report consists of footnotes, or brief notes providing information not covered in the financial statements. For example, the footnotes to an annual report for a health care organization might discuss the amount of charity care provided, the cost of mergers and restructuring, or the extent of inpatient care activities. The annual report also requires an accountant's or auditor's opinion letter in the footnotes. A copy of SouthSide Hospital's FY 2002 Annual Report is in the "Supplemental Tables and Documents" section of the Back-of-Book CD-ROM.

The Income Statement

Probably the simplest yet most meaningful financial question is, "Is the business making money?" For this reason, the income statement, also referred to as the **statement of financial operations**, is an important financial report to review because it focuses on revenues, expenses, and profitability. Income statements differ among organizations, and the name of this report may differ, such as *statement of operations*, *statement of activities*, *revenue and expense summary*, or *statement of revenue and expenses*. Typically the income statement presents at least 2 fiscal years of data, with the most recent time period presented first. In some organizations, the time period may be calendar quarters or months. The focus is on presenting the difference between revenues and expenses to report **net income** (profit) or net loss, thus measuring and reporting the organization's profitability.

Profitability

Recall that revenues generated by the provision of goods and services represent cash payments or the obligation to make payments over time. Revenues less expenses represent profit (or loss), so expenses (costs of inputs) reduce profitability. Chapter 4 discusses concepts and factors related to revenue, including net revenue, which represents gross revenue less any reductions to the full charges or price. Revenues are typically based on volume or utilization and are reported at the time goods or services are provided. However, capitation contract revenues are reported when the contractual coverage begins.

Expenses represent the cost of doing business. As presented in Chapter 4, operating expenses or costs include salaries and wages, supplies, equipment, and other costs related to providing goods or services. Chapter 4 also identifies capital expenses, or costs associated with the purchase of major equipment, renovation, building, or other large, long-term purchases. Financial costs are expenses incurred in obtaining funds to purchase the organization's assets, such as interest on debt.

Expenses may be classified in financial statements in two ways. The **natural classification** method classifies by type of input accruing the expense. For example, a natural classification of expenses might include entries for inputs such as salaries and benefits, medical supplies, or property lease. Line item budgets as described in Chapter 4 are examples of natural classification. The **functional classification** method classifies by the type of output accruing the expense. For example, a functional classification of expenses might include entries for inpatient services, outpatient services, and administration. An operating expense budget summarizing the total costs for each department of an organization is an example of functional classification.

The number and nature of expenses may vary widely on the income statement, depending on what is relevant and of most interest to the organization. Smaller organizations typically report fewer categories of expenses, and larger organizations typically have a more detailed expense report on the income statement. Most users of financial statements desire more detail rather than less, because more insights are obtained if the organization reports revenues and expenses both by type or as a natural classification (for example, salaries vs. supplies) and by a service breakdown or as a functional classification (for example, inpatient vs. outpatient services).

The difference between a pro forma profit and loss (P&L) budget line, which forecasts profit or loss (see Chap. 4), and the income statement is that the pro forma P&L is prepared for managerial accounting purposes and therefore need not be prepared according to standard, approved accounting procedures. The pro forma P&L statement differs from the **P&L statement** in that the pro forma P&L is an estimated or projected difference between revenues and expenses, while the P&L statement is the difference between actual revenues and expenses. A pro forma P&L, a P&L statement, and an income statement may be prepared for an organization or for smaller subunits such as a department or program.

Non-Profit Versus For-Profit Financial Status and Reporting

The type of ownership (in other words, for-profit vs. non-profit status) is important in financial reporting. In the United States, hospitals proliferated as non-profit institutions, and non-profit hospitals and hospital chains continue to dominate the industry, although for-profit hospitals and hospital chains are increasing. According to economic theory, non-profits can address market failures in supplying greatly needed yet unprofitable services such as burn units and emergency departments (which generate high costs not covered by revenues). Because providing these services that address market failures is perceived as beneficial to the community, non-profit hospitals receive favorable tax treatment, which encouraged their growth and dominance.

The favorable tax treatment extended to non-profits because they provide services to the community is a key concept in differentiating these enterprises from for-profits. However, a frequent misunderstanding is that non-profit enterprises do not and need not make a profit. This view of non-profit status is not accurate. To survive and grow, it is as important for a non-profit as a for-profit organization to be profitable. The difference lies in the requirement for non-profits, in order to retain favorable tax treatment, to reinvest all net income (profit) back into the business. Even if the organization or enterprise is non-profit, the financial report must include a performance indicator that represents net income (profit), also reported by non-profits as **net surplus** or **net deficit**.

By contrast, for-profit (investor-owned) enterprises are permitted to pay out some or all of their net income as dividend payments to shareholders, after paying taxes. The proportion of after-tax net income paid out to shareholders is the **payout ratio**. The proportion of net income reinvested in the business is the **retention ratio**. For example, Goodman General Hospital, one of SouthSide Hospital's competitors, is a for-profit with a net income in FY 2001 of $7 million. If $2 million is paid out to shareholders in FY 2001, the amount of net income reinvested, the payout ratio, and the retention ratio are calculated as follows:

$$\text{For-Profit Reinvestment} = \text{Net Income} - \text{Dividends}$$

$$\$5 \text{ million} = \$7 \text{ million} - \$2 \text{ million}$$

$$\text{Payout Ratio} = \text{Dividends}/\text{Net Income}$$

$$28.6\% = \$2 \text{ million}/\$7 \text{ million}$$

$$\text{Retention Ratio} = \text{Reinvestment}/\text{Net Income}$$

$$71.4\% = \$5 \text{ million}/\$7 \text{ million}$$

The dividends plus reinvestment amount must equal the net income, and the payout ratio plus the retention ratio must equal 100%, to account for all of the net income.

For non-profit enterprises, all net income must be reinvested, so in many non-profit reports an entry after the net income entry reconciles net income with the net assets reported in the balance sheet. In other words, for non-profits net income equals reinvestment and is reported on the balance sheet accordingly. For example, SouthSide Hospital, a non-profit, earned $3,253,000 net income in FY 2001, all of which represents funds that will eventually be reinvested into the business.

Table 10-2 presents an income statement for SouthSide Hospital for FY 2001 and 2002 and projected 2003. The figures represent thousands of dollars, so the $126,878 entry for FY 2001 inpatient services is actually $126,878,000. This method of rounding is frequently used to summarize financial data that

TABLE 10-2

SouthSide Hospital, Income Statement, $ thousands, FY 2001–2003

	FY 2001	FY 2002	FY 2003
Patient Revenue			
Inpatient Services	$126,878	$142,063	$159,577
Outpatient Services	52,177	55,711	58,530
Gross Patient Revenue	**179,055**	**197,774**	**218,107**
Deductions from Patient Revenue			
Contractual Discounts	125,726	141,237	158,257
Provision for Charity	2,678	2,955	3,254
Total Deductions from Revenue	**128,404**	**144,192**	**161,511**
Net Patient Revenue	50,651	53,582	56,596
Managed Care Revenue	5,000	5,119	5,170
Other Operating Revenue	160	162	163
Total Operating Revenue	**55,811**	**58,863**	**61,929**
Operating Expenses			
Salaries & Wages	22,077	23,360	24,687
Employee Benefits	4,899	5,183	5,478
Service Contracts & Professional Fees	6,867	6,912	7,102
Supplies	5,744	5,941	6,135
Managed Care IBNR	856	874	914
Depreciation & Amortization	2,727	2,889	2,950
Rents & Leases	186	191	197
Other	2,063	2,084	2,095
Bad Debt	4,102	4,527	4,785
IT Chargeback	929	982	1,025
System Chargeback	12	12	12
System Allocation	832	1,044	1,245
Total Operating Expenses	**51,294**	**53,999**	**56,625**
Non-Operating Revenue	204	183	174
EBIT	4,517	4,864	5,304
Interest & Taxes	1,468	1,985	1,721
Net Income/Loss	$3,253	$3,062	$3,757

represent large amounts. It is always important to note the denominations labeled on financial statements. The formatting and layout of the SouthSide Hospital income statement are typical for this financial report.

Revenues

Gross patient revenue ($179,055,000 for FY 2001) is the sum of SouthSide Hospital's inpatient and outpatient revenues ($126,878,000 + $52,177,000). Contractual discounts of $125,726,000 and charity care amounting to $2,678,000 are deducted from gross patient revenue for a net patient revenue of $50,651,000. Managed care and other operating revenue ($5 million and $160,000) are added to the net patient revenue for a total of $55,811,000 in total operating revenue for FY 2001 (see Table 10-2).

Expenses

The income statement then presents entries for expenses (see Table 10-2). All operating expenses are entered for total FY 2001 operating expenses of $51,294,000. Depreciation and amortization expenses are defined and discussed as part of the balance sheet. The total operating expenses are then subtracted from the total operating revenue ($55,811,000 − $51,294,000), resulting in $4,517,000 **earnings before interest and taxes (EBIT)**, also referred to as **operating profit** or **excess of revenue over expenses from operations**. This entry is made because expenses for interest payments and taxes are not considered operating expenses, as they do not directly contribute to the operations or activities of the organization. In non-profit enterprises EBIT reflects earnings before interest expenses, as non-profits are typically not subject to corporation taxes.

Table 10-2 shows an entry for interest and taxes, as even though SouthSide Hospital is exempt from federal taxation, it does pay some state and local taxes. The interest and tax payments are subtracted from the EBIT and net non-operating revenue is added (for FY 2001 $4,517,000 − $1,468,000 + $204,000), resulting in $3,253,000 net income, or profit. Determining net income is the key purpose of the financial report. The reviewer may then compare revenues, expenses, and profit between FY 2001, 2002, and 2003.

Remember that an organization's net income represents profitability, and that profitability is the most important information provided by the income statement. Net income is also referred to as "the bottom line," or revenues over expenses. A fundamental accounting concept is that the greater the net income (profit), the greater the accounting profitability and the better the organization's financial position. More discussion of non-profit organizations and financial status is in the next section.

Interpretation of the Income Statement

Box 10-1 summarized the purposes of financial statements. These points are applied in interpreting the income statement for SouthSide Hospital. In considering the overall financial health of SouthSide Hospital, note that despite deductions from patient revenue of approximately 72% in FY 2001, 73% in FY 2002, and 74% in FY 2003, the net income remains positive and increases from FY 2001 to FY 2003 (see Table 10-2). This is one indication that SouthSide Hospital is financially healthy.

SouthSide Hospital's income statement reflects the decision to accept heavy contractual discounting on patient charges, probably to maintain patient volume, as the average occupancy rate over FY 2001–2003 is only 53.2% (average daily census of 58.4). It is also clear that the leadership of SouthSide Hospital accepts a limited number of managed care contracts, as shown by the managed care revenue. The impact of these decisions about patient revenue is reported in the lines for total operating revenue and net income.

The non-profit status and community orientation of SouthSide Hospital are shown by the substantial provision for charity that is one of the deductions from patient revenue. The non-profit status is also reflected because there is no entry for dividends to stockholders in the income statement. The priority of SouthSide Hospital is clearly patient care: the overwhelming amount of revenue is patient revenue ($55,811,000 in FY 2001) compared to other sources of revenue ($204,000 in fiscal year 2001). SouthSide Hospital is clearly a non-profit enterprise focused on community service and patient care. It has been able to maintain its profitability over FY 2001–2003.

The Balance Sheet

The balance sheet, also referred to as the **statement of financial position**, provides information about the financial condition of an organization at a given date, not over a specified time period. The balance sheet can therefore offer a "snapshot" view of an organization's financial status, useful because factors such as seasonal demand or rapid growth may cause large changes in financial activities within the course of a fiscal year.

For example, a surge in respiratory disorders typically increases the census of SouthSide Hospital from early November through mid-February. This rise in the census increases revenues as well as expenses beyond the usual patterns seen at SouthSide Hospital, strengthening the financial status over that time period. Increases occur in both cash received and money owed to SouthSide Hospital, as well as in expenses for items such as medical supplies and nursing care required for these additional patients.

Assets are resources held by the organization that possess or create economic benefit. Most assets are **tangible assets** (resources that can be measured, such as units of goods or services or monetary amounts). In some situations, assets are **intangible assets** (resources one cannot measure, such as reputation). The balance sheet is a report about assets (the organization's resources) and the financing required to acquire those assets, which include **liabilities** (claims on assets established by contract) and **equity** (ownership claims on assets). In other words, the balance sheet reports an organization's resources and claims against those resources, or what an organization owns and owes and what its owners (or for non-profits, the community) have invested. The layout of a balance sheet is as follows:

$$\text{Assets} = \text{Liabilities} + \text{Equity}$$

$$A = L + E$$

The balance sheet literally "balances" assets against the liabilities and equity. For example, if Company A has $1,500,000 in assets and $1,250,000 in liabilities, it must have $250,000 in equity. In other words, Company A owns $1,500,000 in assets, for which it owes (or is liable to pay for) $1,250,000, with $250,000 contributed by its owners. Figure 10-1 illustrates the accounting equation for Company A as a pie chart. The following sections discuss the parts of the balance sheet and related concepts in detail.

Current Assets

Current assets (CA, also referred to as **working capital**) include tangible assets such as cash or other resources expected to be converted into cash or exchanged within a fiscal year. **Marketable securities** (highly liquid, low interest-bearing investments), **receivables** (payments due for goods or services provided), **inventory** (supplies kept on hand), and current prepayments are examples of current assets other than cash. Current assets are typically **liquid assets**, or resources that represent cash or that can readily be exchanged for or converted into cash. Assets are recorded in order of their liquidity, from the most liquid to the least liquid.

Cash and Marketable Securities
Cash is, of course, the most liquid current asset. The ending cash balance for SouthSide Hospital for FY 2001 is $1,209,000, which is also the beginning cash balance for FY 2002. Therefore, the change in net cash flow for FY 2002 for SouthSide Hospital is $2,607,000 − $1,209,000, or $1,398,000. It will be important to recall this calculation based on the cash entered in the balance sheet when reviewing the statement of cash flows later in this chapter.

Marketable securities consist of short-term investments that are highly liquid and low risk, including bank savings accounts, U.S. Treasury bills, and money market mutual funds. Cash is converted to

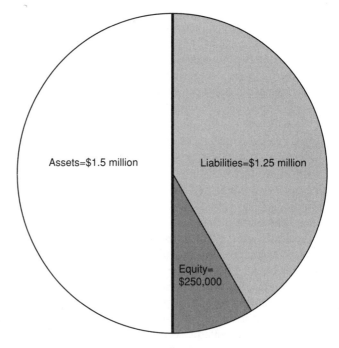

Assets=$1.5 million

Liabilities=$1.25 million

Equity= $250,000

FIGURE 10.1 ■ Company A, Illustration of Accounting Equation (A=L+E) in Balance Sheet.

marketable securities so that it will earn interest. Even though marketable securities typically have low interest rates, the high liquidity is an advantage, and even a low interest rate is better than none. For FY 2001, South-Side Hospital reports $4,679,000 in marketable securities.

Net Accounts Receivable Receivables (also referred to as **accounts receivable** [AR], or **collectibles**) typically represent the largest and most important item for cash management in most health care organizations. **Net receivables** are current assets that represent receivables less any discounts, or the amount the organization actually expects to collect for goods and services provided rather than the entire amount actually due.

⦿ **T A B L E 1 0 - 3**	
SouthSide Hospital, Net Patient Accounts Receivable, $ thousands, 1/31/01	
Net Patient Revenue	**$4,631**
Bad Debt	343
Collections	2,737
Net Patient Accounts Receivable	**$1,551**

Table 10-3 shows a worksheet for calculating net patient accounts receivable for SouthSide Hospital in January 2001. The first entry is for net patient revenue—in other words, all revenue for January FY 2001 less contractual discounts and charity care, totaling $4,631,000. The next entries are for bad debt ($343,000) and collections (cash collected within the month) at $2,737,000. These lines are subtracted from the net revenue to calculate the net patient accounts receivable, or the amount due in payment for goods and services rendered within January 2001, amounting to $1,551,000.

Inventories In hospitals and many other health care organizations, inventories represent the amount of medical supplies kept on hand. There are many factors involved with inventory management and control not discussed in this text. Although there are costs associated with maintaining inventories and keeping items up to date, it is important to be prepared for sudden unexpected demands. The trend is for health care organizations to hold relatively small levels of inventories. One increasingly popular method for managing inventories is the **just-in-time** approach, in which suppliers manage the inventories and deliver supplies just before they are required, thus reducing the costs of storage and unused inventory. Various accounting strategies are used for reporting inventory and are discussed in more advanced texts in health care financial accounting.

Organizations such as medical supply companies or pharmacies that hold large inventories often include footnotes to the balance sheet explaining the accounting practices used to value their inventories. However, in many health care organizations, accountants apply the principle of materiality, so that rather than recording relatively small inventories, they include the value of inventories in an entry for other current assets. SouthSide Hospital lists its FY 2001 supply inventories at $5,795,000.

Prepaid Expenses Prepaid expenses include items such as the lease and utilities that might be paid in advance. SouthSide Hospital includes other current assets that do not fit into the previous categories and that represent too little value to report separately (the materiality principle) for a total of $337,000 in FY 2001. The sum of total current assets for FY 2001 is $15,128,000.

Non-Current Assets

Non-current assets (NCA) include long-term investments, **fixed assets** (also referred to as **real assets** or property, plant, and equipment), which are relatively permanent resources, and other assets (assets that are intangible or fixed assets that do not generate revenue). Long-term investments and fixed assets represent **illiquid assets** (resources that cannot readily be exchanged for or converted into cash). The fundamental rule is that current assets are expected to be converted to cash within a fiscal year and non-current assets are not expected to be converted to cash within a fiscal year.

Long-Term Investments Long-term investments represent financial assets with maturities that exceed 1 year. They are reported on the balance sheet at their current fair market value, which may be higher or lower than their initial cost. Table 10-8 shows that for FY 2001, SouthSide Hospital has $3,683,000 in long-term investments. Although long-term investments are less liquid than short-term investments, they usually earn higher interest rates. Remember that one principle of financial management is to generate returns on available cash rather than allow it to sit idle, so that both short- and long-term investments are important.

Property, Plant, and Equipment Property, plant, and capital equipment are fixed assets that are held over the long term and are unlikely to be readily or quickly converted into cash. The extent of these fixed assets is typically set to handle peak demand. For example, with an average occupancy rate of only 52.8% over FY 2001, SouthSide Hospital's average daily census is 58.1, yet the hospital can accommodate 110 acute care patients at full capacity (in other words, it has 110 beds in service), as in the winter months when respiratory disorders increase the census. Construction in progress is also an entry in the section for property, plant, and equipment.

For FY 2001, SouthSide Hospital reports $56,004,000 in property, plant, and equipment plus $2,144,000 for construction in progress (see Table 10-8). Added together, this equals $58,148,000 in gross fixed assets.

Depreciation It is important to understand the concept of **depreciation** (expensing the cost of a capital asset over its estimated useful life). In most cases people can think of costs as being the same as expenses. However, for fixed assets such as buildings, land, and major capital equipment, accountants spread the original cost of purchasing these assets over their useful lifetime. Therefore, when fixed assets are purchased, the cost is listed in the balance sheet as the cost of property, plant, or equipment. Then the depreciation expense must be calculated to enter into the income statement.

In **straight-line depreciation**, the original cost of a fixed asset, less its salvage value, is divided by the number of years of estimated useful life, and the annual portion is entered as depreciation expense each year. This method is frequently used to calculate depreciation expense. For example, in FY 2001 SouthSide Hospital purchased diagnostic equipment at a cost of $5 million, with an expected useful life of 10 years and a salvage value of $50,000 (this expense is part of the $56,044,000 cost of property, plant and equipment entry in Table 10-8). The calculation of annual depreciation is as follows:

$$\text{Annual Depreciation} = (\text{Original Cost of Fixed Asset} - \text{Salvage Value})/\text{Years of Life}$$

$$\$495,000 = (\$5,000,000 - \$50,000)/10$$

The accountants at SouthSide Hospital therefore expense $495,000 annually for depreciation allocated to the diagnostic equipment for FY 2001 through FY 2010 (this expense is part of the income statement depreciation and amortization entries for FY 2001–2003 in Table 10-2). Straight-line depreciation allocates equal amounts of depreciation expense over the estimated years of useful life of the fixed asset.

One reason for allocating depreciation as an expense over time is that it reduces the negative impact the purchase of fixed assets would have on profitability. Recall from Table 10-2 that the net income of SouthSide Hospital is $3,253,000 in FY 2001. If the entire cost were recorded as an expense at time of purchase, the FY 2001 net income would become a net loss of $1,747,000, as shown in the following calculations:

$$\text{Net Income} = \$3,253,000$$

$$\text{Diagnostic Equipment Expense} = \$5,000,000$$

$$\text{Net Income less Diagnostic Equipment Expense} = \$3,253,000 - \$5,000,000 = \$(1,747,000)$$

Another reason for allocating depreciation as an expense over time reflects the matching principle, in which accountants attempt to match expenses to the revenues they generate. The $5 million spent by SouthSide Hospital in FY 2001 to purchase the diagnostic equipment will generate revenues for the next 10 years, so it makes sense to spread its expense over the same time period.

This method of allocating depreciation is an estimate, as some years the diagnostic equipment might generate more revenue than others (i.e., more diagnostic tests might be run using the equipment), and some years the equipment might lose more in market value (such as later years, when the equipment requires extensive repairs). However, this is not only a fairly simple method but is standard, accepted practice. The revenues and expenses generated by the fixed asset, as well as its cost of purchase, are estimated and averaged over the fixed asset's useful life.

Decisions about the extent of useful life for a fixed asset reflect managerial financial choices, not specific rules. The number of years of useful life over which depreciation is recorded is frequently an estimate or forecast made on the best knowledge currently available from the vendor, experience, and industry standards.

In some cases, health care organizations might choose to use **accelerated depreciation**, or one of several methods in which the depreciation expense is calculated as progressively smaller over subsequent time periods. Accelerated depreciation methods might be selected by for-profit health care organizations to reduce current taxable income and defer taxes to the future. More information on calculating accelerated depreciation may be found in advanced health care finance textbooks.

As the years pass, the income statement reports fixed assets at their original cost of purchase minus **accumulated depreciation**, or the total dollars of depreciation expensed over time (typically year to year) against the original cost of fixed assets. Accumulated depreciation is a **contra-asset account** on the balance sheet because it is a negative asset, so that the higher the accumulated depreciation, the smaller the organization's total assets. For SouthSide Hospital over FY 2001, $31,575,000 in accumulated depreciation is deducted from $58,148,000 in gross fixed assets, for an entry of $26,573,000 in net fixed assets (see Table 10-8).

Assets that suddenly lose value are **written off** (fully expensed so that they no longer appear as assets), such as diagnostic equipment that becomes obsolete before the end of its useful life. However, managerial decisions again come into play. For example, a fixed asset may be written off in the financial statements but may still be used by the organization, or may be sold, renovated, or scrapped. Writing off a fixed asset does not automatically mean that the equipment has become unusable and requires immediate disposal. In addition, the fixed asset may or may not require replacement.

For example, the diagnostic equipment in the above example purchased for SouthSide Hospital at $5 million in FY 2001 would be listed in FY 2003 as shown in Table 10-4. The accumulated depreciation is $495,000 multiplied by 3 years, or $1,485,000 (this is a portion of the total $34,741,000 accumulated depreciation entered in the balance sheet for fiscal year 2003, as shown in Table 10-8). When subtracted from the original $5 million cost, the net asset represents $3,515,000 remaining value (this is a portion of the total $60,191,000 cost of property, plant, and equipment entry for FY 2003). In FY 2005, new technology makes the diagnostic equipment

TABLE 10-4

SouthSide Hospital, Worksheet for Accumulated Depreciation for Diagnostic Equipment, FY 2003[1]

Equipment (Gross Fixed Asset)	$ 5,000,000
Accumulated Depreciation	$ 1,485,000
Net Fixed Asset	**$ 3,515,000**

[1]Purchased in 2001 with annual depreciation of $495,000.

obsolete; it is replaced and there is no entry made for this equipment as an asset in the balance sheet (it is written off).

Other Assets "Other assets" is a category that typically represents fixed assets not used in generating revenues, and intangible assets. An Impressionist painting donated by a wealthy local citizen that is displayed in the lobby and a leather-bound medical book from the 16th century kept in the medical library archives are examples of other assets owned by SouthSide Hospital. The entry for other assets for FY 2001 at SouthSide Hospital is $1,242,000 (see Table 10-8).

A frequently listed intangible asset is **goodwill**, which represents the difference between the **fair market value** (the price paid to the owners) and the **book value** (balance sheet value of owner's equity) of an asset, often obtained via merger or acquisition. It is important to recall the accounting principle of fiscal conservatism, because the value attributed to intangibles such as goodwill can have a large effect on the pro forma P&L and the balance sheet. A substantial change in SouthSide Hospital's reputation or market niche could increase or decrease the amount entered for goodwill.

For example, Goodman General Hospital, one of SouthSide Hospital's competitors, purchased Greatman's Durable Medical Equipment Company, a local business. The price of $4,975,000 paid by Goodman General Hospital represents the fair market value for the business, although the book value (owner's equity) is only $4,783,000. The $192,000 difference represents intangible assets that make Greatman's "worth" more than the fixed assets, inventory, and other items listed as owner's equity. These intangibles include customer loyalty, a reputation for service, and community contacts. Other intangibles that may contribute to goodwill include skilled employees, a good credit rating, and having a market niche by providing unique or otherwise available goods and services.

Until recently it was assumed that goodwill lost its value over time, so it was expensed over time in the same way as depreciation, known as **amortization** (expensing the value of an intangible asset over its life). However, since 2001 it has been accepted practice to keep the full value of goodwill on the balance sheet until evidence indicates the value has been lost or impaired, at which point it is written off.

Total Assets The final entry on the top or left-hand section of the balance sheet is the sum of all current and non-current assets, or total assets. For FY 2001 at SouthSide Hospital, total assets equal $46,626,000 (see Table 10-8). This sum must balance with the total liabilities and equity on the bottom or right-hand side of the balance sheet.

Liabilities and Equity

Liabilities and equity are the categories of items that are recorded on the right side or bottom half of the balance sheet. The categories of liabilities and equity represent the capital raised (in other words, money borrowed or contributed) to acquire the assets recorded on the left side or top half of the balance sheet. Liabilities may be estimated as follows:

$$\text{Total Liabilities} = \text{Total Assets} - \text{Equity}$$

Liabilities are claims against the assets of an organization that are fixed by contract. Bankruptcy is a likely result of **default** (failure to pay interest or principal or maintain financial covenants) on such claims, which may result in **liquidation** (dissolving the business and distributing its assets). By law, if liquidation occurs, assets must first be used to fulfill claims on liabilities, then distributed to shareholders (if a for-profit enterprise) or contributed to charity (if a non-profit enterprise). In recording liabilities, short-term debts or other financial obligations are listed first, then long-term debt or other financial obligations.

Current Liabilities (CL) include debts or other financial obligations that must be paid within the short term (usually within the fiscal year). One current liability entry is **accounts payable (A/P)**, or **trade credit**, which is the amount due to vendors for supplies. Another current liability entry is **accrued expenses**, which comprises expenses that are generated daily, with periodic payment. Employee wages and benefits, interest due on loans, and taxes are examples of accrued expenses. Short-term debt, or debt expected to be repaid within the year, is another current liability. A final type of current liability discussed in this section is **incurred but not reported expenses (IBNR)**. **Net working capital** is the difference between current assets and current liabilities.

Short-Term Debt Typically, short-term debt is used for short-term needs. If the organization requires a loan over a long period of time, it borrows money over the long term. Short-term debt usually carries a higher interest rate then long-term debt because it is typically **unsecured** (does not have collateral, an asset pledged to the lender if the borrower defaults on the loan). When loans are **secured**, the lender can sell the collateral to recover its money if the borrower defaults on the loan. As unsecured loans do not protect the lender from default, the interest rates are typically higher than for secured loans. Another reason that short-term loans typically carry higher interest rates than long-term loans is that the **transaction costs** (administrative, overhead, and other costs related to processing a financial matter) are higher because these costs must be spread over a shorter period of time. For example, the transaction costs for three short-term loans that total $20,000 would be higher than the transaction costs for one 5-year loan for the same amount of $20,000.

Incurred But Not Reported Expenses IBNR expenses are important for health care providers with a large proportion of capitated contracts. Under capitation systems, providers receive payment before the services are provided, so that there may be substantial expenses related to capitation plan enrollees near the end of an accounting period that have not yet been reported (See Chapter 3). To match the timing of the costs of services with the revenue for those services (matching principle), IBNR expenses are reported as a current liability on the balance sheet and an operating expense on the income statement. For example, SouthSide Hospital reports $5 million in managed care revenue in FY 2001 (see Table 10-2), with $856,000 IBNR expense outstanding (see Tables 10-2 and 10-8). The methodology of calculating IBNR expenses is complex, requiring actuarial estimates and budget forecasts based on prior experience.

Table 10-8 shows entries for all of the current liabilities for SouthSide Hospital. Total current liabilities for FY 2001 amount to $8,789,000. The net working capital for SouthSide Hospital for FY 2001 is $15,128,000 less $8,789,000, or $6,339,000.

Non-Current Liabilities

Long-term debt represents debt financing (loans) with remaining maturities greater than 1 year, including debts to banks, bondholders, and some lease arrangements. Long-term debt is a **non-current liability (NCL)**, or liability entry not due within a fiscal year. The **current maturities of long-term debt** represents the portion of long-term debt that must be paid in the coming year. Frequently the borrower must pay a specified portion of the **principal** (amount borrowed) each year, as well as **interest** (a percentage rate representing the price for borrowing). As shown in Table 10-8, long-term debt for FY 2001 at SouthSide Hospital is $9,495,000.

Equity

Equity (also referred to as **owner's equity** [OE]) represents the ownership claim on an organization's assets, or the amount of total assets financed by non-liability capital. Equity may be estimated as follows:

$$\text{Equity} = \text{Total Assets} - \text{Total Liabilities}$$

Different ownership types (for-profit vs. non-profit) result in different terms used for equity. Although the asset and liability sections of the balance sheet are similar regardless of ownership status, the equity section of the balance sheet differs in presentation according to the type of ownership status. The reason for the difference in presentation is that although the substance of the equity section is the same for non-profits and for-profits, the two different ownership types have different forms of equity.

Net Assets of Non-Profits In non-profit enterprises equity is called **net assets** because the earnings must be reinvested in the business. Therefore, any profit a non-profit generates is considered a resource that is reinvested in expansion, renovation, or other organizational improvements. Recall in the earlier section on the income statement discussing non-profit and for-profit status that for non-profits, net income equals the reinvestment amount, and the net income recorded in the income statement is recorded on the balance sheet as net assets. However, given the time lag for payment in health care organizations, on the balance sheet for a large organization such as a hospital, the net income may be incorporated into the cash and the accounts receivable lines.

For example, Table 10-5 presents a simplified worksheet showing how SouthSide Hospital's net income might be converted to net assets for the balance sheet, accounting for the time lag in collections. The FY 2001 $4,517,000 excess of revenue over expenses from operations (EBIT) comes from the income statement (see Table 10-2). The average collection rate of 31.2% indicates that an estimated $1,409,000 was actually collected as cash (31.2% of $4,517,000). The estimated patient accounts receivable of $3,108,000 represents the remainder due for payment ($4,517,000 − $1,409,000).

Table 10-5 then presents the FY 2001 net non-operating revenue for SouthSide Hospital of $204,000 from the income statement (see Table 10-2). As all of this revenue was received as cash, it is added to the collections for the cash entry of $1,613,000 ($204,000 + $1,409,000). The total net assets to record on the balance sheet (or net income, as recorded on the income statement) equals $4,721,000 ($1,409,000 + $204,000 + $3,108,000).

The $1,468,000 in interest and taxes is then subtracted from the total cash and accounts receivable estimate of $4,721,000 to show that the increase in net assets for FY 2001 at SouthSide Hospital is the same as the net income of $3,253,000 (see Table 10-5). These total amounts are the same as for the net income entry in the income statement and for the change in net assets on the balance sheet, but on the balance sheet the net assets are divided between cash and accounts receivables as current assets (see Tables 10-2 and 10-8).

◯ TABLE 10-5

SouthSide Hospital, Worksheet for Estimating Cash and Accounts Receivable Assets for Transferring Net Income to Net Assets, $ thousands, FY 2001

	FY 2001	FY 2002	FY 2003
Excess of Revenue Over Expenses from Operations	$ 4,517	$ 4,864	$ 5,304
Average Collection Rate	31.2%	31.2%	31.2%
Estimated Collections	1,409	1,518	1,655
Estimated Patient Accounts Receivable	3,108	3,346	3,649
Non-Operating Revenue	$ 204	$ 183	$ 174
Estimated Cash	1,613	1,701	1,829
Total Cash & A/R	$ 4,721	$ 5,047	$ 5,478
Less Interest & Taxes	1,468	1,985	1,721
Net Change in Assets (Income/Loss)	3,253	3,062	3,757

In the balance sheet, assets must be balanced by liabilities plus equity. Therefore, the $4,721,000 increase in assets recorded as cash and accounts receivable for SouthSide Hospital over FY 2001 must be balanced by an equal increase in some combination of liabilities and equity on the balance sheet. For example, it is likely that current liabilities would increase with increases in revenues (current assets), because an increase in the census that would increase revenues would also increase the need for items such as supplies and personnel. Any surplus of revenues over expenses would go to equity (net assets or net surplus among non-profits).

In other words, the net income in the income statement must balance with the change in net assets or equity as reflected in the balance sheet (see Tables 10-2 and 10-8). Table 10-6 shows another way of viewing this concept by presenting the net assets portion of the balance sheet for SouthSide Hospital for FY 2001–2002. The increase in net assets of $3,062,000 from the end of FY 2001 to the end of FY 2002 is the same as the amount of net income reported in FY 2002 (see Table 10-2).

Equity in For-Profits Among for-profit enterprises, the change in total equity must balance with net profit or loss. Equity is reported as **stockholders' equity** for for-profit enterprises. The stockholders' equity section of the balance sheet consists of two parts. The **contributed capital** section has entries for **common stock** (shares of stock at its **par** or face value) and **capital in excess of par value** (capital greater than the face value of the stock). The par value of common stock represents the minimum liability of stockholders in the event of bankruptcy, while capital in excess of par represents proceeds from the sale of common stock at a price above par value. The contributed capital section of the balance sheet represents the **capital** or owner's equity in the enterprise contributed directly by stockholders, proprietors, or partners.

The **retained earnings** section represents accumulated earnings reinvested in the business rather than paid in dividends, plus the for-profit reinvestment amount allocated for the current fiscal year. For example, Table 10-7 shows the stockholder's equity portion of the FY 2001 balance sheet for Goodman General Hospital. Although dividend payments may not always be included as an entry, they are listed here for clarity. Retained earnings increased from $20 million at the end of fiscal year 2000 to $25 million at the end of FY 2001, so the amount reinvested into Goodman General Hospital amounted to $5 million for FY

TABLE 10-6

SouthSide Hospital, Balance Sheet, Net Assets, FY 2001–2002

	FY 2001	FY 2002	Change 2001–2002
Net Assets			
Unrestricted	24,550	27,626	3,076
Restricted	3,792	3,778	(14)
Total Net Assets	**$28,342**	**$31,404**	**$3,062**
Total Liabilities & Net Assets	**$46,626**	**$49,453**	2,827

TABLE 10-7

Goodman General Hospital, Balance Sheet, Stockholders Equity Section, $ thousands, December 31, FY 2000–2001

	FY 2000	FY 2001	Change 2000–2001
Dividend Payouts	$2,000	$2,000	0
Retained Earnings	20,000	25,000	**$5,000**
Total Equity	**$22,000**	**$27,000**	5,000
Total Liabilities & Equity	**$122,000**	**$137,000**	15,000

TABLE 10-8A

SouthSide Hospital Balance Sheet, $ thousands, December 31, FY 2001–2003

	FY 2001	FY 2002	FY 2003
Current Assets			
Cash	$1,209	$2,607	$3,577
Marketable Securities	4,679	4,821	4,998
Accounts Receivable	3,108	3,522	3,744
Supply Inventories, at Cost	5,795	5,828	6,287
Prepaid Expenses & Other	337	366	430
Total Current Assets	**$15,128**	**$17,144**	**$19,036**
Long-Term Investments	**$3,683**	**$3,748**	**$3,892**
Property, Plant & Equipment (Fixed Assets)			
Cost of PP&E	56,004	57,544	60,191
Construction in Progress	2,144	4,212	4,531
Gross Fixed Assets	**58,148**	**61,756**	**64,722**
Less Accumulated Depreciation	31,575	34,437	37,336
Net PP&E (Net Fixed Assets)	**S26,573**	**$27,319**	**$27,386**
Other Assets	$1,242	$1,242	$1,242
Total Assets	**$46,626**	**$49,453**	**$51,556**

2001. In other words, Goodman General Hospital, after paying stock dividends of $2 million, retained $5 million to reinvest in FY 2001.

Fund Accounting Entries for **fund accounting** (dividing assets into separate funds with separate accounting records) appear on the balance sheets of many non-profit organizations, representing self-contained individual accounts set up for specific activities, programs, or other purposes. The first and

TABLE 10-8B

SouthSide Hospital Balance Sheet, $ thousands, December 31, FY 2001-2003

	FY 2001	FY 2002	FY 2003
Current Liabilities			
Current Maturities of Long-Term Debt	$69	$78	$89
Notes Payable	728	746	791
Accounts Payable	3,315	3,501	3,653
Accrued Expenses:			
Wages & Benefits	2,453	2,778	2,906
Taxes	171	194	203
Interest Payable	1,197	1,508	1,577
Managed Care IBNR	856	874	914
Total Current Liabilities	**$8,789**	**$9,679**	**$10,133**
Long-Term Debt	**$9,495**	**$8,370**	**$6,262**
Net Assets			
Unrestricted	24,550	27,626	29,511
Restricted	3,792	3,778	5,650
Total Net Assets	**$28,342**	**$31,404**	**$35,161**
Total Liabilities & Net Assets	**$46,626**	**$49,453**	**$51,556**

usually largest category, present in every setting, is the **unrestricted fund** (also referred to as the **general fund** or **operating fund**), which represents assets that are not externally restricted in use. In other words, unrestricted funds may be used by the organization for any legitimate purpose. The unrestricted fund typically consists of revenue, unrestricted donations and grants, and income from the restricted fund when specified conditions are met. The unrestricted fund records entries for working capital or current assets, as well as plant and equipment accounts. A third unrestricted fund entry is **board-restricted accounts**, which are unrestricted accounts because boards are internal decision-making entities that can change their funding restrictions relatively flexibly compared to outside donors and grant funders.

The reason fund accounting is necessary is that donors and grant funders may reserve the authority to limit or designate how their contributions are used. The account records these **restricted assets** (contributions that donors or grant funders require must be used for a designated purpose). In some cases claims against assets and an equity (net asset) balance are included.

Over FY 2001, SouthSide Hospital has $24,550,000 in unrestricted net assets and $3,792,000 in unrestricted net assets, for $28,342,000 total net assets (Table 10-8). When the total current liabilities of $8,789,000 are added to the $9,495,000 in long-term debt (or non-current liabilities) and to the $28,342,000 in total net assets (or equity), total liabilities and net assets equal $46,626,000 for FY 2001. This figure balances or equals the amount for total assets on the top or right-hand side of the balance sheet.

Figure 10-2 illustrates the major categories of the balance sheet for SouthSide Hospital as a pie chart. Again, the current assets, board-restricted accounts, net property, plant, and equipment, and other assets total $46,626,000, equal to the total for current liabilities, other liabilities, long-term debt, and total net assets.

Interpretation of the Balance Sheet

We will use the purposes of financial statements summarized in Box 10-1 to interpret SouthSide Hospital's balance sheet for FY 2001–2003 (see Table 10-8). The balance sheet entries reinforce that the organization is experiencing good financial health. For example, the assets are steadily increasing over time, with steady improvements in property, plant, and equipment and continued investments in construction. Depreciation is climbing steadily but with no extremely large surges that might indicate that a good deal of equipment is becoming obsolete.

The decisions of the managers of SouthSide Hospital appear to have a positive impact on the financial health of the organization. Management appears to be investing in fixed assets that have not reached obsolescence, at least not to a substantial amount. The construction in progress is improving the facility for better community service in the future (see the annual report in "Supplemental Tables and

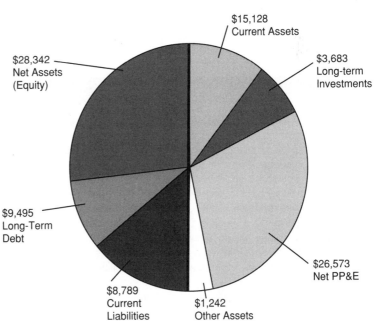

FIGURE 10.2 ■ SouthSide Hospital Balance Sheet, $ thousands, FY 2001.

Documents" in the Back-of-Book CD-ROM. SouthSide Hospital appears to maintain its reputation in the community, given the lack of change in the category for other assets.

The considerable investment in fixed assets underscores the community-oriented perspective, non-profit tax status, and organizational priorities of SouthSide Hospital. It appears to be a management priority to reduce the amount of long-term debt, as it has decreased by $2,108,000 between FY 2001 and FY 2003. The increase in net assets reflects a focus on community-based programs such as breast cancer screening for underserved women; this increases opportunities to receive restricted grant funds.

The Balance Sheet and the Income Statement

Box 10-3 summarizes how the balance sheet and income statement are related to each other. These relationships are mentioned throughout this section. The balance sheet and income statement are also closely related to the statement of cash flows.

The Statement of Cash Flows

Over the short term, the financial condition (and survival) of an organization depends more on cash flow than on profits (see Chap. 4). Bankruptcy can occur with positive income; in other words, profitable enterprises can go bankrupt if they run short of cash. It is therefore essential to forecast cash flow, prepare cash flow budgets (see Chap. 6), and report the flow of cash in and out of the organization.

With accrual accounting (used in most health care organizations), neither revenue nor net income equals cash inflow. In addition, expenses do not equal cash outflow. For example, while depreciation is recorded as an operating expense in the income statements and as a deduction from fixed assets in the balance sheet, it is not actually paid out in cash. Therefore, it is important to review the statement of cash flows (also referred to as the **cash flow statement**), which focuses on financial condition based on cash flow rather than revenues, expenses, or net income. The statement of cash flows provides information about the sources and uses of cash and cash resources. It is a useful management tool that helps prevent liquidity problems, thus protecting the enterprise from cash flow difficulties and the threat of bankruptcy. The following section explains how the statement of cash flows is linked to the balance sheet and the income statement.

BOX 10-3

Linking the Balance Sheet to the Income Statement

- For non-profits, net income equals reinvestment, so a change in net assets on the balance sheet should equal net income in the income statement.
- For for-profits, the amount reinvested in the business equals net income less dividends paid to stockholders, so the change in equity on the balance sheet should equal the retained earnings (net income less dividends) on the income statement.
- Accumulated depreciation is a contra-asset account on the balance sheet because it is a negative asset—the higher the accumulated depreciation, the smaller the organization's fixed and total assets. On the income statement, depreciation is entered as an operating expense.
- IBNR expenses are reported as a current liability on the balance sheet and an operating expense on the income statement.
- Increased revenues increase assets but also generally increase expenses and liabilities, as more inputs are required for higher volume.

The Statement of Cash Flows, Balance Sheet, and Income Statement

The statement of cash flows uses data from both the balance sheet and the income statement to show the relationship between cash flow and earnings. Remember that the basic accounting formula is represented in the layout of the balance sheet:

$$\text{Assets} = \text{Liabilities} + \text{Equity}$$

$$A = L + E$$

This equation can be expanded to show the components of current and non-current assets and liabilities:

Current Assets + Non-current Assets = Current Liabilities + Non-current Liabilities + Owners Equity,

or:

$$CA + NCA = CL + NCL + OE$$

It is then possible to break the equation down by showing the components of current assets:

$$(\text{Cash} + \text{Accounts Receivable} + \text{Inventory}) + NCA = CL + NCL + OE$$

Note that an increase in current liabilities (CL) increases the amount of cash available, and increasing assets such as accounts receivable or inventory reduces the amount of cash available. In other words, the more money owed to an organization (accounts receivable), the less cash it has on hand, and the more it has invested in inventory purchases, the less cash it has available. A key purpose of the statement of cash flows is illustrating the relationship between cash, liabilities, and assets.

Recall the example of Paul Jackson, the Director of Central Supply at SouthSide Hospital, who approved the purchase of 300,000 pairs of sterile latex gloves for patient care. The order was prepaid in February 2001 and received in March 2001, and the gloves were used within the second quarter (April through June) of 2001. Assume the order of 300,000 pairs of sterile latex gloves costs $45,000. Table 10-9 presents the scenario of prepayment of $45,000 for the gloves in February 2001 in the first column of balance sheet figures. In the current assets section, $45,000 in cash (the prepaid amount for the gloves) is reduced, replaced with an equal increase in the amount of prepaid expenses. Within the liabilities and equity section, nothing is entered for accounts payable as the transaction is prepaid (other transactions that might affect prepayment or accounts payable are omitted for simplicity), and total net assets (equity) is $745,000.

TABLE 10-9

SouthSide Hospital, Balance Sheet Scenarios, Central Supply Department Prepaid Expenses vs. Account Payable, $ thousands, February 2000

	Prepaid Scenario	A/P Scenario
Cash	$100	$145
Prepaid Expenses & Other	45	0
All Other Current Assets	745	745
Total Current Assets	**$890**	**$890**
All Other Assets	**$2,030**	**$2,030**
Total Assets	**$2,920**	**$2,920**
Accounts Payable	$0	$45
All Other Current Liabilities	$590	$590
Total Current Liabilities	**$590**	**$635**
Other Liabilities & LT Debt	**$1,585**	**$1,585**
Total Net Assets	**$745**	**$700**
Total Liabilities & Net Assets	**$2,920**	**$2,920**

□ B O X   1 0 - 4

Linking the Balance Sheet to the Income Statement and the Statement of Cash Flows

1. Increases in cash flows from operating activities reflect increases in net income (income statement), depreciation and amortization (income statement), current liabilities (balance sheet), and decreases in current assets (balance sheet).
2. Capital investments are a use of cash, so increases in gross fixed assets decrease cash flow (balance sheet).
3. Financial investments are a use of cash, so increasing marketable securities and long-term investment reduces cash, while increasing notes payable and long-term debt increases cash (balance sheet).
4. The net change in cash should balance as the sum of cash flows from operating activities, capital investing, and financing (statement of cash flows), and as the difference between the beginning and ending cash amounts (balance sheet).

Now assume a second scenario for comparison and to reinforce the relationships between cash, other assets, liabilities, and equity. Paul orders the 300,000 pairs of sterile latex gloves for $45,000 in February 2001, but the vendor bills for payment due the following month. This scenario is illustrated in the second column of balance sheet figures in Table 10-9. The amount of cash and accounts payable both increased by $45,000, while the prepaid expenses dropped by the same amount. Total net assets also dropped by $45,000, as this amount would be payable upon bankruptcy before any remaining assets could be returned to the community (as required of a non-profit in the event of liquidation).

Box 10-4 summarizes the relationships between the balance sheet, the income statement, and the statement of cash flows.

Sections of the Statement of Cash Flows

The statement of cash flows is a report of the cash sources and cash requirements for three categories of financial management: operating activities, investing activities (also referred to as capital investing), and financing activities. The cash flow, or net increase or decrease in cash, is reported for each of these three activities, which appear as sections of the statement of cash flows. The reviewer should evaluate if the business is generating enough cash to cover operating, capital investing, and financial investing expenses.

The statement of cash flows for SouthSide Hospital shown in Table 10-10 reports cash activity for FY 2002 and FY 2003 (to show change in cash flow from year to year, the prior fiscal year's data are required). The SouthSide Hospital income statement and balance sheet show changes in each of the entries for FY 2001–2002 and FY 2002–2003 used in the preparation of the statement of cash flows (see "Supplemental Tables and Documents" on the Back-of-Book CD-ROM).

Cash Flows From Operating Activities The first section of the statement of cash flows reports cash increases or decreases that are directly related to operations. The most important entry is net income, which for FY 2002 is $3,062,000. Net income does not equal cash flow, so a number of adjustments must be made to net income. First, the estimated expense amounts for depreciation and amortization, $2,889,000 in FY 2002, are added back to net income, as they represent non-cash accruals. In other words, no cash payments are ever actually made to accounts for depreciation and amortization, so this entry is an expense but not an actual use of cash. The net income, adjusted for depreciation and amortization, is $5,951,000 for FY 2002.

Adjustments are then made to the working capital, reflecting cash flows related to operations. These are placed in categories of changes in current assets (increases in current assets decrease the amount of cash) and changes in current liabilities (increases in current liabilities increase cash amounts) for easier understanding and interpretation. The first entries are a change in net accounts receivable of $414,000 in FY 2002, a change in inventories of $33,000, and a change in prepaid expenses (such as the lease and utilities) of $29,000. Changes in current liabilities for FY 2002 include $186,000 in accounts payable and a $659,000 increase in accrued expenses.

The changes in current assets are subtracted from the line for net income and non-cash transfers and changes to current liabilities are added for a net amount of cash from operating activities of $6,320,000 for FY 2002. In other words, SouthSide Hospital had a net cash inflow from operating activities of $6,320,000 in FY 2002.

TABLE 10-10

SouthSide Hospital, Statement of Cash Flows, $ thousands, FY 2002 and FY 2003

	FY 2002	FY 2003
Cash Flows from Operating Activities:		
Net Income	$3,062	$3,757
Add Back Depreciation & Amortization	2,889	2,950
Net Income & Non-Cash Transfers	**$5,951**	**$6,707**
Adjustments to Working Capital:		
Changes in Current Assets:		
Change in Net Accounts Receivable	414	222
Change in Inventories	33	459
Change in Prepaid Expenses	29	64
Changes in Current Liabilities:		
Change in Accounts Payable	186	152
Change in Accrued Expenses	659	206
Net Cash from Operating Activities	**$6,320**	**$6,320**
Cash Flows from Investing Activities:		
Capital Expenditures (Change in Gross Fixed Assets)	$(3,608)	$(2,966)
Cash Flows from Financing Activities:		
Change in Notes Payable	18	45
Change in Marketable Securities	142	177
Change in Long-Term Investments	65	144
Change in Long-Term Debt	(1,125)	(2,108)
Net Cash from Financing Activities	**$(1,314)**	**$(2,384)**
Net Change in Cash	$1,398	$970
Cash at Beginning of Year	$1,209	$2,607
Cash at End of Year (Cash Balance)	**$2,607**	**$3,577**

Cash Flows From Investing Activities The second section of the statement of cash flows represents cash flow from investments, also referred to as capital investing. Capital investing represents investments in fixed or non-current assets, not financial investing (which is presented in the third section of the statement of cash flows). Depreciation is already recorded in the non-cash section of the operating cash flows, so it is not included in this section of the statement of cash flows. Therefore, the change in gross fixed assets (not adjusted for depreciation) for FY 2002 from the balance sheet (see Table 10-8) for capital expenditures is recorded.

The change in gross fixed assets for FY 2002 at SouthSide Hospital is a negative $3,608,000, recorded as a negative number as it represents cash outflow. In other words, SouthSide Hospital used $3,608,000 for capital investments over fiscal year 2002.

Cash Flows From Financing Activities The third section of the statement of cash flows records the flow of cash related to financing or financial investments, rather than the capital investments recorded in the second section of the statement of cash flows. The first entry for FY 2002 is $18,000 for the change in notes payable (an increase in notes payable increases the cash amount), then a $142,000 increase in marketable securities (an increase in marketable securities decreases the cash amount). A change of $65,000 is recorded for long-term investments (an increase in long-term investments decreases the cash amount) and a $1,125,000 decrease in long-term debt (an increase in long-term debt increases the cash amount, so the decrease is recorded as a negative, as it decreases the cash amount).

The net cash from financing is a negative $1,314,000 for FY 2002. In other words, SouthSide Hospital used $1,314,000 in cash for financing investments over FY 2002.

Net Cash and Cash Balance

The fourth and final section of the statement of cash flows is the calculation of net cash and the cash balance. The cash amount from operating activities ($6,320,000), the cash amount from investing activities (negative $3,608,000), and the cash amount from financing activities (negative $1,314,000) are added for a net change in cash of $1,398,000 for FY 2002. The cash at the beginning of FY 2002 ($1,209,000, which is the ending balance for FY 2001, as shown in Table 10-8) and the cash at the end of FY 2002 ($2,607,000, also shown in Table 10-8) are also entered in this section. The net change in cash must balance; in other words, the difference between the ending cash balance and the beginning cash balance for FY 2002 must equal the sum of the cash flows from operating activities, investing activities, and financing activities. The difference between the cash at the end of FY 2002 and the beginning of FY 2002 ($2,607,000 − $1,209,000) equals $1,398,000, so that the statement of cash flows balances. Figure 10-3 illustrates the calculations and balance required for the net cash flows in the statement of cash flows for SouthSide Hospital, FY 2002.

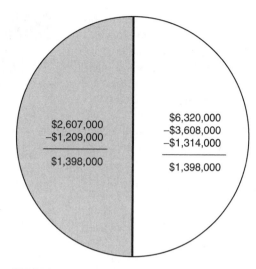

FIGURE 10.3 ■ SouthSide Hospital, Net Cash Flow Balance, FY 2002.

Interpretation of the Statement of Cash Flows

In terms of financial health, the overall cash flow for FY 2002 and FY 2003 is positive; in other words, more cash is coming into the organization than is going out, overall. The management decisions are to spend cash on capital expenditures and on reducing long-term debt (consistent with findings in the income statement and the balance sheet). There has been a substantial increase in cash, which might be better invested in marketable securities. Management should look at this trend and rethink decisions so that cash is not left sitting idle but rather is invested to generate returns.

Conclusion

This chapter introduced financial reporting concepts using the most commonly reviewed financial reports: the annual report, income statement, balance sheet, and statement of cash flows. Critical review of these reports helps in understanding the financial health and performance of a health care organization. Chapter 11 will present further concepts and methods for analyzing financial reports.

■ CRITICAL THINKING EXERCISES

1. Using the budget reports for Freeston ElderCare, and adding your own estimates as needed, prepare an income statement, balance sheet, and statement of cash flows for FY 2001.
2. Interpret the financial statements prepared for Freeston ElderCare. Is this a profitable venture? What managerial decisions and priorities are reflected in the financial statements?

3. Bring financial statements from your health care setting, concealing the identity as appropriate. Interpret these statements and explain how they reflect the tax status, financial health, priorities, and managerial decisions of the organization.

■ R E F E R E N C E S

Baker, J. J., & Baker, R. W. (2000). *Health Care Finance: Basic Tools for Nonfinancial Managers*. Gaithersburg, MD: Aspen.

Cleverley, W. O., & Cameron, A. E. (2002). *Essentials of Health Care Finance*, 5th ed. Gaithersburg, MD: Aspen.

Editors of Career Press (1998). *Business Finance for the Numerically Challenged*. Franklin Lakes, NJ: Career Press.

Finkler, S. A. (1983). *The Complete Guide to Finance & Accounting for Nonfinancial Managers*. Englewood Cliffs, NJ: Prentice-Hall, Inc.

Finkler, S. A., & Kovner, C. T. (2000). *Financial Management for Nurse Managers and Executives*, 2nd ed. Philadelphia: W. B. Saunders.

Folland, S., Goodman, A. C., & Stano, M. (1997). *The Economics of Health & Health Care*, 2nd ed. Upper Saddle River, NJ: Prentice Hall.

Gapenski, L. C. (2002). *Healthcare Finance: An Introduction to Accounting and Financial Management*, 2nd ed. Chicago: Health Administration Press.

Neumann, B. R., Suber, J. D., & Zelman, W. N. *Financial Management: Concepts and Applications for Health Care Providers*, 2nd ed. Owings Mills, MD: National Health Publishing, 1988.

Nowicki, M. (2001). *The Financial Management of Hospitals and Healthcare Organizations*. Chicago: Health Administration Press.

Ottenheimer, J. L. (March 1999). Cutting financial reports down to size. *Journal of Accountancy, 187*, pp. 5–51.

Silbiger, S. (1999). *The Ten-Day MBA*, revised ed. New York: William Morrow and Company.

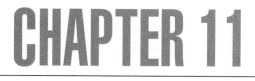

CHAPTER 11

Basic Financial Analysis

▢ Learning Objectives

1. Compare and contrast percent change and common size analysis, and demonstrate how to calculate each of these methods for financial statement analysis.
2. Define and explain the application of at least two financial ratios, showing how each ratio is calculated and interpreted.
3. Identify the purposes and limitations of the use of debt in financial management.

◯ Key Terms

Activity ratios
Asset management ratios
Capital structure ratios
Capitalization ratios
Cash flow coverage (CFC) ratio
Common size analysis
Coverage ratios
Current ratio
Debt management ratios
Debt ratio
Debt-to-assets ratio
Debt-to-capitalization ratio
Debt-to-equity ratio
Degree of operating leverage (DOL)

Fixed asset turnover ratio
Leverage ratios
Liquidity ratios
Long-term capital
Median
Operating leverage
Percentage change analysis
Performance ratios
Profit margin
Profitability ratios
Ratio analysis
Return on equity (ROE)
Return on total assets (ROA)
Total profit margin
Turnover ratios

Chapter 10 covers some fundamental financial accounting and reporting concepts and the basic financial statements used in health care settings. The annual report is not discussed further, as it is prepared primarily for review by the general public rather than for use in financial analysis. This Chapter uses the income statement and balance sheet, presented in Chapter 10, to expand the health care professional's ability to analyze a health care setting's financial performance.

Chapter 10 discusses the assessment of financial condition by presenting the three basic financial statements and their interpretation. This Chapter uses data from the income statement, balance sheet, and statement of cash flows as well as operating data to present concepts and methods for financial statement analysis and operating analysis. SouthSide Hospital continues as the primary example in this chapter.

Financial Statement Analysis

There are three major considerations in analyzing financial performance. The first is to assess the current financial condition and capacity for an organization to perform its mission. Several methods may be used that are discussed in this chapter. The relationship of fixed costs to variable costs and volume may be calculated relative to profitability. Percentages may be calculated based on data from financial statements to compare an organization's financial performance over time, or among other similar health care organizations. Ratios may be calculated from financial statement data for analysis and comparison. Finally, operating analysis using data not usually found in the financial statements (such as volume and productivity measures) may be calculated and interpreted.

In addition, analysis may extend to prior and projected fiscal years or other specified time periods. Analysis of prior and projected time periods not only gives an idea of trends and changes in performance over time, but also allows for the evaluation of the impact of past financial decisions and prediction of the impact of financial decisions on future financial performance. Box 11-1 summarizes methods and approaches to analyzing financial performance.

BOX 11-1

Approaches to Analyzing Financial Performance

- Methods to assess financial condition
  - Financial indicators
  - Percent change analysis
  - Common size analysis
  - Ratio analysis
  - Operating analysis
- Review past management decisions
  - All methods applied to prior FY or time period statements and calculations
- Predict future financial activities
  - All methods applied to projected FY or time period statements and calculations
- Compare an organization to industry standards, internal performance targets, or other similar organizations
  - All methods applied to published or unpublished sources of standards, targets, or analyses of other organizations

Operating Leverage

Operating leverage indicates the proportion of fixed costs for an enterprise compared to its total costs. The higher the proportion of fixed costs (relative to variable costs), the higher the operating leverage, so that a relatively small change in volume causes a relatively large change in profit (net income). Table 11-1 presents a simplified example of the relationships between fixed costs, variable costs, volume, and profit over a given fiscal year.

In this example, the inpatient services of a hypothetical hospital have 20,000 inpatient days (volume measure). The first scenario reports a higher proportion of fixed costs to variable costs ($30 million vs. $10 million, respectively). Total costs equal fixed costs plus variable costs ($40 million) and revenues are $45 million, for a $5 million profit.

Note that when the volume increases by 5%, variable costs and revenues also increase by 5%, because both variable costs and revenues are closely related to volume. Note also that fixed costs, by definition, do not change with changes in volume (particularly relatively small changes such as 5%), so that the total costs increase by only 1%. As a result, with only a 5% increase in volume, given the high fixed costs, profit increases by 35%.

In the second scenario, there is a lower proportion of fixed costs to variable costs ($10 million vs. $30 million, respectively). However, with a volume of 20,000, the total costs again add up to $40 million, and with $45 million in revenue, profits remain at $5 million.

Note that when volume increases by 5% under this scenario of lower fixed costs, total variable costs and revenues again increase by 5% as by definition both are linked to volume. However, because of the higher proportion of variable costs to fixed costs, the total costs increase by 4% and profit increases by only 15%.

Operating leverage is measured using the **degree of operating leverage (DOL)**, calculated using both earnings before interest and taxes (EBIT) and the total contribution margin (from Chap. 8, the total contribution margin represents total revenues less total variable costs). Table 11-2 shows the calculations of the total contribution margin and DOL for SouthSide Hospital's inpatient services for FY 2001–2003. It makes more sense to calculate the operating leverage for inpatient services rather than the entire organization, because charges and costs differ considerably between inpatient and outpatient care, which makes interpretation difficult. For FY 2001 at SouthSide Hospital, inpatient days (volume) totaled 21,217. Total costs for inpatient services are estimated as 84% of the total operating costs plus interest and taxes for SouthSide Hospital, or $44,320,000 for FY 2001 (84% of the sum $51,294,000 + $1,468,000). Total operating revenues for inpatient services are estimated as 83% of the total net operating revenues for SouthSide Hospital,

◯ TABLE 11·1

Inpatient Services Example Comparing Fixed Costs to Variable Costs in Operating Leverage

FY Data	High Fixed Costs			High Variable Costs		
	Volume	5% Increase in Volume	% Change	Volume	5% Increase in Volume	% Change
Inpatient Days (Volume)	20,000	21,000	5%	20,000	21,000	5%
Total Fixed Costs	$30,000,000	$30,000,000	0%	$10,000,000	$10,000,000	0%
Total Variable Costs	$10,000,000	$10,500,000	5%	$30,000,000	$31,500,000	5%
Total Costs	$40,000,000	$40,500,000	1%	$40,000,000	$41,500,000	4%
Total Revenues	$45,000,000	$47,250,000	5%	$45,000,000	$47,250,000	5%
Profit or Loss	**$5,000,000**	**$6,750,000**	35%	**$5,000,000**	**$5,750,000**	15%

⊙ **TABLE 11·2**

SouthSide Hospital, Inpatient Services: EBIT, Contribution Margin & DOL, thousands, FY 2001–2003

	FY 2001	FY 2002	FY 2003
Inpatient Days (actual, not thousands)	21,217	21,326	21,448
Total Inpatient Costs	$44,320	$47,027	$49,011
Total Inpatient Revenues	$46,323	$48,856	$51,401
Less Total Variable Costs	$15,069	$15,989	$16,664
Total Contribution Margin	**$31,254**	**$32,867**	**$34,737**
Less Total Fixed Costs	$29,251	$31,038	$32,347
Profit (Net Income, Change in Net Assets)	**$2,003**	**$1,830**	**$2,390**
Add Back Interest & Taxes	$1,101	$1,489	$1,291
EBIT	**$3,104**	**$3,318**	**$ 3,681**
Degree of Operating Leverage (DOL)	**10.1**	**9.9**	**9.4**

or $46,323,000 for FY 2001 (83% of $55,811,000). Total variable costs for inpatient services are estimated as 34% of the total inpatient services costs, or $15,069,000 for FY 2001.

The total contribution margin for FY 2001 is therefore $46,323,000 less $15,069,000, or $31,254,000 (see Table 11-2). Total fixed costs for inpatient services are $29,251,000. When total fixed costs are deducted from the total contribution margin, the net income or profit for SouthSide inpatient services amounts to $2,003,000 for FY 2001 (see Chap. 8).

SouthSide Hospital's inpatient services EBIT for FY 2001 is $3,104,000, or the amount of profit plus interest and taxes of $1,101,000 (estimated as 75% of the interest and taxes expense for the entire hospital). The degree of operating leverage is calculated by dividing the total contribution margin by EBIT, as follows:

$$\text{Degree of Operating Leverage FY 2001} = \text{Total Contribution Margin} \div \text{EBIT}$$

$$10.1 = \$31,254,000 \div \$3,104,000$$

In other words, a 1% change in inpatient services volume (using the FY 2003 base of 21,217 inpatient days) produces a 10.1% change in profit. For example, if inpatient days for SouthSide Hospital for FY 2001 increased by 1% (to 21,429), net income would increase by 10.1% or would reach $2,205,000, as calculated below:

$$10.1\% \text{ Change in Profit FY 2001} = \text{Base Profit FY 2001} \times 1.101$$

$$\$2,205,000 = \$2,003,000 \times 1.101$$

This represents considerable operating leverage, as a 10% increase in volume would increase profit by over 100%.

Percentage Change Analysis

One way to assess the financial condition of a health care organization is to compare its own performance over time. **Percentage change analysis**, or calculating the percent of change for each item on a financial statement from year to year, is very similar to the method explained for budget variance analysis in Chapter 5. The financial statements analyzed usually include the income statement and the balance sheet. Converting the amount of change for elements in the income statement or balance sheet to a percentage not only enables comparison of an organization's financial performance over time, but also allows similar health care organizations to be compared to each other, or to industry standards. SouthSide Hospital's income statement is used as an example for percent change analysis from FY 2002 to FY 2003.

Table 11-3 shows that in FY 2003 the gross revenue for inpatient services amounts to $159,577,000 compared to $142,063,000 for FY 2002. The amount of change (in this case, an increase) of gross revenue for inpatient services from FY 2002 to FY 2003 is $17,514,000, or $159,577,000 minus $142,063,000. The percent change from FY 2002 to 2003 is calculated as follows:

% Change Inpt. Services Revenue FY 2002–2003 = Change FY 2002–2003 ÷ Revenue FY 2002
12.3% = $17,514,000 ÷ $142,063,000

Table 11-3 shows a percentage change analysis for SouthSide Hospital based on the income statement. The major entries for the income statement are reviewed for FY 2003.

TABLE 11-3

SouthSide Hospital, Income Statement, Percentage Change Analysis, $ thousands, FY 2002–2003

	FY 2002	FY 2003	% change FY 2002–2003
Patient Revenue			
Inpatient Services	$142,063	$159,577	12.3%
Outpatient Services	55,711	58,530	5.1%
Gross Patient Revenue	**197,774**	**218,107**	**10.3%**
Deductions from Patient Revenue			
Contractual Discounts	141,237	158,257	12.1%
Provision for Charity	2,955	3,254	10.1%
Total Deductions from Revenue	**144,192**	**161,511**	**12.0%**
Net Patient Revenue	**53,582**	**56,596**	**5.6%**
Managed Care Revenue	5,119	5,170	1.0%
Other Operating Revenue	162	163	0.6%
Total Operating Revenue	**58,863**	**61,929**	**5.2%**
Operating Expenses			
Salaries & Wages	23,360	24,687	5.7%
Employee Benefits	5,183	5,478	5.7%
Service Contracts & Professional Fees	6,912	7,102	2.7%
Supplies	5,941	6,135	3.3%
Managed Care IBNR	874	914	4.6%
Depreciation & Amortization	2,889	2,950	2.1%
Rents & Leases	191	197	3.1%
Other	2,084	2,095	0.5%
Bad Debt	4,527	4,785	5.7%
IT Chargeback	982	1,025	4.4%
System Chargeback	12	12	0.0%
System Allocation	1,044	1,245	19.3%
Total Operating Expenses	**53,999**	**56,625**	**4.9%**
Non-Operating Revenue	183	174	-4.9%
EBIT	**4,864**	**5,304**	**9.0%**
Interest & Taxes	1,985	1,721	13.3%
Net Income/Loss	**S3,062**	**$3,757**	**22.7%**

Gross revenues for inpatient services increased by 12.3% and for outpatient services by 5.1%, with a 10.3% overall increase in gross patient revenue. However, deductions from patient revenue increased at almost the same rate, 12.0%. The net patient revenue increased by 5.6%, and with increases in managed care and other operating revenues, the total operating revenue increased by 5.2% in FY 2003 (see Table 11-3).

Operating expenses increased overall by 4.9%. Non-operating revenue decreased by 4.9%. EBIT increased by 9.0%, with a decrease in interest and taxes of 13.3%. Net income increased by 22.7% in FY 2003 (see Table 11-3). SouthSide Hospital appears to be controlling its costs compared to revenues and is quite profitable in comparing FY 2002 to FY 2003.

Common Size Analysis

Another method for converting data in the income statement and balance sheet to percentages for comparison over time, among similar organizations, or to industry standards is **common size analysis**. For common size analysis of the income statement, each item is displayed as a percent of total revenues (operating and non-operating); for common size analysis of the balance sheet, each item is displayed as a percent of total assets. SouthSide Hospital's income statement is used as an example.

At SouthSide Hospital for FY 2003, the income statement shows $159,577,000 for gross revenue for inpatient services, with $62,103,000 as total revenues (Table 11-4). The common size analysis for inpatient services revenue is calculated as follows:

$$\text{Common Size Analysis FY 2003} = \text{Inpatient Services Revenue} / \text{Total Revenues}$$

$$257.0\% = \$159,577,000 \div \$62,103,000$$

Table 11-4 shows a common size analysis for SouthSide Hospital based on the income statement for FY 2002–2003. The major entries for the income statement are reviewed for FY 2003. Gross revenue for inpatient services is 257.0% (or about 2.6 times) of total revenues, with outpatient services revenues only 94.2% of total revenues. Gross patient revenue is 351.2% (or about 3.5 times) of total revenues. Deductions from patient revenue are 260.1% (or about 2.6 times) of total revenues, with net patient revenue 91.1% of total revenues. Total operating revenues are 99.7% of total revenues.

Total operating expenses are 91.2% of total revenues, with non-operating revenue only 0.3% of total revenues. EBIT is 8.5% of total revenues, with interest and taxes 2.8% of total revenues. The net income of $3,757,000 is 6.0% of total revenues (see Table 11-4). The common size analysis indicates substantial discounting for inpatient revenues and a lower proportion of operating expenses than operating revenues compared to total revenues.

Ratio Analysis

Of course, the primary purpose of financial statement analysis is to evaluate the fiscal performance of an enterprise. The reviewer asks, "Is this enterprise's financial performance good, poor, improving, or worsening?" To have a basis for evaluation, one more question is required: "Compared to what?" As explained in Chapter 5 regarding the evaluation of budget variances, the reviewer needs to be able to compare data from financial statements with past and projected data and with data from other work units or organizational entities to fully understand what the level of financial performance represents.

Calculating ratios and percents from financial data is helpful in making comparisons (See Math Review at http://connection.lww.com/go/penner). In budget variance analysis, the percent of budget variance is calculated by dividing the budget variance amount by the budget value for the same time period. In working with financial statements, a method often employed is **ratio analysis**, or converting values from financial statements into proportions for analysis and interpretation. Ratios are similar to percents but are composed of numbers from two or more sources. As in using percent budget variances for variance analysis, ratio analysis allows for trend analysis, comparison to industry standards, and benchmarking.

TABLE 11-4

SouthSide Hospital, Income Statement, Common Size Analysis, $ thousands, FY 2002–2003

	FY 2002	Common Size % FY 2002	FY 2003	Common Size % FY 2003
Patient Revenue				
Inpatient Services	$142,063	240.6%	$ 159,577	257.0%
Outpatient Services	55,711	94.4%	58,530	94.2%
Gross Patient Revenue	**197,774**	**334.9%**	**218,107**	**351.2%**
Deductions from Patient Revenue				
Contractual Discounts	141,237	239.2%	158,257	254.8%
Provision for Charity	2,955	5.0%	3,254	5.2%
Total Deductions from Revenue	**144,192**	**244.2%**	**161,511**	**260.1%**
Net Patient Revenue	**53,582**	**90.7%**	**56,596**	**91.1%**
Managed Care Revenue	5,119	8.7%	5,170	8.3%
Other Operating Revenue	162	0.3%	163	0.3%
Total Operating Revenue	**58,863**	**99.7%**	**61,929**	**99.7%**
Operating Expenses				
Salaries & Wages	23,360	39.6%	24,687	39.8%
Employee Benefits	5,183	8.8%	5,478	8.8%
Service Contracts & Professional Fees	6,912	11.7%	7,102	11.4%
Supplies	5,941	10.1%	6,135	9.9%
Managed Care IBNR	874	1.5%	914	1.5%
Depreciation & Amortization	2,889	4.9%	2,950	4.8%
Rents & Leases	191	0.3%	197	0.3%
Other	2,084	3.5%	2,095	3.4%
Bad Debt	4,527	7.7%	4,785	7.7%
IT Chargeback	982	1.7%	1,025	1.7%
System Chargeback	12	0.0%	12	0.0%
System Allocation	1,044	1.8%	1,245	2.0%
Total Operating Expenses	**53,999**	**91.5%**	**56,625**	**91.2%**
Non-Operating Revenue	183	0.3%	174	0.3%
EBIT	**4,864**	**8.2%**	**5,304**	**8.5%**
Interest & Taxes	**1,985**	3.4%	1,721	2.8%
Net Income/Loss	**$3,062**	**5.2%**	**$3,757**	**6.0%**

Tables 11-5 and 11-6 present the same income statement and balance sheet, respectively, as prepared for SouthSide Hospital in Chapter 10. However, to better illustrate the sources of data used in calculating the following ratios used in financial statement analysis, the entries used in calculating ratios are designated with gray backgrounds. In some cases, figures are derived for use in ratio analysis and are highlighted in *italics*. The derived calculation in Table 11-5 is total revenues, calculated as the sum of total operating and total non-operating revenues. The derived calculation in Table 11-6 is total liabilities, calculated as total liabilities and net assets less total net assets.

There are a number of categories and purposes for ratios used in ratio analysis. **Profitability ratios** (also referred to as **performance ratios**) help reviewers understand how well the enterprise generates profits, related to its assets and revenues. **Liquidity ratios** describe an enterprise's capability to turn assets into cash or to cover current debt with cash and other assets available. **Debt management ratios** (also referred to as **capital structure ratios** or **leverage ratios**) show the extent of an enterprise's debt burden, the extent to which investors are financing the enterprise, whether debt payments are covered by current earnings, and the likelihood of the enterprise

◯ TABLE 11·5

SouthSide Hospital, Income Statement, Data Used in Ratio Analysis, FY 2001–2003

	FY 2001	FY 2002	FY 2003
Patient Revenue			
Inpatient Services	$126,878	$142,063	$159,577
Outpatient Services	52,177	55,711	58,530
Gross Patient Revenue	**179,055**	**197,774**	**218,107**
Deductions from Patient Revenue			
Contractual Discounts	125,726	141,237	158,257
Provision for Charity	2,678	2,955	3,254
Total Deductions from Revenue	**128,404**	**144,192**	**161,511**
Net Patient Revenue	50,651	53,582	56,596
Managed Care Revenue	5,000	5,119	5,170
Other Operating Revenue	160	162	163
Total Operating Revenue	55,811	58,863	61,929
Operating Expenses			
Salaries & Wages	22,077	23,360	24,687
Employee Benefits	4,899	5,183	5,478
Service Contracts & Professional Fees	6,867	6,912	7,102
Supplies	5,744	5,941	6,135
Managed Care IBNR	856	874	914
Depreciation & Amortization	2,727	2,889	2,950
Rents & Leases	186	191	197
Other	2,063	2,084	2,095
Bad Debt	4,102	4,527	4,785
IT Chargeback	929	982	1,025
System Chargeback	12	12	12
System Allocation	832	1,044	1,245
Total Operating Expenses	51,294	53,999	56,625
Non-Operating Revenue	204	183	174
EBIT	**4,517**	**4,864**	**5,304**
Interest & Taxes	1,468	1,985	1,721
Net Income/Loss	$3,253	$3,062	$3,757
Total Revenues	*$56,015*	*$59,046*	*$62,103*

paying its debts. **Asset management ratios** (also referred to as **activity ratios** or **turnover ratios**) help reviewers determine how effectively the enterprise is using its assets, and how liabilities are affecting the enterprise.

Some caution should be exercised in using ratio analysis, especially when comparing one institution to another. It is important to consider whether one institution resembles another across many aspects, such as size, patient mix, and inpatient versus outpatient services. There are also differences, allowable under financial accounting standards and regulations, in the way financial statements are reported that may cause ratios to differ.

Many ratios exist in each of these categories for use in financial statement analysis. This chapter presents a few of the ratios in each category that are more commonly used in financial statement analysis for health care settings. This introduction should enable further learning of the calculation and interpretation of other ratios used in one's work setting.

Profitability Ratios

The **profit margin** (also referred to as the **total profit margin**) is a profitability ratio that helps managers evaluate expense control. For a given amount of revenue, the lower the expenses, the higher the

TABLE 11-6

SouthSide Hospital Balance Sheet, Data Used in Ratio Analysis, $ thousands, December 31, FY 2001–2003

	FY 2001	FY 2002	FY 2003
Current Assets			
Cash	$1,209	$2,607	$3,577
Marketable Securities	$4,679	$4,821	$4,998
Accounts Receivable	3,108	3,522	3,744
Supply Inventories, at Cost	5,795	5,828	6,287
Prepaid Expenses & Other	337	366	430
Total Current Assets	**$15,128**	**$17,144**	**$19,036**
Long-Term Investments	**$3,683**	**$3,748**	**$3,892**
Property, Plant & Equipment (Fixed Assets)			
Cost	56,004	57,544	60,191
Construction in Progress	2,144	4,212	4,531
Gross Fixed Assets	**58,148**	**61,756**	**64,722**
Less Accumulated Depreciation	31,575	34,437	37,336
Net PP&E (Net Fixed Assets)	**$26,573**	**$27,319**	**$27,386**
Other Assets	1,242	1,242	1,242
Total Assets	**$46,626**	**$49,453**	**$51,556**
Current Liabilities			
Current Maturities of Long-Term Debt	$69	$78	$89
Notes Payable	728	746	791
Accounts Payable	3,315	3,501	3,653
Accrued Expenses:			
Wages and Benefits	2,453	2,778	2,906
Taxes	171	194	203
Interest Payable	1,197	1,508	1,577
Managed Care IBNR	856	874	914
Total Current Liabilities	**$8,789**	**$9,679**	**$10,133**
Long-Term Debt	**$9,495**	**$8,370**	**$6,262**
Net Assets			
Unrestricted	24,550	27,626	29,511
Restricted	3,792	3,778	5,650
Total Net Assets	**$28,342**	**$31,304**	**$35,161**
Total Liabilities & Net Assets	**$46,626**	**$49,453**	**$51,556**
Total Liabilities (Total Debt)	*$78,284*	*$18,049*	*$16,395*

net income and profit margin, generally speaking. Remember in the example of operating leverage in Table 1-1 that when volume and revenues are kept constant, a smaller percent increase in total costs results in a larger percent increase in profits. The profit margin is calculated by dividing the net income by the total revenues.

For example, SouthSide Hospital has $55,811,000 in total operating revenues and $204,000 in net non-operating revenues for FY 2001 (see Table 11-5), for $56,015,000 total revenues. SouthSide Hospital's FY 2001 net income is $3,253,000. The profit margin for FY 2001 is calculated as follows:

$$\text{Profit Margin} = \text{Net Income}/\text{Total Revenues}$$

$$5.8\% = \$3,253,000/\$56,015,000$$

Each dollar of revenues generated by SouthSide Hospital in FY 2001 produced 5.8 cents of profit and required 94.2 cents of expenses compared to the industry average (median) of 5.0% (Table 11-8). SouthSide Hospital's profit margin for FY 2001 is just a little better than the industry average.

The **return on total assets (ROA)** is a profitability ratio that measures the ability to control expenses and to use assets to generate revenue. The higher the ROA, the more productive the assets. The ROA is calculated by dividing the net income by the total assets. For FY 2001, SouthSide Hospital has a net income of $3,253,000 and total assets of $46,626,000 (see Table 11-5). The FY 2001 ROA is calculated as follows:

$$ROA = Net\ Income \div Total\ Assets$$

$$7.0\% = \$3,253,000 \div \$46,626,000$$

Each dollar of total assets owned by SouthSide Hospital in FY 2001 generated 7 cents in profit, well above the industry average of 4.8%. It appears that the assets of SouthSide Hospital are well managed.

The **return on equity (ROE)** is a profitability ratio that is particularly useful in reviewing the financial analysis of for-profit enterprises, as it measures the utilization of investor-supplied capital. In the financial analysis of non-profits, the ROE indicates how well community-supplied capital is utilized. The ROE is calculated by dividing the net income by total equity. For example, SouthSide Hospital's net income for FY 2001 is $3,253,000 and its total net assets (the non-profit equivalent of equity) are $28,342,000 (see Tables 11-5 and 11-6). The ROE is calculated for FY 2001 as follows:

$$ROE = Net\ Income \div Total\ Equity\ (Total\ Net\ Assets)$$

$$11.5\% = \$3,253,000 \div \$28,342,000$$

SouthSide Hospital is able to generate 11.5 cents of income for each dollar of net assets, well above the industry average of 8.4%.

Increased liabilities, as occurs with debt financing (discussed in the section on debt management ratios), increase the ROE, as shown in Table 11-7. In this example based on a given fiscal year, a health care organization generates $3.5 million in net income and in the first scenario reports $25 million in equity compared to $50 million in liabilities that finances $75 million in assets. The ROE is 14.0% ($3.5 million/$25 million).

In the second scenario, the net income and total assets remain the same, but the liabilities have increased by $10 million in debt financing, so equity is reduced to $15 million (remember, liabilities plus equity must equal assets, so an increase in liabilities, holding assets constant, reduces equity). The resulting ROE is 23.3% ($3.5 million/$15 million), higher than in the first scenario.

Liquidity Ratios

The **current ratio** is a liquidity ratio that measures an enterprise's liquidity, as an indicator of the extent to which short-term claims are covered by liquid assets. The current ratio is calculated by dividing the current

◯ TABLE 11-7

Example of Increased Liabilities (Debt Financing) on ROE Over a Given FY

Scenarios	Net Income	Equity	ROE	Liabilities	Assets
Less Debt Financing	$3,500,000	$25,000,000	14.0%	$50,000,000	$75,000,000
More Debt Financing	$3,500,000	$15,000,000	23.3%	$60,000,000	$75,000,000

assets by current liabilities. For example, SouthSide Hospital has $15,128,000 in current assets for FY 2001 and $8,789,000 in current liabilities (see Table 11-6). The FY 2001 current ratio is calculated as follows:

$$\text{Current Ratio} = \text{Current Assets} \div \text{Current Liabilities}$$

$$1.72 = \$15,128,000 \div \$8,789,000$$

The current ratio shows that the liquidation of SouthSide Hospital's current assets at book value provides $1.72 of cash for every dollar of current liabilities compared to the industry average of $2.00 (Table 11-8). In other words, for FY 2001, current assets could be liquidated at 58.1% of book value and would cover current liabilities (current creditors), as shown by the following calculations:

$$\% \text{ of Book Value} = 1 \div \text{Current Ratio}$$

$$58.1\% = 1 \div 1.72$$

$$\text{Current Assets} = \$15,128,000$$

$$\text{Liquidation at \% Book Value} = \text{Current Assets} \times \% \text{ Book Value}$$

$$\$8,789,000 = \$15,128,000 \times 58.1\%$$

$$\text{Current Liabilities} = \$8,789,000$$

○ TABLE 11-8

SouthSide Hospital, Selected Financial Ratios & Industry Standards, 2001–2002

Ratio	Formula	FY 2001	FY 2002	Industry Average (Median)*
Profitability Ratios:				
Profit Margin	Net Income ÷ Total Revenues	5.8%	5.2%	5.0%
Return on Assets (ROA)	Net Income ÷ Total Assets	7.0%	6.2%	4.8%
Return on Equity (ROE)	Net Income ÷ Total Equity	11.5%	9.8%	8.4%
Liquidity Ratios:				
Current Ratio	Current Assets ÷ Current Liabilities	1.72	1.77	2.0
Days Cash on Hand	Cash + Marketable Securities/([Expenses - Depreciation - Provision for Uncollectibles] ÷ 365)	48.3	58.2	30.6
Debt Capitalization Ratios:				
Debt Ratio (Debt-to-Assets Ratio)	Total Debt ÷ Total Assets or 1 - Equity Ratio	39.2%	36.5%	43.0%
Equity Ratio	Total Debt ÷ Total Equity or 1 - Debt Ratio	60.8%	63.5%	57.0%
Debt Coverage Ratio:				
CFC Ratio	(EBIT + Lease Payments + Depreciation Expense) ÷ ([Interest Expense + Lease Payments + Debt Principal] ÷ [1-T])	1.8	1.7	2.3
Asset Management (Activity or Turnover) Ratios:				
Fixed Asset Turnover (Utilization) Ratio	Total Revenues ÷ Net Fixed Assets	2.1	2.2	2.2
Days in Patient Accounts Receivable	Net Pt. AR/(Net Patient Revenue ÷ 365)	22.4	24.0	64.0

*Industry averages from Gapenski, 2002.

Days cash on hand is another liquidity ratio that indicates the amount of cash that is readily available for day-to-day monetary requirements. It is calculated by the following formula, with the data presented in Table 11-9:

$$\text{Days Cash on Hand} = (\text{Cash} + \text{Marketable Securities}) \div (\text{Expenses} - \text{Depreciation} - \text{Provision for Uncollectibles}) \div 365$$

Table 11-9 reports $1,209,000 in cash for SouthSide Hospital for FY 2001 and $4,679,000 in marketable securities, for a total of $5,888,000. Total expenses for FY 2001 are $51,294,000. Because the income statement deducts charity care from revenues (see Table 11-5), only the entry for bad debt is used in the calculations to represent provision for uncollectibles, an amount of $4,102,000. Depreciation for FY 2001 is $2,727,000. Expenses less depreciation less bad debt total $44,465,000 for FY 2001; divided by 365 days in a year, this amounts to $122,000. The $5,888,000 in cash and marketable securities is divided by $122,000 for 48.3 days cash on hand on average for FY 2001. SouthSide Hospital's days of cash on hand is substantially higher than the industry average of 30.6 days (see Table 11-8).

Debt Management Ratios

As noted previously, debt management ratios show the ability of a health care organization to manage and pay its debts. The owners (or in the case of non-profit organizations, the community) take out the loan, so that debt management is closely related to equity. It is important to measure and analyze debt management because debt increases the organization's financial risk, cost of capital, and claims on assets in the event of bankruptcy and liquidation.

Debt increases the organization's financial risk because regardless of profits or losses, debts are obligations requiring repayment or claims on assets. In addition, debt increases the cost of capital because interest must be paid to the creditor as well as the principal. An organization using debt financing must carefully forecast its revenues to be reasonably sure that the future earnings are adequate to cover the debt expense as well as all other expenses, or it risks default.

On the other hand, equity financing typically does not result in claims on assets, because in the event of bankruptcy and liquidation, the claims of creditors are paid out before the claims of owners or investors. Equity financing also typically does not require repayment. However, it may be difficult for health care organizations to raise capital via equity financing. In the first place, many health care organizations are non-profits, so they cannot sell stock or allow private investors or owners to invest in the business. For-profit health care organizations may have poor returns on their stock given limited profits, so they may use debt financing because the capital needed may not be available via equity financing.

If earnings from investments financed with debt are greater than the interest paid on the loan, the return on equity increases (or is "leveraged up"). In many cases, health care organizations use long-term

○ **TABLE 11-9**

SouthSide Hospital, Worksheet to Calculate Days Cash on Hand, $ thousands, FY 2001–2002

	FY 2001	FY 2002
Cash	$1,209	$2,607
Marketable Securities	$4,679	$4,821
Cash + Marketable Securities	**$5,888**	**$7,428**
Total Expenses	51,294	53,999
Provision for Uncollectibles (Bad Debt)	4,102	4,527
Depreciation	2,727	2,889
Expenses-Depreciation-Bad Debt	**44,465**	**46,583**
Expenses-Depreciation-Bad Debt/365	**$122**	**$128**
Days Cash on Hand	**48.3**	**58.2**

debt to finance fixed assets. These fixed assets, whether a new structure, major renovation, or state-of-the-art equipment, are typically expected to maintain and increase earnings or "pay for themselves" by attracting volume and generating revenue. However, it may be difficult to match the costs of debt with the revenues from investments such as fixed assets financed by the debt.

For security reasons, creditors prefer low debt ratios and pay attention to the amount of equity capital provided to the enterprise. If the owners (or community) provide only a small amount of total financing, there is greater risk on default of loans should bankruptcy and liquidation occur. However, owners of for-profit enterprises may seek higher debt in order to increase their return on equity, or because they do not want to give up control by selling stock. Managers of non-profit organizations may seek higher debt to provide more services to the community. Therefore, debt management should help maintain a reasonable balance between financing by creditors and owners.

It is also important to understand how debt may or may not be defined. In this discussion of debt management ratios, debt is defined as total debt, which represents all liabilities, including current liabilities, long-term debt, and lease obligations. In other words, in this discussion of debt management ratios, debt is represented by the sum of all entries on the right side or bottom section of the balance sheet, except equity. Other organizations may vary on how debt is defined for the purposes of financial analysis. For example, many organizations use the **debt-to-capitalization ratio**, in which long-term debt is divided by **long-term capital** (long-term debt plus equity), to show the proportion of debt utilized for permanent capital. As in many of the concepts presented in this text, it is important to learn how debt is defined and analyzed in one's own health care setting.

Two types of ratios are used to analyze debt management. The first include **capitalization ratios**, which indicate the extent to which assets are financed by debt. Balance sheet data are used to compute capitalization ratios. The second type of ratios are **coverage ratios**, which show how well reported profits cover fixed financial charges such as interest. Income statement data are used to compute coverage ratios.

The **debt ratio** (**debt-to-assets ratio**) is a debt capitalization management ratio that indicates the extent to which debt is used to finance assets. Remember that in this discussion of debt management ratios, total debt is defined as total liabilities, which equal $18,284,000 for FY 2001 at SouthSide Hospital, and total assets are $46,626,000 (see Table 11-6). The debt ratio is calculated for FY 2001 as follows:

$$\text{Debt Ratio} = \text{Total Debt} \div \text{Total Assets}$$
$$39.2\% = \$18,284,000 \div \$46,626,000$$

Each dollar of assets for FY 2001 was financed by 39.2 cents of debt, somewhat less than the industry average of 43% (see Table 11-8). In other words, SouthSide Hospital utilizes debt somewhat less than the industry average.

The **debt-to-equity ratio** is a debt capitalization management ratio that provides lenders with information on how much capital creditors have provided to the organization per dollar of equity capital. The debt ratio and the debt-to-equity ratio are inverse transformations of each other; in other words, debt ratio may be calculated as 1 minus the debt-to-equity ratio, and the debt-to-equity ratio may be calculated as 1 minus that debt ratio. For FY 2001 at SouthSide Hospital, total net assets (total equity) is $28,342,000 (see Table 11-6). The debt-to-equity ratio is calculated for FY 2001 as follows:

$$\text{Debt-to-Equity Ratio} = \text{Total Debt} \div \text{Total Equity}$$
$$60.8\% = \$18,284,000 \div \$28,342,000$$

In FY 2001, SouthSide Hospital's creditors contributed 60.8 cents for each dollar of equity capital, compared to the industry average of 57% (see Table 11-8). In other words, SouthSide Hospital uses equity financing a little more than the industry average.

The **cash flow coverage ratio (CFC ratio)** is a debt coverage management ratio that shows how well cash flow covers fixed financial needs. Data for calculating the CFC ratio are from the income statement, except lease payments and debt principal. The CFC ratio is calculated according to the following formula, with data for FY 2002–2001 for SouthSide Hospital presented in Table 11-10:

○ TABLE 11-10

SouthSide Hospital, Worksheet for Calculation of Cash Flow Coverage Ratio, $ thousands, FY 2001–2003

	FY 2001	FY 2002
EBIT	$4,517	$4,864
Lease Payments	186	191
Depreciation	2,727	2,889
Subtotal	**$7,430**	**$7,944**
Interest	$1,468	$ 1,985
Lease Payments	186	191
Debt Principal	2,500	2,418
Subtotal	**S4,154**	**$4,594**
CFC Ratio	**1.8**	**1.7**

CFC Ratio = (EBIT + Lease Payments + Depreciation Expense) ÷ ([Interest Expense + Lease Payments + Debt Principal] ÷ [1 − Taxes])

Table 11-10 shows that for SouthSide Hospital for FY 2001, EBIT equals $4,517,000. Lease payments are $186,000 for FY 2001 and depreciation is $2,727,000, for a subtotal of $7,430,000. Interest payments are $1,468,000, lease payments are $186,000, and debt principal is $2,500,000 for FY 2001, for a subtotal of $4,154,000. Dividing the first subtotal of $7,430,000 by the second subtotal of $4,154,000, the FY 2001 CFC ratio is 1.8. In other words, SouthSide Hospital's cash flow for FY 2001 covers its fixed financial requirements by 1.8 times, or it has 80% more cash than is required by its fixed financial obligations, not as high as the 2.3 industry average (see Table 11-8).

Note that the (1 − Taxes) portion of the equation was ignored in the calculation. This is because SouthSide Hospital is a non-profit, tax-exempt organization. The taxes included in the income statement line for interest and taxes (see Table 11-5) are minimal, as SouthSide Hospital pays only a few state and local taxes. For-profit enterprises must repay debt principal with after-tax income, so the (1 − Taxes) term is required to calculate the pre-tax income required to cover fixed financial obligations.

Asset Management (Activity) Ratios

The **fixed asset turnover ratio** shows how well property, plant, and equipment are utilized to generate profits and provide services, using data from both the income statement and the balance sheet. The fixed asset turnover ratio is calculated by dividing total revenue, which equals $56,015,000 for FY 2001 for SouthSide Hospital, by net fixed assets, which equal $26,573,000 (see Tables 11-5 and 11-6):

Fixed Asset Turnover Ratio = Total Revenue ÷ Net Fixed Assets

2.1 = $56,015,000 ÷ $26,573,000

Each dollar of fixed assets at SouthSide Hospital generated $2.10 in revenue for FY 2001, very close to the industry average of $2.20 (see Table 11-8).

Days in patient accounts receivable is an asset management ratio that may also be used as a liquidity ratio, using data from both the income statement and the balance sheet. This measure is of interest because

☐ **B O X   1 1 · 2**

Financial Ratio Analysis

Profitability (Performance) Ratios:

■ Total Profit Margin (Profit Margin)
 –Net Income ÷ Total Revenues expressed as a percent
 –Data are from the income statelment
 –A measure of expense control—for a given amount of revenues, the higher the net income and profit margin, the lower the expenses
■ Return on Total Assets (ROA)
 –Net Income ÷ Total Assets expressed as a percent
 –Data are from the income statement and the balance sheet
 –Measures the ability to control expenses and to use assets to generate revenue—the higher the ROA, the more productive the assets
■ Return on Equity (ROE)
 –Net Income ÷ Total Equity expressed as a percent
 –Data are from the income statement and the balance sheet
 –Especially meaningful analyzing for-profit businesses—shows the utilization of owner-supplied capital
 –For non-profits, indicates how well community-supplied capital is utilized

Liquidity Ratios:

■ Current Ratio
 –Current Assets ÷ Current Liabilities expressed as number of times
 –Data are from the balance sheet
 –Indicator of extent to which short-term claims are covered by liquid assets
■ Days Cash on Hand
 –Cash + Marketable Securities ÷ (Expenses less Depreciation less Provision for Uncollectibles) ÷ 365 expressed in days
 –Data are from the income statement and the balance sheet
 –Must also review the cash budget: current ratio and days cash on hand may provide conflicting results

Debt Management (Capital Structure or Leverage) Ratios:

■ Debt Capitalization (indicates the extent to which assets are financed by debt)
 –Debt Ratio (Debt-to-Assets Ratio):
  ● Total Debt ÷.Total Assets or 1 − Debt to Equity Ratio expressed as a percent
  ● Data are from the balance sheet
  ● Shows the extent to which debt is used to finance assets
 –Debt to Equity Ratio:
  ● Total Debt ÷ Total Equity or 1 − Debt Ratio expressed as a percent
  ● Data are from the balance sheet
  ● Tells lenders the extent of risk to creditors
■ Debt Coverage (shows how well reported profits cover fixed financial charges)
 –Cash Flow Coverage (CFC) Ratio:
  ● (EBIT + Lease Payments + Depreciation Expense) ÷ ([Interest Expense + Lease Payments + Debt Principal] ÷ [1-T])
  ● Data are from the income statement, except estimated debt principal
  ● Indicates the margin by which cash flow covers fixed financial needs

continued

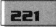

Asset Management (Activity or Turnover) Ratios:

- Fixed Asset Turnover (Utilization) Ratio
  - –Total Revenue ÷ Net Fixed Assets expressed as number of times
  - –Data are from the income statement and the balance sheet
  - –Measures how productively fixed assets are utilized
- Days in Patient Accounts Receivable
  - –Net Patient Accounts Receivable ÷ Average Daily Patient Revenue expressed in days
  - –Data are from the income statement and the balance sheet
  - –Important to collect receivables as soon as possible

it is important to collect receivables as soon as possible in order to maintain adequate cash flow and reduce the amount of uncollectibles. The days in patient accounts receivable is calculated by dividing the patient accounts receivable (which for FY 2001 at SouthSide Hospital equals $3,108,000 [see Table 11-6]) by the average daily patient revenue ($50,651,000 ÷ 365 or $139,000 [see Table 11-5]):

$$\text{Days in Patient Accounts Receivable} = \text{Net Patient Accounts Receivable}/\text{Average Daily Patient Revenue}$$

$$22.4 \text{ Days} = \$3,108,000 \div \$139,000$$

On average, SouthSide Hospital shows 22.4 days in patient accounts receivable, far lower than the industry average of 64 days (see Table 11-8). It appears that patients and their insurers pay their bills to South-Side Hospital far more quickly than the industry average.

Box 11-2 summarizes the classification, name, calculation, and interpretation of all of the financial ratios discussed in this chapter.

Operating Analysis

Operating analysis uses operating data that may not be found in financial statements. These indicators help reviewers understand the productivity of the enterprise. Data required to calculate some of these indicators are presented in Table 11-11. Dividing the total patient days for SouthSide Hospital's inpatient services by 365 days in the year (21,217 ÷ 365), the average daily census (ADC) of 58.1 is calculated for FY 2001. Remember that the ADC is a volume measure, discussed in Chapters 4 and 7.

One indicator using the ADC is the occupancy rate, or the percent of occupied beds; it is calculated by dividing the ADC by the number of beds available (see Chap. 4). For example, in FY 2001 SouthSide Hospital has an ADC of 58.1 and 110 beds available. SouthSide Hospital's FY 2001 occupancy rate of 52.8% is somewhat greater than the industry average (median) of 48.6% (Table 11-12).

Another indicator is the change in occupancy, which allows for comparison over time and among similar health care facilities. The change in occupancy rate requires both the reported fiscal year (or other specified time period) occupancy rate data and data for the preceding fiscal year (or other specified time period). Using

◯ TABLE 11-11

SouthSide Hospital, Worksheet for Calculating ALOS, FY 2001–2002

	FY 2001	FY 2002
Inpatient Days	21,217	21,326
ADC	58.1	58.4
Discharges	4,466	4,632
ALOS	4.8	4.6

FY 2001–2002 data from SouthSide Hospital, the change in occupancy is calculated as follows:

$$\text{Change in Occupancy} = (\text{Reported Year Occupancy} - \text{Preceding Year Occupancy}) \div \text{Reported Year Occupancy}$$
$$0.5\% = (53.1\% - 52.8\%) \div 53.1\%$$

SouthSide Hospital's FY 2001–2002 change in occupancy of 0.5% is greater than the industry average of negative 0.15% (see Table 11-12).

Average length of stay (ALOS) is a productivity measure calculated by dividing the total number of inpatient days by the number of discharges, expressed as days (some facilities divide the total hospital days by admissions rather than discharges, as presented in Chap. 5). For example, SouthSide Hospital's FY 2001 inpatient services days are 21, 217 with 4,466 discharges (see Table 11-11). ALOS for FY 2001 is calculated as follows:

$$\text{ALOS FY 2001} = \text{Total Inpatient Days} \div \text{Discharges}$$
$$4.8 \text{ days} = 21,217 \div 4,466$$

SouthSide Hospital's FY 2001 ALOS of 4.8 days is somewhat higher than the industry average of 4.59 days (see Table 11-12). In other words, inpatients are hospitalized somewhat longer at SouthSide Hospital than on average.

The average age of plant is a measure to show how old a health care organization's fixed assets are. Average age of plant is calculated by dividing the accumulated depreciation by the depreciation expense, expressed as years. For example, SouthSide Hospital's accumulated depreciation for FY 2001 is $31,575,000 (see Table 11-6) and the depreciation expense is $2,727,000 (see Table 11-5). Average age of plant for SouthSide Hospital for FY 2001 is calculated as follows:

$$\text{Average Age of Plant FY 2001} = \text{Accumulated Depreciation FY 2001} \div \text{Depreciation Expense FY 2001}$$
$$11.6 \text{ years} = \$31,575,000 \div \$2,727,000$$

○ TABLE 11-12

SouthSide Hospital, Operational Indicators & Industry Averages, FY 2001–2002

Indicator	Formula	FY 2001	FY 2002	Industry Average (Median)
Occupancy Rate	Average Daily Census (ADC) ÷ Beds in Service	52.8%	53.1%	48.6%*
Change in Occupancy	(Reported Year Occupancy – Preceding Year Occupancy) ÷ Reported Year Occupancy	—	0.5%	−0.15%*
Average Length of Stay (ALOS)	Total Hospital Days ÷ Discharges expressed as days	4.8	4.6	4.59 days*
Average Age of Plant	Accumulated Depreciation ÷ Depreciation Expense expressed in years	11.6	11.9	9.1 years[†]

*Industry averages from Griffith & Alexander, 2002.

[†]Industry average from Gapenski, 2002.

BOX 11-3

Operating Analysis Indicators

- Occupancy Rate
  - Average Daily Census (ADC) ÷ Beds in Service
- Change in Occupancy
  - (Reported Year Occupancy − Preceding Year Occupancy) ÷ Reported Year Occupancy
- Average Length Of Stay (ALOS)
  - ALOS = Total Hospital Days ÷ Admissions, or
  - ALOS = Total Hospital Days ÷ Discharges
- Average Age of Plant
  - Accumulated Depreciation ÷ Depreciation Expense expressed in years
  - Measure of the average age in years of fixed assets

SouthSide Hospital's fixed assets are older than the industry average of 9.1 years, probably requiring more capital expenditures in the future (see Table 11-12).

Conclusion

This chapter presents methods for analyzing several of the most commonly encountered financial reports in order to better assess the financial performance of health care organizations. Box 11-3 summarizes the indicators used in operating analysis that are discussed in this chapter. Box 11-4 provides sources for financial ratio standards for hospitals, physician practices, skilled nursing facilities, and other health care organizations. Box 11-5 provides Internet sources for information on financial reports and ratios.

BOX 11-4

Sources of Financial Ratio Standards for Health Care Organizations

Campbell, C. R., Schmitz, H.H., & Waller, Linda C. (1998). Financial management in a managed care environment. Albany, NY: Delmar.

Cleverley, W. O. (Spring 2001). Financial dashboard reporting for the hospital industry. Journal of Health Care Finance, 27(3); 30–40.

Cleverley, W. O., & Cameron, A. E. (2002). Essentials of health care finance, 5th ed. Gaithersburg, MD: Aspen.

Gapenski, L. C. (2002). Healthcare finance: an introduction to accounting and financial management, 2nd ed. Chicago: Health Administration Press.

Griffith, J.R., & Alexander, J. A. (January/February 2002). Measuring comparative hospital performance. Journal of Healthcare Management, 47(1), 41–57.

Nowicki, M. (2001). The financial management of hospitals and healthcare organizations. Chicago: Health Administration Press.

RMA (Risk Management Association) (2000/2001). Annual statementstudies. Philadelphia: RMA.

■ C R I T I C A L   T H I N K I N G   E X E R C I S E S

1. Using the balance sheet prepared for Freeston ElderCare, calculate the percent change and common size analyses for FY 2003. How would you interpret these analyses?
2. Project an income statement and a balance sheet for Freeston ElderCare for FY 2004, and calculate a percent change analyses comparing FY 2003 to FY 2004. What is your interpretation?
3. Bring financial statements and information regarding fixed and variable costs from your health care setting, concealing the setting's identity as appropriate. If not available, use the financial statements available in this chapter. Calculate the degree of operating leverage, percent change analysis, common size analysis, financial ratios, and operating ratios using your data and best estimates. Interpret your analyses. If possible, compare the financial ratios to industry standards.

■ R E F E R E N C E S

Baker, J. J., & Baker, R. W. (2000). *Health care finance: basic tools for nonfinancial managers.* Gaithersburg, MD: Aspen.

Campbell, C. R., Schmitz, H. H., & Waller, L. C. (1998). *Financial Management in a Managed Care Environment.* Albany, NY: Delmar.

Center for Healthcare Industry Performance Studies (2002). *Almanac of hospital financial & operating indicators.* Columbus, OH: Center for Healthcare Industry Performance Studies.

Cleverley, W. O. (Spring 2001). Financial dashboard reporting for the hospital industry. *Journal of Health Care Finance, 27*(3), 30–40.

Cleverley, W. O., & Cameron, A. E. (2002). *Essentials of health care finance,* 5th ed. Gaithersburg, MD: Aspen.

Editors of Career Press (1998). *Business finance for the numerically challenged.* Franklin Lakes, NJ: Career Press.

Finkler, S. A. (1983). *The complete guide to finance & accounting for nonfinancial managers.* Englewood Cliffs, NJ: Prentice-Hall, Inc.

Finkler, S. A., & Kovner, C. T. (2000). *Financial management for nurse managers and executives,* 2nd ed. Philadelphia: W. B. Saunders.

Gapenski, L. C. (2001). *Understanding healthcare financial management,* 3rd ed. Washington, DC: AUPHA Press.

Gapenski, L. C. (2002). *Healthcare finance: an introduction to accounting and financial management,* 2nd ed. Chicago: Health Administration Press.

Griffith, J. R., & Alexander, J. A. (January/February 2002). Measuring comparative hospital performance. *Journal of Healthcare Management, 47*(1), 41–57.

Keller, G., Warrack, B., & Bartel, H. (1990). *Statistics for management and economics: a systematic approach*, 2nd ed. Belmont, CA: Wadsworth.

Neumann, B. R., Suber, J. D., & Zelman, W. N. (1988). *Financial management: concepts and applications for health care providers*, 2nd ed. Owings Mills, MD: National Health Publishing.

Nowicki, M. (2001). *The financial management of hospitals and healthcare organizations*. Chicago: Health Administration Press.

RMA (Risk Management Association) (2000/2001). *Annual statement studies*. Philadelphia: RMA.

Silbiger, S. (1999). *The ten day MBA*, revised ed. New York: William Morrow and Company.

CHAPTER 12

Writing a Business Plan

- **Components of the Business Plan**
  Problem or Need Identification
  Product Definition
  Market Analysis
  Budget Estimates
  Financial Analysis
  Timeline
  Conclusion and Feasibility Statement
- **Conclusion**

Learning Objectives

1. Describe the components included in most business plans, and their purpose.
2. Explain why a budget is an essential component of a business plan.
3. Identify at least two types of financial analysis useful in developing a business plan.

Key Terms

Market share
Principal proponent

This chapter, along with Chapter 13, brings together many of the skills and concepts regarding budgeting and financial analysis. Business plans enable health care professionals to make a convincing case to get resources such as staff and equipment identified as a need in their department or unit. Business plans can be used to support expanding programs or to recommend starting a new business or venture. In addition, business plans can demonstrate the impact of staff cuts or program downsizing or the financial risk or unprofitability of a proposed program or business. The sample business plan found in Appendix C can be used as a guide for formatting, content, and length. SouthSide Hospital is the setting for the sample business plan, which proposes funding and staffing for a new cardiac catheterization laboratory.

The design, formatting, level of detail required, and length of business plans may differ somewhat across various health care settings, so it is important to learn the formal or informal guidelines and the accepted procedures in one's work setting. It is also important to consider the size and scope of the program proposed by the business plan. The scope might be as small as requesting an additional crash cart for the nursing unit, or as large as building a wing for the medical center. In some settings or for some purposes, a brief memo may suffice as a business plan; in other cases, business plans may require 50 or more pages of text and extensive data tables and analyses.

The business plan directly reflects on the credibility and expertise of the presenting person or entity, so it requires careful proofreading for accuracy, clarity, flow, and grammar. Statements and figures must be accurate, with sources provided so the reader can verify assertions. The numbers and calculations used in the plan must be checked carefully; when possible, calculations should be explained so they are clear to the reader and can be replicated.

The writing and presentation of data must be clear to the reader; jargon should be avoided, acronyms explained, and, as necessary, terminology defined. The CEO, vice-president, bank president, or other potential funder reading the business plan may not be familiar with clinical terminology or acronyms but must be able to understand the case made for financing what the plan requests. A business plan with grammatical errors and misspelled words reflects a lack of attention that easily leads to rejection. For all of these reasons, it is important to critically read and re-read drafts of the plan, and, if possible, to have one or more critical reviews of the plan, with revisions, before it is officially submitted.

The business plan should have a logical flow, with headings and subheadings, depending on the length and level of detail, and transition sentences to bridge between sections. The points made should logically build upon and link to one another; for example, the problem to be addressed should be linked to the program or other intervention developed, which should be linked to the market analysis, and the resources needed for the program or other intervention should be linked to the budget (Chap. 6 presents budget preparation concepts). Any additional financial analyses should be linked to the rest of the plan and should make sense to the reader.

In many cases more than one person will review the business plan, and these are busy people who may want the information in the business plan distilled into one or two pages and a budget page. It is therefore important to include an executive summary of the business plan, no more than one or two pages in length, that clearly, accurately, and succinctly summarizes the key points of the business plan. An overall budget table (including a pro forma P&L statement if the program generates revenues) no more than one or two pages in length should accompany the executive summary.

Business plans may propose a new product or service. For example, in Chapter 6, the budget proposal developed for an activities program could easily be rewritten as a business plan. Business plans may propose the expansion of an existing program or service; for example, the budget justification report regarding the expansion of Freeston's hospice program in Chapter 5 could be rewritten as a business plan.

Health care professionals or managers may write business plans as **principal proponents**, when their staff and setting benefit directly from the plan's approval. For example, Martha, nurse manager for the pediatric intensive care unit (PICU), writes a business plan to replace the nearly obsolete monitors on the PICU with up-to-date technology. On the other hand, health care professionals or managers may prepare business plans in supportive roles. For example, Jeff, director of the Radiology Department, develops a business plan for the physician radiologists to obtain more state-of-the-art examination equipment. Although Jeff and his staff of radiology technicians do not directly benefit if the equipment is obtained, there are substantial indirect benefits because physician satisfaction and diagnostic capability increase.

Components of the Business Plan

Business plans are typically developed in steps and include certain components. The first step in developing a business plan, and the first section in most business plans, is problem or need identification, followed by product definition, or describing the service or product to be developed. A market analysis follows, then budget estimates, additional financial analysis, and a conclusion that includes a feasibility statement.

Problem or Need Identification

The first step in preparing a business plan is to identify the problem or need to be addressed. This is also the first section of the business plan; after all, readers considering funding a venture must first be convinced that the proposal is necessary. Although it may seem simple enough to identify problems in health care settings, it is useful to carefully consider the extent to which a problem or need meets the following criteria for addressing in a business plan. The following questions are often useful to ask:

- Is this a problem that can be solved by a new program or other intervention? For example, cardiac catheterization technology has substantially improved over recent years, which makes it worth consideration for the business plan at SouthSide Hospital.
- What is the political context of the problem? For example, if the CEO of the medical center mandates that staffing must be cut by 5% over the coming year, then requests for staffing increases, even in a well-drafted business plan, may not be politically feasible.
- How well does the business plan fit with the organizational mission, values, and goals? The better the fit, the more likely the business plan will receive attention and support. For example, SouthSide Hospital is a center for excellence in cardiac care, which is a very good fit with a business plan to upgrade cardiac catheterization services.
- Where does this problem rank compared to other departmental and organizational priorities? Even for a relatively small request, considerable time and effort may be spent in preparing and reviewing a business plan. Be sure to use time and resources to best advantage, focusing on the most important issues.

The Cardiac Catheterization Project Committee (CCPC) at SouthSide Hospital uses demographic and epidemiologic data regarding population age and estimated rates of cardiac problems, as well as interviews with cardiologists, to show the need for improved cardiac catheterization capabilities.

Product Definition

Frequently, clinicians do an expert job of problem or need identification, but it is sometimes more difficult to clearly describe the product: the program, service, or other intervention that is proposed. It is important to describe the specific product clearly so the reader knows exactly what is planned. Does the unit require a specific piece of equipment, added staffing, or more space? Is new construction or remodeling required?

It is often useful to propose or compare alternative ways in which the product could be provided. For example, The manager of a psychiatric unit sees a need for one or two detoxification beds where patients in acute alcohol or illicit drug withdrawal could be monitored more closely than in the psychiatric adult care unit. The manager proposes two alternatives for providing this product:

- Designate a patient room adjacent to the psychiatric adult care nursing station as a detoxification unit and train the unit's staff in detoxification policies and procedures
- Train the emergency room staff and admit these patients to the emergency department's 24-hour care beds

The use of alternative scenarios frequently leads to a cost-effectiveness analysis, in which the costs and feasibility of these alternatives are compared in the business plan. In the sample business plan for the cardiac catheterization laboratory at SouthSide Hospital, the alternative is to continue the next 4 years with the same equipment and space, and the profitability of the two alternatives is compared.

Market Analysis

A market analysis is an important piece of a business plan, but it is new to many health care professionals and managers who have not had a lot of experience looking at the overall business and marketing environment. A market analysis identifies the estimated market share, clients and client mix, payors and payor mix, the strengths and weaknesses of actual and potential competitors, and the demand for a product or service. Further, the market analysis discusses anticipated change in any or all of these environmental factors and considers any other trends that might affect the product or service. For example, the market analysis for the cardiac catheterization laboratory business plan provides information on potential competitors for cardiac catheterization procedure referrals.

Market share is the estimated percentage of the entire market for a product or service that is managed by a provider or organization. For example, if 20% of all patients requiring total hip replacement in a given market area come to ABC Hospital, then ABC Hospital has 20% of the market share. The market share allows for comparison among competitors. It is important to consider whether the product or service proposed in the business plan is something for which there is already considerable competition. Is this a new product or service that is not offered in the market area, or is the business plan attempting to increase the organization's competitive position?

The business plan should clearly identify the clients and client mix for the proposed product or service. Who is likely to demand or use this product or service? What demographic characteristics are clients likely to share, including age, income, employment status, gender, and ethnicity? These demographic characteristics are likely to influence the anticipated payors and payor mix; for example, older persons are likely covered by Medicare, employed populations may have private health insurance, and poorer or severely, chronically ill persons may be covered by Medicaid. In the cardiac catheterization laboratory business plan, the growth in persons over age 65 in SouthSide Hospital's service area supports the feasibility and success of the proposal.

In addition to estimating the current and potential market share, it is necessary to examine the strengths and weaknesses of actual and potential competitors for the proposed product or service. What is the reputation of other providers in delivering this product or service? Is there adequate access for clients who demand this product or service? How would the proposed price or fee compare with that of competitors? Is it possible to market the product or service to large purchasers, such as employee groups, unions, or government programs? The demand for the product or service must be addressed: are clients or purchasers interested? What is the volume (the number of clients or units of the product or services) estimated for the coming year?

After identifying the problem or need, defining the product, and reviewing the market analysis, further planning for the product or service typically continues if there is a strong need, a product that could be provided to meet the need, and a market analysis indicating a strong demand and a competitive edge. Further business planning may end at this stage if the need is not compelling, there is no profitable or feasible way to meet the need, or the market analysis shows there is little demand or strong competition in the context of the overall environment.

Budget Estimates

The next step is to develop an operating expense budget and a capital expense budget for the proposed program or service. If the program or service generates revenues, a revenue budget is also required. These budget estimates should be as accurate as possible. Budget estimates should include direct costs (space, personnel and non-personnel expenses) and indirect costs such as administrative overhead. The business plan for SouthSide Hospital's cardiac catheterization laboratory presents a capital budget, an operating expense budget, and a pro forma P&L statement that includes entries for revenue and overhead.

At this step, the decision to continue, end, or revise the business plan requires evaluating the pro forma P & L statement. If revenues exceed costs, business planning is likely to continue; if costs exceed revenues, particularly in fiscal years following start-up, business planning is likely to be dropped or the business plan revised.

In some cases, the profitability of the venture may not be clear. It may be advisable in such cases to do more detailed and in-depth study of the proposed product or service's marketability and profitability. Estimation of alternative scenarios may also be helpful, for example, under various possible competitive positions, levels of demand, or amounts of volume that might be generated. In this way, the impact of a "worst-case" versus expected versus a "best-case" scenario can be anticipated and compared as part of the decision-making process.

Financial Analysis

Following the development of a market analysis and operational budget, it is frequently useful to conduct a financial analysis that builds on the budget estimates and provides further support for carrying out the business plan (or, in some cases, helps determine the plan is not feasible). Break-even analysis (see Chap. 8), cost-benefit analysis, and cost-effectiveness analyses (see Chap. 9) are examples of calculations that may be used. If the overall purpose of a proposed project is to save money, a cost-benefit analysis or a cost-effectiveness analysis might make more sense than a break-even analysis. If the major purpose is to generate profits, a break-even analysis including a profit target might be advisable.

Timeline

It is essential to develop a specific and realistic timeline to implement the product described in the business plan. Very large projects, such as new construction, may require more than 1 fiscal year for completion, but most smaller programs or services are generally completed within a fiscal year. In some cases it is useful to estimate alternative best-case, worst-case, and most-likely scenarios for the timeline to allow planning for unexpected events. The timeline for the business plan for the cardiac catheterization laboratory goes from business plan submission on October 8, 2001, through beginning patient care services in the newly renovated facility on April 29, 2002, approximately 7 months total.

BOX 12-1

Business Plan Components and Process

1. Problem or need identification
2. Product definition
3. Market analysis
   - ✓ Continue or end here. If continued:
4. Budget estimates
   - ✓ Continue, revise, or end here. If continued:
5. Additional financial analysis
   - ✓ Continue, revise, or end here. If continued:
6. Timeline
7. Conclusion and feasibility statement
   - ✓ Accept, reject, or revise the business plan.

Conclusion and Feasibility Statement

As with most reports, the final section briefly summarizes and wraps up the business plan, concluding with a statement regarding the overall feasibility of the business plan. There is an inherent bias and motivation, of course, to try to make one's proposed product or service as attractive as possible, and to overlook facts and figures that point to the unprofitability and infeasibility of the project. However, it may well be far more valuable to the organization (and to the manager responsible for the business plan) to recommend dropping a proposed product or service should the evidence indicate the project is unfeasible. The sample business plan for the cardiac catheterization laboratory points out some potential threats to the plan but concludes that the plan is feasible.

Conclusion

This chapter describes the components of a business plan and demonstrates how to use skills in budgeting and financial analysis in developing a business plan. Box 12-1 summarizes the components and process used in developing a business plan. Chapter 13 extends this discussion, focusing on the components and development of a health program grant proposal. Box 12-2 provides Internet resources for writing business plans.

BOX 12-2

On-line Sources for Information on Writing a Business Plan

BusinessTown.com—Business Planning: http://www.businesstown.com/planning/creating.asp
CCH Business Owner's Toolkit—Planning Your Business:
  http://www.toolkit.cch.com/text/P02_0001.asp
Indian Health Service Business Plan Workgroup:
  http://www.ihs.gov/NonMedicalPrograms/businessplan/index.asp
The Management Library—Business Planning: http://www.managementhelp.org

CRITICAL THINKING EXERCISES

1. Using a topic of interest or an idea for a program, product, or service derived from your work setting, prepare a business plan including all of the recommended components. Discuss the feasibility of this plan.
2. Instead of using a topic or idea as suggested in the first exercise, rewrite the Chapter 5 budget justification report regarding the expansion of Freeston's hospice program, or the Chapter 8 break-even analysis for a cardiac rehabilitation program as a business plan.

REFERENCES:

Cardiac Catheterization Laboratory Standards, published by the American College of Cardiology: *http://www.acc.org*
American Heart Association: *http://www.americanheart.org*
Brooks, J. K., & Stevens, B. A. (1987). *How to write a successful business plan.* New York: Beta Enterprises, Inc.
Eichenberger, J. (May 1998). Project management, Part III: Budgets for projects. *AAOHN Journal, 46*(5), 268–270.
Finkler, S. A., & Kovner, C. T. (2000). *Financial management for nurse managers and executives*, 2nd ed. Philadelphia: W. B. Saunders.
Grandinetti, D. (1998). Need cash for a new venture? Start here. *Medical Economics, 75*(5), 111–119.
Sahlman, W. A. (July/August 1997). How to write a great business plan. *Harvard Business Review, 75*(4), 98–108.

CHAPTER 13

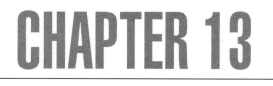

Grant Writing: Getting Funding From an Outside Source

☐ Learning Objectives

1. List at least three types of health program grant proposals, and explain how they differ from each other.
2. Describe the components of health program grant proposals and their purpose.
3. Write a health program objective that is specific, achievable, and measurable within a specified time frame.

○ Key Terms

Business grant proposals
Capability statement
Capital improvement grants
Competitive grants
Demonstration grant proposal
Fiduciary agency
Health program grant proposal
In-kind contribution
Letter of transmittal
Memorandum of understanding (MOU)
Needs assessment
Ongoing activity grants
Operational assistance grants
Planning grant proposal
Problem definition

Program description
Program objectives
Request for application (RFA)
Request for proposal (RFP)
Research grant proposal
Seed money
Soft money
Sole source grants
Solicited grant
Special project grant
Technical assistance grant proposal
Technical grant proposal
Training grant proposal
Unsolicited grants

More and more, health care is moving to the community, a setting in which grant funding is frequently available and needed. For example, programs focusing on health care screening, education, and prevention may be eligible for foundation or government funds. Financial skills such as budget preparation are as applicable to writing a health program grant proposal as a business plan. Skills in budget control and monitoring, financial analysis, and financial reporting are useful in managing grant funding. This chapter discusses definitions and purposes of grant proposals, identifies ways to locate sources for funding, covers the key components of health program grant proposals, provides insights on evaluating health program grant proposals, and offers tips for grant renewals. The sections typically included in health program grant applications are described. A sample grant proposal is included in Appendix D.

Types of Grant Proposals

There are various categories of grant proposals, so it is important to be clear about definitions and approaches. One category of grant proposals frequently seen in health care is the **research grant proposal**, which focuses on the investigator's topic and methodology for study or evaluation. Research proposals are not the focus of this chapter, and readers interested in developing research proposals should consult research methods texts for such information.

The category of grant proposal covered in this chapter is the **health program grant proposal**, a positive, convincing report that outlines a plan for a specified health care program or service and maximizes the opportunity for funding. It typically focuses on planning or providing a specific service or set of services (in other words, a program) to a target population in need of care.

Health program grant proposals may request funding to plan for services. This type of health program proposal, a **planning grant proposal**, provides funding (typically for no more than 1 to 2 years) to assess community needs, plan the program, and network with community providers, advocates, agencies, and experts to address the problem and implement and maintain the proposed program. For example, the Healthy Start program provides up to $50,000 over 1 to 2 years for collaborative planning for the health of children in eligible schools.

Other types of grant proposals include **training grant proposals**, which provide staff training and education, and **technical assistance grant proposals**, which assist in developing, implementing, and managing the activities of a community organization. For example, the Healthy Start program provides up to $300,000 over 3 to 5 years for operational grants. These grants are used to train staff and provide technical

TABLE 13-1

Types and Purposes of Health Program Grant Proposals

Type	Purpose
Planning	Requests funding a community needs assessment, program planning, and networking to develop and enhance community-level coordination, collaboration, and partnership in addressing the health problem
Training	Asks for funding to provide staff training and education
Technical assistance	Justifies funding for developing, implementing, and managing the activities of a community organization
Demonstration	Requests funding for model programs, services, or methodologies
Capital improvement	Applies for funding to build or renovate buildings or to acquire capital equipment
Operational assistance	Requests funding to help fund overhead and maintain the day-to-day activities of the organization

assistance in the development of health programs for children attending eligible schools. An increasingly popular type of health program proposal is the **demonstration grant proposal**, which funds state-of-the-art or model programs, services, or methodologies.

Planning grants are frequently linked to technical assistance or demonstration grants. Typically, an agency applies for planning grant funds to assess need, design a program, and establish community collaboration. Once that stage is complete, it applies for health program funding to implement the plan.

Capital improvement grants, which provide funding to build or renovate buildings and to acquire capital equipment, are fairly rare in the health arena. **Operational assistance grants**, which fund overhead expenses and the day-to-day support of the organization implementing the program, are also unusual. Funders typically expect applicants to fund their own operational and capital expenses from sources other than grants.

Table 13-1 summarizes the major types of grant proposals and their purposes.

Purposes of Health Program Grant Proposals

Health program grant proposals serve several purposes. The grant proposal is a written plan describing a health care program; it specifies available and needed resources, activities required to carry out the program, and budget requirements, all within a given time frame. Even if the grant proposal is not funded as requested, a well-written proposal provides a blueprint for implementing the program, regardless of the source of funding.

The grant proposal makes a request for specific resources, as well as a promise of performance within the budget that is funded. Contracts are frequently used by government funders. Although other funders may regard grants as somewhat less formal than a contract, grant proposals should be viewed as contracts to the extent that the proposal states a given service or program will be provided for a given sum of money.

Primarily, however, the grant proposal is an instrument of persuasion. By identifying one or more community needs that require the proposed program, the grant proposal should convince the funder that a serious problem or gap in services exists. It should also show that the proposed program is the best way to address this problem or gap in services, and that the agency submitting the proposal is the best qualified to provide the proposed program.

Other Types of Grants

Special project grants typically fund new, special, pilot, or demonstration projects. Funding for special project grants is often referred to as **seed money** because it serves to start a project or program; the agency receiving the grant is expected to maintain the program on its own. By contrast, grants funding ongoing activities (**ongoing activity grants**) may extend for 3 to 5 years or even longer to fund selected programs continuously.

Depending on the policies of the funder, grant proposals may be **solicited grants** (grants that are formally and periodically requested by the funding agency). Frequently such a solicited request is referred to as a **request for proposal (RFP)** or a **request for application (RFA)**. In these health program grant funding announcements, application and funding criteria are specific and detailed, and a proposal must target and address these criteria to qualify for funding. There usually is a specific deadline for proposal submission. Government funders typically use the RFP or RFA approach, with application forms, guidelines, and deadlines for submitting proposals. However, most proposals are for **unsolicited grants**: foundations frequently have some policies around funding (for example, funding only children's programs, or only in a particular geographic area) but accept proposals without a lot of formal criteria, if any, and allowing submission at any time of the year rather than adhering to specific deadlines.

Technical grant proposals focus on the program's objectives, activities, methods, organization, and staffing. By contrast, **business grant proposals** describe the budget, pricing, and all other financial information. In most cases, these are two sections of the same grant proposal rather than two separate proposals.

Health program grant proposals frequently restrict funding to direct service provision as provided by the program described in the grant proposal, with little or no funding allowed for operating or capital expenses. Some funders may allow the purchase or rental of equipment directly related to program operation, but rarely fund building, renovation, or major capital equipment expenses. A number of funders allow a percentage of funds to the sponsoring organization for overhead; this practice is more common among governmental funders than private foundations. However, funders typically restrict operational assistance funding, expecting instead that applicants will be able to maintain the day-to-day operations of their organization independent of the grant funding.

Grant funding also varies depending on the amount of competition. **Sole source grants** occasionally occur when one and only one organization in the community demonstrates the ability to carry out a program and is selected without competing with other organizations. Even in the case of sole source funding, though, a proposal is still required. More frequently, grant funding is competitive (**competitive grants**), with several agencies vying for the funding. Increasingly, funders are encouraging or even requiring interagency planning, coordination, collaborative efforts, and partnerships as a criterion for grant funding to reduce duplication of programs and to make better use of the scarce funding available.

Funding Sources

There are many sources for grant funding, although it is sometimes difficult to find the exact match between the funding needed and the funding available for specific health care programs. One way to classify funding sources is government versus private. Federal, state, and local agencies and programs fund grants, typically via an RFP or RFA process in which funding is available for applicants submitting proposals by a given deadline for specified activities meeting specific guidelines. An example of an RFP issued by a government agency is shown in Box 13-1.

Private funders are typically represented by charitable foundations, such as The Robert Wood Johnson Foundation. Foundations may solicit grant proposals via an RFP or RFA process but in many cases use a much less structured and formal approach in which the proposal need only meet the foundation's requirements for funding to be reviewed.

To locate funders that can be targeted for grant proposals, foundation centers and public libraries frequently have directories of government and private funding sources. Although traditionally hard-copy government catalogs and directories such as *The Foundation Directory* were the key ways to locate grant funders, most grant funders can now be located on the Internet. One suggestion in locating as many potential funders as possible is to do an Internet search, combining the search term "grant" with the key words for the program, such as "grant + mammography + Hispanic women."

Key Components of Proposals

Although funders may vary in their specific requirements for the contents of grant proposals, and the page length may also vary accordingly, this chapter presents all the components that are likely to be required by the funder, or at least helpful to consider and address in submitting a grant proposal. These components include a letter of transmittal, items that promote clarity, and a convincing introduction. Nearly all health

---

BOX 13-1

Example of a Request for Proposal (RFP), Government Funder

TITLE: Alcohol Education Project Grants (NIH Guide, Sept. 10, 1999, PAS-99-165)

AGENCY: National Institute on Alcohol Abuse and Alcoholism (NIAAA)

SCOPE: Broad ranges of educational approaches are included within the context of this announcement. Examples of anticipated activities include: (1) Educational activities directed to patients, their families, and the general public which impart knowledge gained through research on alcohol-related health issues, including those related to screening, treatment, and prevention; (2) Educational activities directed toward enhancing the knowledge of primary and secondary school educators and/or students on alcohol-related problems; and (3) Educational activities directed toward college students and college-age individuals, which apply knowledge gained through research in addressing the particular alcohol issues confronting this age group.

DEADLINE: Ongoing.

CONTACT: Application Kits: (301) 435-0714. Programmatic Information: [personal name and direct phone number excluded]

Source: Rural Information Center Health Service. (September 15, 2002). Federal Grant Opportunities Relevant to Rural Health. Beltsville, MD: National Agricultural Library. http://www.nal.usda.gov/ric/richs/grants.htm

program grant proposals require problem definition and the results of a community needs assessment, program objectives, and a clear description of the program and its activities.

The proposal nearly always must describe the resources available to the agency, the resources that are needed, and a budget that itemizes, explains, and totals the amount of funding requested. Increasingly, both government and private funders want to see a plan for evaluating the program as part of the grant proposal. Typically funders review and evaluate the qualifications that the applicant provides in a capability statement. It is often advisable to conclude a proposal with a brief statement regarding plans for ongoing funding and maintenance of the program, should it prove to meet expectations.

The proposal is likely to be reviewed by more than one person in the funding agency. Moreover, some parts of the proposal may be read by some reviewers and other parts by other reviewers. Thus, it is not only acceptable but also frequently necessary to repeat certain information in several parts of the proposal, such as contact information and a proposal summary.

Letter of Transmittal

Even if not specifically required, it is customary to include a cover letter or **letter of transmittal** when sending the proposal to the funding agency. This letter is frequently the first part of the proposal the funding reviewer sees, so make sure it sets the tone for the proposal and introduces the agency and specific contacts sending the proposal. The letter of transmittal should be brief, neat, clear, and accurate and should be written on the official letterhead of the applicant. The grant proposal must be sent to the right contact person in the right department of the funding agency.

The letter of transmittal should include the name, address, and phone number of the applicant and clear and specific contact information. The funder should know whom to contact in the agency regarding any questions or further discussion of the proposal, and how this person can be reached. A brief summary of the proposal should make up the body of the letter, including a brief explanation of why this particular funder was selected for the proposal. The letter may be concluded by reviewing the applicant's interest, capability, and experience.

Items Promoting Clarity

The primary purpose of a health program grant proposal is to present a convincing statement for funding for a proposed program, and a clearly written and logically organized proposal will help the reviewer read and understand the proposal, increasing the chances that funding will be provided.

The title page includes the title of the proposal, the date it was submitted, the name and address of the funding agency and of the agency submitting the proposal, along with contact information. The proposal should be organized logically, beginning with the introduction and continuing through the various sections as outlined in this chapter or as specified by the funder. Proposals longer than six to eight pages should be accompanied by a one- or two-page summary of the proposal, with a paragraph summarizing each major section. Proposals longer than six to eight pages should use headings and, if necessary, subheadings that clearly indicate the sections of the proposal. Proposals longer than 20 to 25 pages should include a table of contents so reviewers can quickly locate sections of the proposal that are of interest. All of these features will help the reader to grasp the message in the proposal.

The proposal requires careful proofreading and revision; if possible, an outside reader should be invited to review the proposal and make critical comments, particularly related to clarity. One should avoid jargon and colloquialisms and spell out acronyms the first time they are used, unless it is certain they will be understood. For example, CHF should be spelled out as "congestive heart failure (CHF)" the first time the term is used, with "CHF" used thereafter, unless it is certain that the persons reviewing the grant is familiar with the acronym.

If appendices are used, they should be identified and discussed in the proposal. The appendices should be numbered in the order in which they are mentioned in the proposal. For example, if a table of needs assessment results is first mentioned in the proposal, it is identified as Appendix 1; if next a budget table is mentioned, it is identified as Appendix 2; and so on.

Proposal Introduction

Just like the letter of transmittal, the introduction should establish the tone and theme of the proposal. It should capture the attention and interest of the reviewer, increasing the likelihood that the entire proposal will be reviewed and funded. The introduction should begin with the title and name of the applicant organization and the name of the funding source. It should be clear what RFP, RFA, or funder interest the proposal addresses. The introduction should briefly describe the geographic area of the program, the target population to be served, the purpose and significance of the program, and the basic approach and major activity of the program.

Problem Definition and Needs Assessment

Following the introduction, the applicant needs to discuss the proposed program. This section should define the problem, document the need for the program in the target population, and discuss the purpose and benefits of the program. The program's model, rationale, or conceptual framework can be presented and compared to other approaches.

The **problem definition** describes the nature, extent, and seriousness of the problem in enough detail to convince the funder of the problem's importance. For example, if the problem is a communicable disease, the problem definition should include a discussion of the disease process, mortality and harmful sequelae attributed to the disease, costs of the disease, and trends in incidence and prevalence.

The overall aims or goals of the program should then be discussed. Details of the program should be given later in the proposal; for the purposes of this section, the proposal should focus on the benefits, not the mechanics, of the program, in a brief and specific way. If applicable, this section should then discuss the model, rationale, or conceptual framework upon which the program is based. A review of relevant literature comparing programs based on similar or different models or frameworks may be useful. Another approach is to critique similar programs based on other models or frameworks and point out why the model or framework selected would be more effective.

Documenting Need

By now the funder should have at least an introductory understanding of the problem the proposed program addresses and the overall goals and approaches the program will use. A **needs assessment** can help the applicant clearly and convincingly present the extent and seriousness of need for the program in the target community.

There are various ways to document need. One approach is to present quantitative data, such as statistical or epidemiologic findings, or demographic information. These data must be accurate, relevant, and clear to the reader. Explain any data used in the proposal, ensure that the data are accurate, and clearly identify the sources of data. Include data only when it is relevant to the needs assessment and the proposal; do not include tables of data merely to serve as "filler." The results of relevant surveys to assess community needs can be quite helpful. These surveys may have been funded by a related planning grant. Quantitative data should report and reinforce evidence of the extent and seriousness of the need, such as the extent of demand, the characteristics of the target group, and the number of persons who are unserved or underserved by current programs.

Qualitative data may include observations or stories indicating and supporting the existence of need. For example, in a proposal for a program to reduce tobacco use by teenagers, a content analysis of local cigarette billboards may be helpful. Anecdotes may be quite helpful and convincing: for instance, a teenage girl's story of how easy it is to buy cigarettes, or the reasons why she and her peers decided to start smoking and now wish they could stop.

Documentation of need may include a discussion of the limitations of existing programs, comparing differences between the proposed program and existing programs. If the limitations of existing programs were discussed earlier in the proposal in comparing and contrasting the proposed program's model or framework to that of existing programs, this information need not be repeated, but it may be helpful to briefly remind the reviewer of that earlier discussion.

Objectives

The proposal's **program objectives** are clearly stated, measurable tasks intended to achieve a goal within a specific time frame. Program objectives should be limited in number, realistic to achieve, measurable, set within an appropriate time frame, and linked to program activities and the program evaluation plan. Program objectives must be clearly related and linked to the problem definition, needs assessment, and program goals and the proposal's resource needs and budget.

Many beginning grant writers try to do too much in their proposals. For each program objective specified in the proposal, there must be associated program activities and measures to evaluate the achievement of the objective. The more objectives proposed, the more difficult it may be to demonstrate success. Therefore, use three to seven key program objectives (unless the proposal involves a highly complex, long-term program with considerable funding expected). Setting such a limit will help the grant writer include only the objectives that are most important to meet the identified needs.

Program objectives should be reasonably realistic, depending on the specific problem, target population, resources and capability, program design, and any other factors that affect success. Funders may question the capability of a program to meet a given need at a 100% level, so set objectives that seem reasonable given the potential obstacles involved. On the other hand, avoid setting the bar too low; indicate a high enough expectation for achievement that the funder could expect a demonstrated improvement or impact on the problem being addressed. Be aware of success rates, quality indicators, and other measures of achieving objectives commonly reported for this kind of problem.

Although it is frequently difficult to measure whether health program objectives have been achieved, particularly in areas such as prevention, awareness, and education, it is also difficult to convince a funder that objectives have been achieved without measures that can be used in evaluation reports. Numbers of clients and client contacts, survey scores, numbers of clients completing a given program, immunization levels for given age groups, and other measures can be used to help quantify objectives.

The objectives should have a specific time frame related to the funding cycle and guidelines. If the grant funding is for a fiscal year, objectives should be completed within that year. If funding guidelines specify that any start-up must be completed by the end of the second month of funding, objectives related to start-up activities should not stretch beyond this deadline.

Finally, program objectives should be linked to program activities and to the plan for program evaluation. After all, program activities are the methods used to reach program objectives, and the evaluation plan is the design used to measure and report the extent to which program objectives are achieved. One way to link program objectives, program activities, and program evaluation is to use a three-part design for writing program objectives in the proposal:

- Objective: specific, achievable, measurable, time frame
- Activities: two to five specific activities that will achieve the objective
- Evaluation: two to five ways that progress in achieving the objective will be identified and measured

Although this method may not meet the requirements or be useful for all health program grant proposals, and although it may seem a bit tedious to write objectives according to this outline, this approach is very helpful in clearly identifying and linking program objectives, activities, and evaluation methods. Particularly for a smaller program, this approach reduces or even eliminates the amount of additional writing needed for the sections on program activities and evaluation, since the program activities and the evaluation plan are outlined in the discussion of the objectives. In larger grant proposals, or when this approach seems awkward, program activities and evaluation may be included in separate sections. Some beginning grant writers find it helpful to use this approach as a starting point for their proposals because they can organize their ideas about addressing the problem they have identified.

Box 13-2 presents an example of a program objective that links program activities and program evaluation.

Program Description

A **program description** is just that: a description of the program and its activities. Clearly discuss the program's methods and operations. Indicate how, not just what, activities will be done to achieve objectives. For example, if teen clients in a smoking prevention program are to design artwork to display on the outside of city buses, how will this be accomplished? Clearly link activities to objectives, within a specified timetable.

Resources and Resource Needs

This section of the health program grant proposal first describes the resources that are available for use by the proposed program, then identifies the resources that are needed. The resource needs can then be itemized and costed out in the program proposal budget and discussed in terms of funding needs. It is necessary to describe the organizational structure of the agency applying for the grant, including the number of employees, number of clients, annual budget, board of directors, and physical space. This section then identifies the organizational administration and persons responsible for decision making, coordination, and accountability; including an organizational chart, if relevant, in the appendix. If the proposed program will be part of a larger operation, one must explain how the new program will fit into the organization as a whole.

This section discusses available staffing, physical facilities, and equipment in relation to the proposed program. Resources that are already available and that will be contributed by the applying organization are

---

☐ **B O X 1 3 · 2**

Example of Program Objective Linking Program Activities and Program Evaluation

---

Objective I: Community outreach for mammograms for women in the Woodside neighborhood will be provided to at least 150 women over the fiscal year the program is funded (4–6 weekly, 16–24 monthly, 48–72 quarterly).

Activities to achieve Objective I:

a. Weekly 6-hour visits to the ABC supermarket using the mobile mammography van in the Woodside neighborhood, examining 4–6 clinically and financially eligible women per visit.
b. Public awareness of the mobile mammography van via a free public service broadcast on XYZ radio for the first 3 months of the program.

Evaluation of Objective I:

a. Count of eligible clients examined weekly, monthly, quarterly, and annually, with at least 75% of the target number examined (3–4 weekly, 12–18 monthly, 36–54 quarterly, 112 annually).
b. Public service broadcast on XYZ radio for August through October of the program year.

---

frequently referred to as **in-kind contributions**. Funders typically look favorably on organizations that show a strong willingness to contribute to the implementation of their proposed programs or services. It is important to describe staff members in terms of qualifications, responsibilities for program activities, and the amount of time they will contribute to the proposed program. Physical facilities typically include office, clinic, classroom, or other space needed by the proposed program, its clients, and its staff. Equipment may include vehicles, office equipment, or other equipment needed for program implementation.

Increasingly, funders want to encourage the development of community partnerships and collaborative efforts to help reduce duplication of services, make the best use of scarce funding resources, and ensure that communities work together, rather than in opposition, to resolve problems and meet needs. For this reason, many health program grant proposals are strengthened by including a description of agency partnerships, coalitions, and successful collaborative efforts. Letters of support, in which agencies and influential individuals in the community endorse the applicant's efforts, provide evidence of good interagency and community relationships but are not always clear regarding the extent of collaboration.

It is frequently helpful to include in the appendix a **memorandum of understanding (MOU)** documenting the contributions that collaborating agencies will provide to the proposed program; discuss these MOUs in the resources section. For example, if the local chapter of the Lung Association agrees to provide 5,000 pediatric asthma awareness brochures to the proposed school-based pediatric asthma program, the MOU, on the Lung Association's official letterhead, briefly discusses their support of the program, their contribution, and its estimated dollar value. Although MOUs are not guarantees that these promises of contributions will be honored in full, they are strong indications of collaborative support and typically are a substantial source of resources. Many funders strongly approve of MOUs, and some funders, such as the Healthy Start Program, require them. The use of MOUs is increasingly important in grant proposals that focus on addressing community-level problems that require interagency collaboration and coordination.

Resource needs represent the staffing, physical space, equipment, supplies, and any other resources not provided via an in-kind or MOU contribution. This section must be linked to the objectives and program activities and should logically relate to the budget section. For example, if an objective specifies mobile community outreach for mammograms and the program activities include the use of a van equipped to perform these examinations, the van might be available from the organization applying for the grant as an in-kind contribution, but resource needs might include fuel, maintenance, and supplies.

Budget and Explanation

The budget presents and explains estimated expenses and revenues for the proposed program in dollars. It is often simpler and clearer to prepare a budget table with the line item details for expenses and, if applicable, revenues, and to include this budget table in the appendix. Key items and highlights of the overall budget may then be discussed in the budget section of the proposal. In continuing the example of the mammography van, the budget section would discuss the amount and rationale for budget estimates for fuel, maintenance, and supply expenses that were identified in the resource needs section of the proposal.

A two-step process may be very useful in preparing a proposed expense budget. In the first step, the applicant identifies the resource needs and converts them to expense budget line items within categories of personnel and the non-personnel categories of equipment and supplies. One must link associated dollar figures to the line items and total the expense budget. In the second step, the applicant must critically review each line item with an eye toward reducing the expense as much as possible, or even eliminating it. It is essential to re-evaluate how to increase the amount of in-kind contributions available, and re-examine potential community contributions via MOUs. In the example of the van, possibly a local service station would provide an MOU that it will donate some fuel or provide fuel at a discount. The agency submitting the proposal might increase its in-kind contribution to cover the maintenance of the van and mammography equipment. A local chapter of the American Cancer Society might provide an MOU donating some of the supplies, such as paper gowns. This is an effective technique for reducing an initial expense budget while cultivating partnerships and agency support.

Budget estimates should be as accurate as possible, so the budget is realistic and justifiable to the funder. Proposal reviewers frequently have considerable familiarity with programs and typical expenses and revenues and are likely to recognize when grant writers overbudget ("pad") or underbudget. Overbudgeting may seem like a good strategy for several reasons: the extra resources would cover unanticipated expenses or organizational needs such as a staff position; funders are likely to fund less than the budget requested; and program management appears efficient, as the manager can more easily remain within the budget. However, funders are likely to recognize this strategy and cut the funding award accordingly, or to favor competing proposals that show more accurate budget estimates and demonstrate a more cost-effective approach.

Underbudgeting may also appear to be a good strategy, as it appears that the proposed program is run more cost-effectively than competing programs. Again, however, funders are likely to recognize underbudgeting and to question the capability of the agency submitting the proposal if the budget estimates are not realistic. It is best to develop and present the most accurate and realistic budget estimates possible.

In some cases, despite the best efforts to present a realistic and accurate budget, the funding agency offers funding far below that which is necessary to implement or maintain the proposed program. After reviewing budget figures and repeating the process of determining whether line items might be further reduced by additional in-kind contributions and community support, the available funding might still not be adequate to implement or maintain the proposed program. At that stage, it is advisable to diplomatically refuse unrealistic expense budget cuts, with a careful re-explanation of the expense budget. In many cases, other funding sources are available, and a search for these sources and re-application of the proposal to a new funding source may eventually provide support for the proposed program.

Evaluation Plan

While an evaluation plan is not always mandatory, it is becoming increasingly important as funders focus on the achievement of objectives outlined in the proposal. Even if this section is not included in the proposal itself, drafting an evaluation plan while preparing the proposal will facilitate internal monitoring and management should the program be funded. Further, writing a program proposal with evaluation in mind is likely to improve the selection and description of objectives. The first step in developing a convincing and effective evaluation is to establish objectives that are specific, realistic, measurable, and contained within a specific time frame. When objectives are written according to these criteria, indicators may be established to determine whether the objectives were achieved.

A timeline for evaluation should be part of the evaluation plan. This timeline should include periodic monitoring, not just at the end of the funding year. Program evaluation for monitoring purposes should probably take place at least monthly, with quarterly reports and a final end-of-the-year report. Some funders require periodic evaluation reports.

For example, the objectives for the mobile mammography van specify the screening of at least 150 eligible clients over the year the program is funded. It is frequently not realistic to expect to achieve objectives at a 100% level. For this reason, the grant writer, using experience, established standards, or funding guidelines, should set reasonable indicators of success at some point below 100%, yet at a level that would reasonably satisfy funders that the program is worthwhile. The associated indicator for success is determined to be 75% of this objective, or screening at least 112 women.

In many cases, it is difficult to evaluate program objectives. In some cases, intangible outcomes such as improving the quality of life for a home-bound person with Alzheimer's makes it difficult to measure the achievement of objectives. In other cases, there may be unmeasurable outcomes, such as a client's lifetime HIV risk-reduction behavior following an HIV prevention course. The evaluation plan should identify variables influencing successful outcomes, such as completed assessments of the home and the caregiver for the person with Alzheimer's, or the client's completion of an HIV risk-reduction course.

Identify data requirements and sources for the data needed to evaluate the program. It is important to describe measurement instruments, such as standardized questionnaires or equipment. If it will be necessary to develop a measurement instrument, such as a client satisfaction survey, this section should discuss a time frame and plan for development, pretesting, and refinement of the instrument.

Indicate the methods that will be used to collect data, including sampling methods, if applicable. The applicant must explain data reporting and analysis, with an overview of the content of the evaluation reports. Staffing and management of evaluation must be described so it is clear to the funder that staff and management are designated to be accountable for performing and reviewing the evaluation.

Capability Statement

The **capability statement** presents a convincing description of the qualifications of the agency and participating staff in implementing the proposed program. It should summarize the abilities, competence, resources (size and budget), personnel, experience, achievements, viability, reputation, and philosophy of the applicant. As relevant, the applicant's origins and history, particularly as related to the proposed program should be briefly discussed. The applicant must provide evidence of adherence to standards, community endorsements, and ongoing support such as partnerships. Any other relevant information regarding capability, such as previous success in programs with the same or similar populations should be included.

Plans for Future Funding

Increasingly, funders want to see planning and development strategies for maintaining programs beyond the proposal's funding period. Frequently, funders provide seed money to start the proposed program, while expecting applicants to develop plans and strategies for ongoing program operation. As a result, applicants should describe ongoing program operation plans and strategies (for example, efforts to develop ongoing community partnerships, or fund-raising strategies). There may be plans to introduce fees for services,

TABLE 13-2

Recommended Components of Health Program Grant Proposals in Suggested Order

Component	Purpose
Letter of transmittal	Cover letter for proposal; establishes the tone and theme and provides contact information
Summary or abstract	Summarizes the proposal
Title page, headers, table of contents	Helps keep the proposal clear and well-organized
Introduction	Establishes the tone and theme of the proposal, reinforces clarity, and provides contact information
Problem definition	Convincingly describes and discusses the extent and importance of the health problem
Needs assessment	Documents the target population's need for the health program
Program objectives	Presents methods to achieve program goals that are limited in number, achievable, measurable, set within a time frame, and linked to program activities and the program evaluation plan
Program description	Describes the program that is designed to meet program objectives
Resources	Identifies resources available within the applying organization (in-kind contributions) and from outside partnering organizations (MOUs)
Resource needs	Identifies resources beyond those available, which are linked to the proposal budget and funding request
Budget	Itemizes personnel and non-personnel costs, linked to program objectives and resource needs
Evaluation plan	Details a plan to evaluate the extent to which program objectives are met
Capability statement	Justifies why the applicants (both individual and organizational) are qualified to carry out the proposed program
Plan for future funding	Explains how the program will be supported beyond the proposal's funding period

or to obtain approval for reimbursement by payors such as Medicaid or insurers. If the proposed program is based within a larger agency such as a non-profit organization or a health department, plans for increasing agency support beyond the proposed funding period should be discussed.

Table 13-2 summarizes the key components of health program grant proposals in their suggested order of inclusion.

Evaluating Proposals

All the recommendations provided for grant writing may be applied to the evaluation of health program proposals. Typically, health program proposals are evaluated on the basis of clarity, completeness, responsiveness, internal consistency, external consistency, understanding of problem and services, capability and effectiveness, efficiency and accountability, and realism.

Grant Renewals

Grant funding is sometimes referred to as **soft money**, or income that may or may not be available; this captures the uncertainty of the grant funding situation. Even if funding has been approved for more than 1 year, funding typically is on a yearly basis, and the applicant must provide an annual report and re-apply for continued funding. Grant recipients must adhere to the funder's requirements and implement effective reporting mechanisms that provide evidence that funding requirements were met. It is important to maintain

---

☐ B O X 1 3 · 3

On-line Sources for Information on Grant Writing

Comprehensive International Program of Research on AIDS (CIPRA) planning and organizational grant-writing: http://www.niaid.nih.gov/daids/cipra/r03.htm
Federal Register: http://www.access.gpo.gov/fr/index.html
Foundation Center: www.fdncenter.org
Grantmakers in Health: http://www.gih.org/
Office of Minority Health Resource Center: http://www.omhrc.gov/OMHRC/funding.htm
NIH Guide for Grants and Contracts: http://grants1.nih.gov/grants/guide/index.html

---

positive relationships with the funding agency, and diplomatically resolve any misunderstandings, miscommunications, or differences that might arise.

The applicant must ensure that the program is managed effectively. Many of the principles of financial management are covered in other chapters of this text, including budgeting and financial reporting. Although principles of program management are beyond the scope of this text, there are many resources helpful to health program managers, such as Breckon (1997). In many settings, the applicant enlists the assistance of a **fiduciary agency**, which assumes the responsibility for financial management of the grant and handles activities such as writing reimbursement checks and paying bills, salaries, and wages. The fiduciary agency may be an umbrella organization (for example, a school district office managing the Healthy Start program grant awarded to one of its schools), or it may be an agency outside the overall organization. In either case, the fiduciary agency typically requires payment of a given percentage of the grant award for its services.

Careful recordkeeping, evidence of outcomes and program success, and strategies for expanding or revising the program are elements to consider in successful grant renewal.

Conclusion

This chapter describes various types of health program proposals and their purpose. The components of a typical health program proposal are provided, with information on seeking funding and evaluating proposals. Box 13-3 provides Internet resources for grant writing and seeking grant funding for programs in health care settings.

■ C R I T I C A L   T H I N K I N G   E X E R C I S E S

1. Think about a new program or service that would benefit from grant funding in your work setting or a health care setting of interest. Identify at least three potential funders for this program or service. Narrow your selection to a single funder you believe would be most likely to fund your proposal, and explain your rationale for targeting this funder. Who is the best contact in this funding agency?

2. Identify what you believe would be the three easiest and the three most difficult elements to prepare if you were writing a health program proposal for the work or selected health care setting identified in Exercise 1. In other words, would the needs assessment, program description, and budget be easiest or

most difficult, or the objectives, evaluation plan, or capability statement? Compare your assessment with that of other students and discuss.

3. Using the selected health care setting from Exercise 1, prepare a draft grant proposal and exchange it with another students (or show it to an outside reader) for feedback on clarity, formatting, and capability. How does this help you revise and rethink your final proposal?

■ R E F E R E N C E S

Bauer, D. G. (1999). *The "How to" grants manual: Successful grant-seeking techniques for obtaining public and private grants*, 4th ed. Phoenix, AZ: Oryx Press.

Breckon, D. J. (1997). *Managing health promotion programs*. Gaithersburg, MD: Aspen.

Gitlin, L. N., & Lyons, K. J. (1996). *Successful grant writing: strategies for health and human service professionals*. New York: Springer.

Graham, B. (March 21, 2001). *Business planning for grassroots nonprofits*. The Management Center Best Practices Conference, Oakland, CA.

Kibel, B. M. (May 27, 1999). *Outcome engineering: an overview*. Workshop sponsored by Bay Area Health Ministries, Fairfield, CA.

Oakland Unified School District. (2000). *Healthy Start support services application for funding. Planning grant application*. Oakland, CA.

Oakland Unified School District. (2001). *Healthy Start support services application for funding. Operational grant application*. Oakland, CA.

Sugiwaka, H., & Odero-Winegar, M. (1999). *Suggested example for writing health program objectives*. Unpublished, from course paper in Masters of Nursing Community Health Program at Holy Names College, Oakland, CA.

U.S. Dept. of Health & Human Services. (Sept. 17, 1999). Framework for program evaluation in public health. *MMWR, 48*(RR-11), entire publication. *http://www2.cdc.gov/mmwr/mmwrsrch.htm*

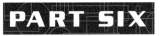

PART SIX

International Perspectives and Future Trends

CHAPTER 14

International Health Economics Issues

⬛ Learning Objectives

1. Compare and contrast at least two types of national health care systems, identifying strengths and limitations of each.
2. Compare the performance of the U.S. health care system to that of at least two other nations, including factors such as population age and health care spending per capita or as a percent of GDP.
3. Identify at least two global problems or issues related to health care economics, finance, and budgeting.

◯ Key Terms

Gross domestic product
International dollar
National health insurance
National health service

Pluralistic health system
Rationing
Socialized health service

Why should we discuss the economics of health care in countries other than our own? One reason is to review other health care systems and approaches. Another reason is to make comparisons between the United States and other countries across measures such as national and per capita expenditures. An additional reason is that globalization is an external economic factor that can influence health care economics and financing.

Learning about international health care economics also provides insights regarding concerns that many nations share. Recall in Chapter 1 that three major expectations of health care providers and consumers are high quality, access, and cost control. These expectations are shared by providers and consumers around the world, not just Americans. This chapter gives a brief overview of international health care systems, economic comparisons in health care, and health care economics concerns shared by the United States and other countries.

Health Care Systems

Table 14-1 shows three major types of health care systems prevalent in the major industrialized nations. The first type, the **pluralistic health system**, is what exists in the United States. It combines government and non-government providers and funders but does not provide universal guarantees of health care coverage for its citizens and residents. The pluralistic system, an incredibly complex and fragmented set of insurers and providers, evolved over time from an earlier, almost entirely private approach to health care in the United States. Medicare and Medicaid programs, established in the 1960s as part of the Johnson administration's War on Poverty efforts, provide funding to cover the health care of persons age 65 and older and some poor and uninsured persons and families. Many employed persons are able to purchase health insurance for themselves and their families through group plans offered by their employers (often with employers paying some of the costs). Other persons do not meet government or non-government insurance criteria and are uninsured unless they are able and willing to pay for private health insurance.

Many industrialized countries in Europe, as well as Canada and Japan, have some type of **national health insurance**, in which the government guarantees health coverage for all its citizens but does not necessarily own or employ the health care providers. For example, Canadians are covered by national health insurance mandated by the Canadian government, but private-sector physicians and other health professionals are not directly employed by the government. In Canada, hospital operating costs are funded via the national health insurance system, so hospital budgets must be approved by the provincial government,

◯ TABLE 14-1

National Health Systems

Type of System	Pluralistic	National Health Insurance	National Health Service
Principal features	Some uninsured citizens & foreign residents; government & non-government providers; multiple government & non-government funding streams.	Universal coverage; government & non-government providers; often national & provincial budgets	Universal coverage; largely government providers; funding largely government with some self-pay
Typical problems	Uninsured populations	Health care rationing	Health care rationing
Examples of countries	United States	Canada, Japan, many European nations	Great Britain

Source: Adapted from V. G. Rodwin, in Kovner & Jonas, 1999.

which does allow for some governmental control over the hospital's size and scope of services. Many of the European nations with national health insurance systems have similar control over hospital capacity and costs. One problem is that of rationing (discussed in more depth later in this chapter), often manifested by waiting lists for elective or non-emergency health care services due to limits on capacity.

Great Britain has a **national health service**, not only guaranteeing health coverage for all its citizens but also owning and employing many of the health care providers. Although the number of private providers in Great Britain is growing as the number of persons willing to pay out-of-pocket for health care grows, most health care is provided through publicly owned and operated hospitals, clinics, and other settings. Rationing of some health care services is a problem under national health service systems, which is one reason for the growing popularity of private providers so people can "jump ahead" in the line rather than remaining on a waiting list for care.

The **socialized health service** system was established in the former U.S.S.R. and its satellite countries and now exists in Cuba. The socialized health service allows for little or no privately owned or employed providers and requires its citizens, who are guaranteed universal coverage, to seek services solely through government providers. Many people believe that if a government mandates universal health care coverage, then health care must become socialized, but this is not the case. The predominant system among the industrialized nations is for the government to mandate universal health care coverage but allow private entrepreneurship in the provision of health care services.

Economic Comparisons: Industrialized Nations

Table 14-2 shows health expenditures as a percent of **gross domestic product (GDP)**, or the total value of domestic goods and services produced by a country per year, the percent of the country's population age 65 and older, and total health care employment per thousand for nine industrialized nations that are members of the Organization for Economic Cooperation and Development (OECD). The United States shows the highest level of health expenditures as a percent of GDP, 12.9%, with the median at 8.4%. Germany shows the highest percent of persons age 65 and older, 16.8%, with the median at 14.1%. The rate of health employment is also highest in Germany, at 42.3 per thousand, with France at the median level of 26.4 per thousand.

In comparing the economic performance of the United States to other industrialized countries, Table 14-2 shows that although the proportion of elderly persons (who typically incur more health care costs than younger persons) and the rate of

○ **TABLE 14-2**

Health Spending, Population Age, and Health Employment in Selected OECD Countries, 1999

Country	% of GDP Spent on Health*	% of Population age 65+	Total Health Employment per thousand[†]
Australia	8.6%	12.2%	31.2
Canada	9.3%	12.4%	25.2
France	9.3%	15.9%	26.4
Germany	10.3%	16.8%	42.3
Japan	7.5%	16.7%	21.2
Mexico	5.3%	5.3%	6.7
New Zealand	8.1%	11.7%	—
Spain	7.0%	16.6%	15.7
United Kingdom	6.9%	15.7%	29.9
United States	12.9%	12.3%	32.6
Median	**8.4%**	**14.1%**	**26.4**

Source: OECD, OECD Health Data 2001.

* Australia, Germany, Japan, Mexico & Spain are 1998 data.

[†] Canada & France are 1994 data; Germany 1997 data; United States 1993 data.

health care employment is not the highest among the countries, the percent of GDP for health care expenditures in the United States is the highest among other nations. The greater ability of countries with national health plans to reduce funding streams and establish greater bargaining power for goods and services such as pharmaceuticals are factors in the differences in spending between the United States and other countries.

A 2001 health care survey conducted by the Commonwealth Fund compared experiences of adults with the health care system in Australia, Canada, New Zealand, the United Kingdom, and the United States. Waiting times for non-urgent (elective or non-emergency) surgery was longest in the United Kingdom and shortest in the United States. However, adults in the United Kingdom reported the fewest problems with health care access related to cost, while adults in the United States reported the highest rate of problems with health care access related to cost. Twenty-six percent of the U.S. respondents reported they did not fill a prescription over the past year due to cost, with the next highest reported by Australians (19%). Twenty-four percent of the U.S. respondents reported that they did not see a physician for a medical problem over the past year due to cost, with the next highest reported by New Zealanders (20%). Twenty-two percent of the U.S. respondents reported that they did not get a test, treatment, or follow-up care over the past year due to cost, with the next highest reported by Australians (15%). Twenty-one percent of the U.S. respondents reported problems paying medical bills, with the next highest reported by New Zealanders (11%). Reported disparities in health care access were even greater for low-income respondents, particularly in the United States. For most indicators, the United States ranked the lowest among the other industrialized countries surveyed in health care equity, access, and financing (Schoen, et al., 2002).

Issues in Developing Nations

Developing nations have some health care system issues that compound problems in providing high quality and access while controlling costs. The developing nation has a very small health care budget, possibly supplemented by financial donations, resulting in chronic, serious resource shortages. A relatively high proportion of this budget is often spent on personnel costs and capital budget, with very little investment in the maintenance of health care facilities. There are significant gaps in the availability and use of technology, even for interventions such as antibiotics that are common in industrialized nations.

Preparation, support, and working conditions for health care workers in developing countries are frequently far from adequate. There are often few resources available for training, education, and continuing education, resulting in shortages of trained, up-to-date personnel. In some developing countries there is an over-supply of physicians, resulting in increased health care costs even though overall health conditions do not improve. Inadequate pay and benefits and poor working conditions for physicians and other health care professionals often provide strong incentives for them to move to wealthier, industrialized nations to meet their shortages of health care workers, thus leaving the developing nations with even fewer resources. Box 14-1

☐ BOX 14·1

Disparities in Global Health Care Financing

"The resources devoted to health systems are very unequally distributed, and not at all in proportion to the distribution of health problems. Low and middle income countries account for only 18% of world income and 11% of global health spending ($250 billion or 4% of GDP in those countries). Yet 84% of the world's population live in these countries, and they bear 93% of the world's disease burden."

—World Health Organization (WHO). *The World Health Report 2000*, pg. 7.

contains a quote from a recent global report on health citing some dramatic disparities in resources between many developing and industrialized countries.

Table 14-3 compares a number of developing and industrialized countries using selected indicators for health expenditures and health status. The OECD nations (considered to be industrialized) listed in Table 14-2

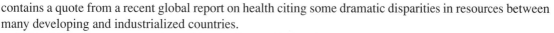

TABLE 14-3

Comparison of Selected Nations on Health Care Expenditures and Population Indicators, 1999

Countries by WHO Region	Population 000's, 1999	Expenditures as % of GDP	Total Per Capita Expenditures, 1997*	% Age 60+ 1999	Male Life Expectancy at Birth, 1999	Female Life Expectancy at Birth, 1999
African Region						
Eritrea	*3,719*	*3.4%*	*$6*	*4.6%*	*46.6*	*46.5*
Kenya	29,549	4.6%	$171	*4.4%*	*47.3*	*48.1*
Region of the Americas						
Canada	30,857	8.6%	$1,783	16.7%	**76.2**	81.9
Ecuador	12,411	4.6%	$75	6.8%	67.4	70.3
Mexico	97,365	5.6%	$240	6.8%	71.0	77.1
Nicaragua	*4,938*	8.0%	$35	*4.6%*	64.8	68.8
United States	**276,218**	**13.7%**	**$4,187**	16.4%	73.8	79.7
Eastern Mediterranean Region						
Egypt	67,226	3.7%	$44	6.3%	64.2	65.8
Pakistan	152,331	4.0%	*$17*	4.9%	62.6	64.9
European Region						
France	58,886	**9.8%**	$2,369	20.5%	74.9	**83.6**
Germany	82,178	**10.5%**	**$2,713**	**22.7%**	73.7	80.1
Spain	39,634	8.0%	$1,071	**21.6%**	75.3	82.1
South-East Asia Region						
India	**998,056**	5.2%	$23	7.5%	59.6	61.2
Indonesia	**209,255**	*1.7%*	$18	7.3%	66.6	69.0
Western Pacific Region						
Australia	18,705	7.8%	$1,730	16.1%	**76.8**	**82.2**
Japan	126,505	7.1%	**$2,373**	**22.6%**	**77.6**	**84.3**
Lao People's Democratic Republic	5,297	3.6%	*$13*	5.2%	*54.0*	*56.6*
Malaysia	21,830	*2.4%*	$110	6.5%	67.6	69.9
New Zealand	*3,828*	8.2%	$1,416	15.5%	73.9	79.3

Source: WHO, World Health Report 2000.

Three highest values in **bold**, three lowest values in *italics* for each indicator.

Data vary in completeness & reliability—see World Health Report 2000 notes on tables.

*Estimates at the official exchange rate, US $.

☐ **B O X   1 4 - 2**

The International Dollar

Given that the purchasing power of the currency of various nations may differ, the international dollar is calculated based on purchasing power parities (PPP), or conversions of currency that takes into account the differences in price levels between various nations.

are included in Table 14-3 for comparison purposes. For each indicator, the values for the three highest-ranking countries are indicated in **bold**, and for the three lowest ranking countries in *italics*. Box 14-2 provides an explanation of the **international dollar**, a unit of currency that takes the price levels of various countries into account.

As shown in Table 14-3, although the United States ranks the highest in health care expenditures as a percent of GDP and per capita expenditures, it is not the highest in its population age 60 years and over or in life expectancy. Compared to the 13.7% of GDP for health care in the U.S., developing countries commonly expend less than 6% of their GDP on health care.

Health Care Rationing

As mentioned earlier, many countries use health care **rationing** (mandatory policies limiting health care expenditures) as a way to control their health care costs. As the burden of health care costs has increased worldwide, some industrialized nations as well as many developing nations employ some form of rationing. Table 14-4 summarizes two of the most commonly used approaches to health care rationing among industrialized and developing nations.

○ **T A B L E   1 4 - 4**

Approaches to Health Care Rationing

Approach	Strict controls limiting the health care budget to an affordable level	Establish controls based on specific priorities determined by preset criteria
Target	Does not target specific diseases or interventions	Often provides an affordable "basic" or "essential" package of interventions
Principal features	Most common approach; most frequently used in countries with national health budgets	Social, political, and cost-effectiveness criteria used to determine priorities
Typical problems	Resources managed according to politics, often favoring the higher income citizens at the expense of the poor	Providers respond to demand for services outside the approved package; limitations to cost-effectiveness criteria
Examples of countries	Pre-1990 National Health System in the U.K., some European Union countries, some developing nations	The Netherlands, New Zealand, Norway, Sweden, Oregon (U.S.), Mexico, Bangladesh, Columbia, Zambia

Source: Adapted from WHO, World Health Report 2000.

The first approach, which is the more commonly used, is simply to limit the national budget for health care to what is considered an affordable level, without targeting specific diseases (such as HIV/AIDS) or interventions (such as cardiac catheterizations) for budget priorities or budget cuts. One problem with this approach is that the resource allocation decisions are often controlled by the parties in power, so that these decisions favor the relatively wealthier and more powerful citizens at the expense of those who are poorer and less powerful.

The second approach is to base the national (or state, in the case of Oregon) health care budget on specific priorities targeting diseases or interventions, using preset criteria. For example, a country may establish priorities for the vaccination of all children at the expense of the purchase of life-support or dialysis equipment largely used by the elderly. One advantage of this approach is its potential to incorporate "rationality" into rationing by using social and cost-effectiveness criteria in addition to political criteria.

The second approach, using specific priorities, also poses potential problems in its application. When consumers demand services not included in the approved "package," providers still face strong ethical and financial incentives to provide them regardless of the policy mandate. For example, if government policy does not fund dialysis for the elderly, providers may charge out-of-pocket fees for consumers who can pay and provide dialysis on a private basis, or find other ways of subsidizing this service. Another problem with the second approach is that cost-effectiveness criteria have limitations (see Chap.9) and may be politicized.

In short, there is no "absolute" method of rationing care that also meets everyone's expectations of high quality and access while controlling costs. However, in a time when health care resources cannot increase to meet all demand, rationing is an attempt to control and, if possible, improve the delivery of services.

Global Concerns

Nursing shortages are a concern in many industrialized and developing countries. Changing immigration laws to recruit more foreign nurses to countries facing shortages may not be an effective long-term solution, given the global nature of nursing shortages. The global nursing shortage is expected to worsen; factors common to many countries include declining job satisfaction, an aging workforce, and reduced retention in hospital settings. Similar problems exist regarding physicians, with industrialized countries such as the United States attracting many foreign physicians.

Global aging is another concern in many industrialized and developing countries. As of 1998, there were about 580 million persons worldwide age 60 and older; approximately 355 million of them lived in developing countries. It is projected that by 2020 there will be close to 1 billion persons worldwide age 60 and older; more than 700 million of them will reside in developing countries. Persons over age 60 are expected to represent 25% of Europe's population by 2020, 31% of Japan's population, and 23% of North America's population.

The federal government in the United States is debating how to address concerns about financing the Medicare program for American elderly. In 2000, Japan introduced a national old-age nursing care insurance plan financed by the government and by contributions from persons over age 40. Nine major countries in the OECD, besides the United States, have adopted patient classification systems similar to the Medicare DRGs as part of their health care reimbursement systems to better control costs.

Consumer and provider complaints about the quality of health care are increasing in many industrialized and developing countries. Issues include better reporting and reduction of medical errors, reducing waiting times for health care services, and increasing consultation time between physicians and patients.

Access to specialty physician care was a common concern in the Commonwealth Fund's 2001 survey. In the United States and New Zealand, the reason for problems with specialty access was cost; for Australia, Canada, and the United Kingdom, reasons were both cost and waiting times.

☐ **B O X   1 4 - 3**

On-line Sources for International Health Care Economics

Health Canada, Canada: http://www.hc-sc.gc.ca/
National Health Services (NHS), United Kingdom: http://www.york.ac.uk/inst/crd/
Organization for Economic Cooperation and Development (OECD): http://www.oecd.org/
Pan American Health Organization (PAHO): http://www.paho.org/
World Health Organization (WHO): http://www.who.int/

The majority of respondents in all countries in the Commonwealth Fund's 2001 survey indicated that their health care system requires fundamental change. Proposals for health care reform are also under development in Japan. Issues of improving health care quality and access while reducing cost are becoming more of a concern at a global level.

Conclusion

This chapter introduces concepts of health care economics, finance, and budgeting in countries other than the United States and compares the health care performance of other countries to the United States. Box 14-3 provides Internet resources for further information on international health care issues.

■ C R I T I C A L   T H I N K I N G   E X E R C I S E S

1. Locate and critique a website that focuses on international health issues or health issues in a country other than the United States. What problems of health care quality, access, and cost does it discuss or address?

2. Based on your own experience as a provider and consumer of health care goods and services in the United States, discuss how you would rate this country in health care quality, access, and cost. How do you think the United States compares to other countries?

■ R E F E R E N C E S

Aiken, L. A., Clarke, S. P., Sloan, D. M., et al. (2001). Nurses' reports of hospital quality of care and working conditions in five countries. *Health Affairs, 20*(3), 43–53.

Forgione, D. A., & D'Annunzio, C. M. (Winter 1999). The use of DRGs in health care payment systems around the world. *Journal of Health Care Finance, 26*(2), 66–78.

Imai, Y. (2002). *Health care reform in Japan.* Economics Department Working Paper No. 321. Paris: Organization for Economic Cooperation & Development (OECD). *http://www/oecd.org/eco*

Pan American Health Organization (PAHO). (1998). *Health in the Americas, Vol. I.* Scientific Publication No. 569. Washington, DC: World Health Organization (WHO).

Peterson, C. (Jan. 31, 2001). Nursing shortage: Not a simple problem, no easy answers. *Online Journal of Issues in Nursing, 6*(1), Manuscript 1. Available: *http://www.nursingworld.org/ojin/topic14/tpc14_1.htm*

Reinhardt, U. E., Hussey, P. S., & Anderson, G. F. (May/June 2002). Cross-national comparisons of health systems using OECD data, 1999. *Health Affairs, 21*(3), 169–181.

Rodwin, V. G. (1999). Comparative analysis of health systems: An international perspective. In A. R. Kovner & S. Jonas (Eds.) *Health care delivery in the United States* (6th ed., pp. 116–151) New York: Springer.

Rosseter, R. (Last update: March 1, 2002). *Nursing shortage fact sheet.* Washington, DC: AACN. *http://www.aacn. nche.edu/Media/Backgrounders/shortagefacts.htm*

Schoen, C., Blendon, R. J., DesRoches, C. M., & Osborn, R. (May 2002). *Comparison of health care system views and experiences in five nations, 2001: Findings from the Commonwealth Fund 2001 International Health Policy Survey.* Publication #542. New York: The Commonwealth Fund.

World Health Organization (WHO). (2000). *Health systems: improving performance.* The World Health Report 2000. Geneva, Switzerland: WHO. *http://www.who.int/whr/2000/en/report.htm*

World Health Organization (WHO). (Revised September 1998). *Population aging: a public health challenge.* Fact Sheet No. 135. Geneva, Switzerland: WHO. WHO home page *http://www.who.ch/*

CHAPTER 15

Future Trends and Keeping Updated

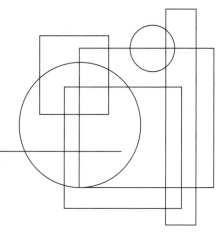

Learning Objectives

1. Identify at least two questions to apply to issues of health care policy that affect economics, finance, or budgeting.
2. Identify at least two future trends in health care economics, finance, or budgeting, and discuss the potential impact (positive or negative) of each.
3. Identify at least two approaches to keeping updated on health care economics, finance, or budgeting that will affect your discipline and work setting.

Key Terms

Centenarian
Equity

Parity
Universality

This text has discussed health care economics, managed care, budgeting, financial reporting and analysis, steps in writing business plans and grant proposals, and international health care issues. A final question is, "where are we headed from here?" Information about health care economics and financing quickly becomes outdated, particularly in this time of rapidly changing policies to address rising costs and demand. This chapter discusses possible future directions and trends in health care related to economics and financing, and suggests ways for health care professionals to keep up to date on relevant economic and financial issues. A discussion of policy questions that might be applied in following future trends is followed by a brief review of possible trends in the immediate future, concluding with suggestions for keeping abreast of health care economics and financing over time. The focus of this chapter is on policies relevant to health care professionals in the United States, although the concepts may be applied to the policies of other industrialized and developing nations.

Health Policy Questions

As shown in Table 15-1, Roberts and Clyde (1993) pose seven policy questions that may be used as a framework for tracking future trends in health care and relating these trends to health economics and financing. Table 15-1 also includes possible trends for the immediate future, discussed later in this chapter. (A copy of Table 15-1 is adapted as a worksheet for future use as Table E-1 in Appendix E.)

Roberts and Clyde's (1993) policy questions include the three expectations of health care consumers and providers: cost, high quality, and access. In Table 15-1 cost is listed as the first question, as it is seen to be the most relevant to future trends in health economics and financing, as well as being related to any health care trend or policy. For example, one may anticipate ongoing requirements for measuring and reducing costs as costs continue to rise. It is essential to think about the impact of policies, plans, and decisions affecting the cost and change in cost of health care goods and services. Cost control is also a fundamental expectation of health care consumers and providers. One implication is that budgeting skills will become increasingly important for persons working in health care fields.

◯ T A B L E 1 5 · 1

Policy Questions for Tracking Future Trends in Health Care

Policy Question	Future Trends
Cost	Ongoing need for improved cost measures; rising costs; cost concerns influence all policy questions
Quality	Increased application of quality management concepts & techniques; improved outcomes measures; increased emphasis on outcomes research & tracking
Access	Parity vs. disparity; design of entitlement programs; demise of charity care
Universality	Debates about expanding coverage or national health coverage
Equity	Controversy about health care rationing & priority setting
Efficiency	Increased emphasis on productivity; increased application of other industry models; computerization
Choice	Willingness to pay for choice; demand for choice vs. limited resources
Prevention	Increased concerns about bioterrorism; better methods disease detection; CBA, CEA and outcomes research

Source: Adapted from Roberts & Clyde, 1993.

Quality and access are the next policy questions posed by Roberts and Clyde; these are also fundamental expectations of health care consumers and providers. Problems in analyzing these issues include difficulties in measuring both quality and access. However, resource allocation decisions based on health economics and financing are likely to affect both the quality of care available and access to health care. Increased application of quality management concepts and techniques is likely in health care, with improved clinical outcomes measures linked to costs of care, as the result of increased emphasis on outcomes research and tracking. Issues likely to arise related to access include debates about **parity** (relative equality of resource allocation to various disease entities, populations, or interventions), the design of entitlement programs to allow increased access, and the demise of charity care related to reductions in reimbursements.

Universality (relatively equal access for all persons) and **equity** (burden of cost fairly distributed based on the ability to pay) are related policy questions (Roberts & Clyde, 1993) shown in Table 15-1. Both universality and equity would be substantially influenced by health economics and financing policies. For example, expanding health care coverage and establishing some form of national health coverage are universality issues that may arise in the future. Equity issues include health care rationing and priority setting.

Chapter 2 discusses choice, another policy question, as an important incentive for both health care consumers and providers. Chapter 2 points out that managed care mechanisms reduce both consumer and provider choice. It is anticipated that consumers will continue to demand choice in health care and will demonstrate willingness to pay for choice, but this demand will be countered by the forces of limited resources.

Prevention is the final policy question in Table 15-1. It is likely that increased concerns about bioterrorism will lead to prevention strategies in the future. One may also predict continued improvement in disease detection and increased use of cost-benefit analysis, cost-effectiveness analysis, and outcomes research related to prevention efforts and the evaluation of prevention programs. Recent outbreaks of Severe Acute Respiratory Syndrome (SARS) worldwide and monkeypox in the midwest are examples of new and emerging diseases requiring control.

Keeping Updated on Future Trends

The following section discusses a few health care issues likely to affect trends in health care economics and financing over the next 5 years or so. However, any publication on health care trends will quickly become outdated because changes occur continuously. Health professionals concerned about the economics and financing of health care must take the initiative to keep updated on issues, policies, and decisions.

Many resources are available to keep updated on health economic and financing issues. Following the news and reading specialized newsletters such as policy updates from the Kaiser Family Foundation highlight policies and legislation in this area. Professional organizations and advocacy groups such as the American Medical Association, the American Public Health Association, and the AARP (American Association of Retired Persons) frequently publish press releases, position statements, and policy recommendations related to the economics and financing of health care. Journals such as *Health Affairs* publish articles regarding health care economics and financing.

Non-profit and academic health economics and policy research centers, such as the Center for Studying Health System Change and the George Washington University National Health Policy Forum, prepare reports analyzing trends. Government sources, increasingly available over the Internet, are also helpful resources, including the Bureau of the Census and the Centers for Medicare & Medicaid Services (CMS), formerly the Health Care Financing Administration.

A periodic review of the kinds of resources mentioned above is part of every health professional's responsibility for keeping updated on policies, proposals, and decisions that affect health care economics and financing. In addition, training and updates available in the work setting can be valuable sources of information. Changes in health care economics and financing are as continuous as changes in clinical issues and interventions. Box 15-1 provides some Internet resources for keeping updated in the areas of health care economics, finance, and budgeting.

Future Trends

This section presents a few specific issues relevant in the United States that are likely to affect policies and decisions about health care economics and financing in the future. Some of these issues are the same as the global concerns presented in Chapter 14, such as an aging population and the nursing shortage.

☐ **B O X   1 5 - 1**

On-line Sources for Future Trends in Health Care Economics, Finance, and Budgeting

Alliance for Health Reform: http://www.allhealth.org/
Center for Healthcare Strategies: www.chcs.org
Center for Studying Health Systems Change:
http://www.hschange.com
National Health Policy Forum: www.nhpf.org
United States Census: www.census.gov

Aging Population

One highly predictable trend is the continuing and increasing growth of the elderly as a proportion of the overall population. In 2000 there were about 35 million persons age 65 or older in the United States, approximately 13% of the total U.S. population. The generation of "baby boomers" begins to turn 65 in 2011, and by 2030 the number of persons age 65 or older is expected to double to about 70 million, or about one in five Americans.

Even more important to future trends in health economics and financing is the rapid growth in the population of Americans age 85 and older, who have more health problems and require more health services. In 2000 there were about 4 million persons in the United States age 85 or older, a population segment expected to increase to as many as 19 million by 2050. The number of **centenarians** (persons age 100 and older) is also growing rapidly.

Table 15-2 summarizes per capita health care expenditures (insured and out-of-pocket) for Medicare beneficiaries age 65 and over by selected age groups from 1992 through 1999. Health care costs are not only

---

○ **T A B L E   1 5 - 2**

Average Health Care Expenditures among Medicare Beneficiaries Age 65 or Older, in 1999 Dollars, by Age Group, 1992–1999

Age Groups	1992	1993	1994	1995	1996	1997	1998	1999
65 to 69	$5,816	$5,467	$6,365	$5,698	$6,204	$5,793	$5,418	$6,711
70 to 74	$6,085	$6,810	$7,064	$7,804	$7,135	$7,626	$7,717	$8,099
75 to 79	$7,459	$8,676	$8,709	$8,895	$9,960	$9,251	$8,853	$9,241
80 to 84	$10,070	$10,903	$11,442	$12,219	$11,911	$12,317	$11,790	$10,683
85 or older	$15,232	$15,629	$16,946	$17,396	$17,420	$17,493	$17,119	$16,596
All	**$7,757**	**$8,261**	**$8,835**	**$9,108**	**$9,249**	**$9,228**	**$8,991**	**$9,352**

Note: Data include both out-of-pocket expenditures and expenditures covered by insurance.

Source: Medicare Current Beneficiary Survey in Older Americans 2000, www.agingstats.gov

rising over time, but also increase even more rapidly as people become older. In 1999, health care expenditures were $6,711 for persons age 65 to 69 years and $16,596 for persons age 85 and over. As a result, projected increases in the elderly population and in elderly persons age 85 and over will lead to increases in health care costs. Elderly Americans are a strong voting bloc and exert advocacy for interests such as Medicare, so they are likely to support increased funding to address rising costs for their care.

Health Care Labor Imbalances

Another future trend is the continuing problem of labor shortages and surpluses in health care that will affect health care economics, budgeting, and financing. One example is the current and projected shortage of professional nurses (RNs). The U.S. Bureau of Labor Statistics forecasts that over 1 million new nurses will be needed by 2010. A 21% increase is projected in the need for nurses nationwide from 1998 to 2008, compared with a 14% increase for all other occupations. A steady increase in the demand for nurses is expected over the years to come, based on a growing population, a growing elderly population, and more advanced technology requiring RN skills.

Two factors affecting the supply of RNs is a decline in the number of RN graduates and an aging RN workforce. Enrollments in RN programs declined from the mid-1990s to 2000. In addition, enrollment in ADN (associate degree nursing) programs is declining more rapidly than in BSN (baccalaureate nursing) programs. This intensifies supply problems, as barriers to entry are greater for BSN nurses than those prepared in ADN programs, as BSN programs are typically about 4 years in length, about twice that of ADN programs.

The decline in new nursing graduates, increases in the average age of recent nursing graduates, and the aging of the existing RN labor pool are all factors contributing to an aging RN workforce. New RN graduates are now 33 years old on average, and the proportion of RNs under age 30 declined from 25% in 1980 to 9% in 2000. Projections indicate that 40% of all RNs will be over age 50 by 2010. This will accelerate supply shortages as nurses reach retirement age.

Future trends of labor imbalances are not limited to the RN workforce; another example is that of licensed pharmacists. Demand has recently grown and is expected to continue to grow rapidly for pharmacists based on rapid growth in prescription volume and the expansion in the role of the pharmacist in delivering health care services. However, barriers to entry limit the supply, as educational preparation is at the doctoral level and access to the workforce by foreign applicants is limited. Another factor is the increased entry of women into the pharmacy workforce, from only 13% in 1970 to 46% in 2000; women are more likely to work part-time rather than full-time. Surveys report increasing vacancy rates and difficulties in hiring qualified, experienced pharmacists in hospitals and other health care settings.

Growth in Technology Use

Advances in technology generally increase health care costs. Improved technology typically increases the intensity of health care services provided. For example, better diagnostic techniques for cardiac disorders increase the likelihood that patients will be scheduled for cardiac treatment and follow-up, thus increasing overall costs. Technologies that reduce the per-unit (per intervention or per patient) intensity and costs frequently lead to an increased volume of services, increasing the overall costs. For example, cataract surgery is now successfully performed as a brief outpatient intervention, but many more patients are scheduled for cataract surgery than in the past, when extended hospitalization was required for recovery.

The cost of technology as a percent of total health care spending in the United States increased from 12% in 1994 to 39% in 1999. It is projected that between 2001 and 2005, the growth in personal care expenditures will be 6% to 7% annually, with technology making up about 25% to 33% of this increase. Moreover, expenditures on prescription drugs in the United States rose an estimated 15.5% for hospitals and clinics and 18.5% in outpatient settings from 2001 to 2002. Prescription medication costs are rising faster than any other segment of health care.

Access to Health Care

Even in a time of economic growth, low unemployment, and increases in the number of insured persons, access to care did not improve (except for children) in the United States from 1997 to 2001. About one in seven Americans reported some difficulty getting needed health care in 2001, which was about the same as for 1997. Nearly 16 million Americans reported they were unable to get the medical care they needed in 2001, with another 26 million reporting they delayed needed care in the previous 12 months. Cost of care was the leading cause for not receiving or delaying needed medical care. The probability of an uninsured American not obtaining needed medical care is about three times that of an insured person.

Rising health care costs and an economic downturn have led to expected reductions in health care coverage for poor Americans as well as retired employees. As of January 2003, 49 states and the District of Columbia reported plans to control the growth of Medicaid spending. Interventions include reducing Medicaid benefits and eligibility. Citing rising health care costs, over half of over 400 large, private-sector U.S. employers surveyed in 2002 planned to increase health insurance premiums and co-payments for retirees over the next 3 years. Nearly one in four of these employers did not intend to provide health insurance coverage for their future retirees.

These findings intensify concerns about future trends in health care access, given the recent economic downturn and related shortfalls in state budgets that will affect health care programs for under- and uninsured Americans. Rising health care costs and increasingly restrictive health care plans are also expected to increase access problems in the near future. For low-income working families most affected by health care access problems, possible solutions include increased government funding to address the disparities in coverage, employer mandates to provide health insurance, or some form of national health coverage.

Medicare Reimbursement

Other current issues with future implications related to health care access are congressional debates over Medicare reimbursement. One issue under debate is a Medicare prescription drug benefit to help cover the rising costs of prescription medications for American senior citizens. Another related issue is a proposed "give-back" bill that would repeal cuts authorized in 1997 in Medicare reimbursement to providers such as physicians and hospitals. Congress is not expected to pass either a Medicare drug benefit bill or a Medicare "give-back" bill by the end of 2003. The Medicare Payment Advisory Commission (MedPAC) has recommended freezing Medicare payments to physicians, hospitals, and home health agencies over FY 2003. As a result, one may expect increasing concerns about senior citizens' access to prescription drugs and health care services over 2003, although the elderly and interests such as physicians and hospitals are also expected to exert political advocacy in this arena.

National Health Care Coverage

Earlier in this chapter, universal health coverage was mentioned as a way to meet the access needs of working families. A national health plan might also have the advantage of increasing the bargaining power for costly technologies and prescription drugs, costs that are mounting given the rising number of elderly citizens in America. Yet another advantage of a national health plan would be to set overall budgets and priorities for providing universal access within limits determined by social, political, and cost-effectiveness criteria.

Universal health coverage is being discussed in some health care and political settings. A number of health plan executives, among them Bruce G. Bodaken, the chief executive of Blue Shield of California, and Dr. William W. McGuire, chief executive of the UnitedHealth Group, are calling for universal health insurance. Bodaken has recommended a statewide universal health plan for California, while McGuire has asked the U.S. Congress to include all Americans in a health care plan. Sen. John B. Breaux of Louisiana is working on a universal health plan proposal that would require all Americans to purchase private health insurance, with some government subsidies and adjustments for income.

However, the history of efforts to implement a national health care plan in the United States reflects strong resistance from interest groups such as physicians, hospitals and other health industries, as well as citizens fearful of increased taxation and government control of health care. The United States is a country based on a capitalist philosophy, in which market forces are generally considered superior to governmental intervention. Previous attempts to establish universal health coverage, such as under the Truman and the Clinton administrations, have met with overall rejection and failure. Any consideration of national health coverage is highly controversial and is not on the current horizon of federal policy issues.

Implications for Readers

This discussion of future trends in health care economics, finance, and budgeting has implications for readers regarding the concepts and skills presented in this text. In terms of budgeting, future trends indicating growing concerns about costs and access indicate an increased focus on the ability of health professionals to manage and control resources. As a result, budgeting skills are expected to increase in importance throughout the health care professions.

Recent corporate financial scandals in health care and non-health care industries have placed an increased focus on fiscal responsibility. Health care institutions are expected to face more comprehensive and intense financial review, with increased regulation of accounting practices. Skills in reviewing and analyzing financial reports will be increasingly helpful to health professionals who want to critically examine and understand the financial operations of their organization and work setting.

Although economic wealth is not the only factor in health care spending, it is an important factor at personal, organizational, and national levels. To the extent that health care is valued at any of these levels, it will be pursued to the extent that the economic situation allows. Responsible fiscal practices based on knowledge and understanding of economic, financial, and budgeting concepts therefore enhance the ability to provide health care quality and access while controlling costs.

Conclusion

This chapter presents concepts and strategies for identifying and evaluating future trends in health care economics, finance, and budgeting and for keeping updated regarding these topics.

■ CRITICAL THINKING EXERCISES

1. Identify at least three professional organizations providing support or information relevant to your discipline or work setting about health care economics, budgeting, or finance. Share contact information and discuss.

2. Use the worksheet provided in Appendix E to identify future trends in health care economics, finance, and budgeting relevant to your discipline and work setting. Discuss the potential impact of these future trends.

■ REFERENCES

Blum, D. (Last updated June 3, 2002). *E-text on health technology assessment (HTA) information resources, Chapter 7.* Agency for Healthcare Research and Quality (AHRQ). Bethesda, MD: U.S. National Library of Medicine, National Institutes of Health, Department of Health & Human Services. *http://www.nlm.nih.gov/nichsr/ehta/chapter7.html*

Brock, F. (Jan. 5, 2003). Why a centrist (no fooling) wants universal insurance. *The New York Times*, Section 3, p. 7.

Decker, F. H., Dollard, K. J., & Kraditor, K. R. (2001). Staffing of nursing services in nursing homes: Present issues and prospects for the future. *Seniors Housing & Care Journal, 9*(1), 3–26.

Department of Health & Human Services (DHHS). (December 2000). *The pharmacist workforce: A study of the supply and demand for pharmacists. Report to Congress.* Washington, DC: Department of Health & Human Services, Health Resources and Services Administration, Bureau of Health Professions. *http://bhpr.hrsa.gov/healthworkforce/pharmacist.html*

Department of Health & Human Services (DHHS). (July 2002). *Projected supply, demand, and shortages of registered nurses: 2000–2020.* Washington, DC: Department of Health & Human Services, Health Resources and Services Administration, Bureau of Health Professions, National Center for Health Workforce Analysis. *http://bhpr.hrsa.gov/healthworkforce/rnproject/default.htm*

Federal Interagency Forum on Aging-Related Statistics. (August 2000). *Older Americans 2000: Key indicators of well-being.* Federal Interagency Forum on Aging-Related Statistics. Washington, DC: U.S. Government Printing Office. *http://www.agingstats.gov/*

Freudenheim, M. (Dec. 7, 2002). Some tentative first steps toward universal health care. *The New York Times* On-line: http://www.nytimes.com/2002/12/07/business/07CARE.html?pagewanted=print&position=top

Gabel, J., Levitt, L., Pickreign, et al. (October 2001). Job-based health insurance in 2001: Inflation hits double digits, managed care retreats. *Health Affairs, 20*(5), 180–186.

Gilmartin, M. J. (2001). Economic issues in health care. In J. L. Creasia & B. Parker (Eds.) *Conceptual foundations: the bridge to professional nursing practice* (3rd ed., pp. 228–255). Philadelphia: Mosby.

Heffler, S., Smith, S., Won, G., Clemens, M. K., Keehan, S., & Zezza, M. (March/April 2002). Health spending projections for 2001–2011: The latest outlook. *Health Affairs, 21*(2), 207–218.

Henry J. Kaiser Family Foundation & Hewitt Associates. (December 2002). *The current state of retiree health benefits. Findings from the Kaiser/Hewitt 2002 Retiree Health Survey.*

Joint Commission on Accreditation of Healthcare Organizations (JCAHO). (2002). *Health care at the crossroads: strategies for addressing the evolving nursing crisis.* Oakbrook Terrace, IL: JCAHO.

Kaisernetwork.org (Sept. 3, 2002). *Congressional Quarterly Audio Report 9/3/2002.* Capitol Hill Analysis. Transcript_090302_CQ. Menlo Park, CA: Henry J. Kaiser Family Foundation. *http://www.kaisernetwork.org/health_cast/uploaded_files/Transcript_090302_CQ.pdf*

Levit, K., Smith, C., Cowan, C., Lazenby, H., & Martin, A. (January/February 2002). Inflation spurs health spending in 2000. *Health Affairs, 21*(1), 172–181.

Mohr, P. E., Mueller, C., Neumann, P., et al. (Feb. 28, 2001). *The impact of medical technology on future health care costs, final report.* Prepared for: Health Insurance Association of America and Blue Cross and Blue Shield Association. Bethesda, MD: Project HOPE, Center for Health Affairs.

Napper, M. (Last updated Aug. 21, 2002). *E-text on Health Technology Assessment (HTA) Information Resources, Chapter 11.* Health Economics Information. Bethesda, MD: U.S. National Library of Medicine, National Institutes of Health, Department of Health & Human Services. *http://www.nlm.nih.gov/nichsr/ehta/chapter11.html*

Pear, R. (Jan. 19, 2003). Commission to urge freezing some Medicare payments. *The New York Times*, Section 1, p. 18.

Roberts, M. J. with Clyde, A. T. (1993). *Your money or your life: the health care crisis explained.* New York: Doubleday.

Rosseter, R. (Last updated March 1, 2002). *Nursing shortage fact sheet.* Washington, DC: AACN. http://www.aacn.nche.edu/Media/Backgrounders/shortagefacts.htm

Shah, N. D., Vermfulen, L. C., Santell, J. P., et al. (Jan. 15, 2002). Projecting future drug expenditures, 2002. *American Journal of Health-Systems Pharmacy, 59*, 131–142. *http://www.ahrq.gov/research/may02/0502RA12.htm#head2*

Smith, V.K., Gifford, K., & Ramesh, R. (Jan. 13, 2003). *Medicaid spending growth: a 50-state survey update for fiscal year 2003.* Health Management Associates & V. Wachino, Kaiser Commission on Medicaid and the Uninsured.

Strongin, R. J. (October 2001). *Emergency preparedness from a health perspective: preparing for bioterrorism at the federal, state and local levels.* Washington, DC: The George Washington University National Health Policy Forum.

Strunk, B. C., & Cunningham, P. J. (March 2002). *Treading water: Americans' access to needed medical care, 1997–2001.* Tracking Report No. 1. Washington, DC: Center for Studying Health System Change.

Strunk, B. C., & Reschovsky, J. D. (August 2002). *Working families' health insurance coverage, 1997–2001.* Tracking Report No. 4. Washington, DC: Center for Studying Health System Change.

Toner, R., & Stolberg, S.G. (Aug. 11, 2002). Decade after health care crisis, soaring costs bring new strains. *The New York Times,* pp. 1, 18.

U.S. Census Bureau. *Statistical abstract of the United States: 2002. http://www.census.gov/statab/www/*

Wagner, W. (Last updated Aug. 21, 2002). *E-text on health technology assessment (HTA) information resources, chapter 15.* Identifying and tracking new and emerging health technologies. Bethesda, MD: U.S. National Library of Medicine, National Institutes of Health, Department of Health & Human Services. *http:// www.nlm.nih.gov/nichsr/ehta/chapter15.html*

APPENDIX A

A Cost-Benefit Analysis Evaluating Adult Outpatient Asthma Education February 8, 2003 Patient Education Committee of the Healthy Ways Clinic and the Healthy Ways Hospital Financial Office

Asthma is an inflammatory disorder of an individual's airway that is chronic and may persist into adulthood. Symptoms include coughing, wheezing, chest tightness, and hypersensitivity to substances such as pollen or perfume. This breathing disorder may result in death; patient education is a way to help adults control their asthma and reduce risk as well as acute care costs. Studies have shown that asthma education helps adults reduce their symptoms and use of emergency care, and improves compliance with treatment.

This is a cost-benefit analysis (CBA) evaluating FY 2002 Healthy Ways Clinic's Adult Asthma Education Program (AAEP), conducted by the Patient Education Committee of the Healthy Ways Clinic in collaboration with the Healthy Ways Hospital Financial Office. The asthma education classes are a disease management effort that began operation January 2, 2002, as a series of year-round, weekly classes for adult outpatient asthmatics that last for 2 hours per class. Participants attend a class session scheduled from 5:30 p.m. to 7:30 p.m. every Tuesday except holidays.

The classes are conducted by certified respiratory therapists, employed by Healthy Ways Clinic, under the supervision of an RN Coordinator. All instructors are trained in asthma management and patient education techniques; only one instructor is scheduled per class. Class size is limited to no more than 10 patients who may bring a family member or companion. Teaching approaches include lectures to the group, one-on-one personalized instruction, small group work, and peer support. Each participant is also assessed using physiological measures, a review of medication compliance and a standardized health survey to obtain a baseline Quality-Adjusted Life Year (QALY) score during the class session attended.

AAEP Costs

The FY 2002 budget for the AAEP is $10,500 (note that the actual budget was only $10,341 because variable costs were lower than projected). Funding for the adult asthma classes is shared by Medical Services (25%), Allergy Services (25%), and the Emergency Care Department (25%) of Healthy Ways Hospital; the

TABLE A-1

Healthy Ways Clinic, Budget for Adult Asthma Classes, FY 2002

Item	Cost per Class	Cost per Attendee	Annual Cost
Fixed Costs:			
RN Coordinator@ $30/hr for 1 hr/wk	$30	$6	$1,530
RT @ $20/hr for 3 hrs/wk	$60	$12	3,060
Clerical @ $12/hr for 3 hrs/wk	$36	$7	1,836
Trainer training	29	$6	1,500
Trainer materials	6	$1	325
Snacks & beverages	15	$3	765
Variable Costs:			
Patient education materials	$26	$5	1,325
Total	**$203**	**$40**	**$10,341**

remaining 25% of funding is from Healthy Ways Clinic. All of these departments, particularly Emergency Care, are impacted by adult patients in acute asthmatic distress; this analysis demonstrates that each of these departments generated benefits (cost savings) over FY 2002 from their $2,625 contribution to the AAEP.

Fixed costs for the adult asthma classes include staff time for the instructors, program coordinator, and clerical support. Other fixed costs include instructor training, instructor materials, and refreshments served each class session. Variable costs consist of educational materials provided to each patient attending the class. Indirect costs (overhead expenses) are excluded, as Healthy Ways Clinic is open during the times the classes are scheduled, so any additional housekeeping, security, or other indirect costs are assumed to be negligible. Table A–1 below presents a detailed breakdown of the adult asthma education expense budget (the program does not generate revenues).

AAEP Participation

Table A–2 provides summary information about class attendance at the AAEP over FY 2002. Healthy Ways Clinic physicians, including family practitioners and allergy specialists, were requested to refer symptomatic adult asthma patients to the AAEP for classes beginning January 2, 2002. Average class attendance is about 4–5 participants, improving somewhat over the second half of FY 2002. Over the first half of FY 2002, 119 patients attended the asthma management course, with a total of 261 attendees for FY 2002. Data were not available on the number of patients referred by Healthy Ways Clinic physicians, so it was not possible to report enrollment rates.

AAEP Benefits

The benefits of the asthma classes are measured in several ways, some of which are converted to dollar values, as shown in Table A–3. Tangible benefits that can be

TABLE A-2

Summary Information for AAEP Participation, FY 2002

	1st 6 Months FY 2002	FY 2002
Attendance	119	261
Average Attendance/Class	4.6	5.1
Number of Classes	26	51

Cost Savings Estimates for AAEP, FY 2002[1]

	Baseline	Completion	Sample Study Savings	Sample Study Savings per Class	Sample Study Savings per Attendee	Estimated Annual Savings
MD visits	46	28	18	0.69	0.72	187.9
MD costs @ $85/visit	$3,910	$2,380	$1,530	$58.85	$61.20	$15,973
ER visits	7	3	4	0.15	0.16	41.8
ER costs @ $320/visit	$2,240	$960	$1,280	$49.23	$51.20	$13,363
Hospital Days	6	4	2	0.08	0.08	20.9
Hospital Costs @ $1200/day	$7,200	$4,800	$2,400	$92.31	$96.00	$25,056
Total Medical Costs	**$13,350**	**$8,140**	**$5,210**	**$200**	**$208**	**$54,392**
Average QALY scores	0.83	0.87	0.04	—	—	—
QALY productive hours	45,464	47,611	2,146	82.55	85.8	22,406
QALY costs @ $5/hour	$227,322	$238,053	$10,731	$412.73	$429.24	$112,032
Total	**$240,672**	**$246,193**	**$15,941**	**$613.12**	**$637.64**	**$166,424**

[1] Annualized based on data from 6-month retrospective and prospective review of medical records and quality of life survey for random sample of 25 attendees between January 2 and June 26, 2002.

converted to dollar values include reductions in physician visits, ER visits and hospital days related to asthma symptoms or complications. Data were collected from a review of patient medical records for 25 randomly sampled AAEP participants who attended an asthma management class between January 2 and June 26, 2002. A 6-month retrospective chart review from the date the participant attended their asthma management class provided the baseline data. A 6-month prospective chart review from the date the participant attended the asthma management class provided the AAEP completion data.

As shown in Table A-3, physician visits are estimated at $85 per visit, ER visits at $320 per visit, and hospitalization at $1,200 per hospital day. Over the first 6 months of FY 2002, the 25 randomly sampled participants in the AAEP experienced a reduction in physician visits for asthma symptoms or complications from 46 to 28 visits, with an estimated $1,530 reduction in physician visit costs for the 25 study participants. ER visits were reduced from 7 to 3 visits, with an estimated $1,280 reduction in ER costs for the 25 study participants. Hospital days were reduced from 6 to 4 days, with a $2,400 reduction in hospital costs for the 25 study participants.

The sample study medical cost savings per class are estimated by dividing the total sample study savings by 26 (the most conservative estimate for 6 months of weekly classes). On average, each asthma management class is estimated to save $58.85 in physician visit costs, $49.25 in ER visit costs, and $92.31 in hospital costs. Sample study attendee medical costs savings are estimated by dividing the overall cost savings by 25 (the number of attendees in the study). Each person attending the AAEP class is estimated to save $61.20 in physician visits, $51.20 in ER visits, and $96.00 in hospitalization costs.

The sample study medical cost savings were annualized for all participants over FY 2002 by multiplying the estimated per-attendee savings by 261 total attendees. On an annual basis, the AAEP generated an estimated $15,973 in physician visits, $13,363 in ER visits, and $25,056 in hospital costs. The total savings in medical costs generated by the AAEP are estimated at $54,392.

The 15–D Health–Related Quality of Life Index was used to survey participants during the asthma management class. The 25 AAEP participants who were randomly sampled for a study of medical costs were also contacted by telephone 6 months after attending the asthma management class for a follow-up Quality of Life survey. Baseline and completion data focused on symptoms and functioning related to asthma were analyzed for the 25 participants who completed the AAEP course the first 6 months of FY 2002. These data are used to calculate QALY scores, then converted to dollar values by assuming that individuals average 12 productive hours per day, with each productive hour valued at $5 as a conservative average.

Given that there are 8,760 hours in a year (365 × 24), if half of those hours are productive they total 4,380 hours. As the retrospective and prospective chart reviews for these participants was limited to 6 months, the productive hours for the baseline and completion are 2,190 hours. A person with a QALY score of 0.75 would report a 25% loss in productivity, or only 1,642.5 (2,190 × 0.75) productive hours over the 6-month period. This represents a loss of 547.5 productive hours (2,190−1,642.5). At a value of $5 per hour, the dollar loss due to asthma symptoms is $2,737.50 (547.5 × $5).

The table presents summary data for the QALY scores and value of productive hours from baseline to completion for the 25 sample participants attending an AAEP class the first half of FY 2002. QALY scores improved for these attendees from 0.83 to 0.87. Overall, the participants showed a 2,146 hour increase in productive hours, related to better management and control of asthma symptoms. When valued at $5 per hour and annualized, the total QALY savings are estimated at $112,032.

Intangible benefits (not included in the analysis) include increased patient satisfaction and an enhanced reputation for both Healthy Ways Clinic and Healthy Ways Hospital. Patients also report they can better manage their families, job responsibilities, and other aspects of their lives now that their asthma is under control. Physicians report satisfaction with increased patient compliance and fewer emergency calls.

TABLE A-4

Cost-Benefit Analysis, AAEP, FY 2002[1]

	Estimated per Class	Estimated per Attendee	Estimated Annual
Program Costs:	$203	$40	$10,341
Medical Cost Savings	$200	$208	$54,392
QALY Cost Savings	$413	$429	$112,032
Total Benefits	**$613**	**$638**	**$166,424**
CBA:			
Medical Savings Net Benefits	$(2)	$169	$44,051
Total Program Net Benefits	$410	$598	$156,083
Medical Costs B/C Ratio	1.0	5.3	5.3
Total Program Benefits B/C Ratio	**3.0**	**16.1**	**16.1**

[1] Annualized based on data from 6-month retrospective and prospective review of medical records and quality of life survey for random sample of 25 attendees between January 2 and June 26, 2002.

Net Benefits and B/C Ratios

Table A9–4 presents the results of the CBA of the AEPP for FY 2002 annualizing the 6-month data over the entire year. Results are estimated per class session, per attendee, and for FY 2002. Results are presented that omit the QALY savings in productive hours from calculations, and that include the QALY savings.

As shown in Table A9–4, the FY 2002 cost of the AAEP is $10,341 (in line with the budget of $10,500). The cost per class session is calculated by dividing the annual cost by 51 weekly sessions per year, amounting to $203. The estimated cost per attendee is estimated by dividing the annual cost by the 261 participants, amounting to $40. Program benefits, as shown in Table A9–4, are first calculated by focusing on the savings in medical costs (MD visits, ER visits and hospital days) as presented in the table. Medical cost savings total $200 per class, $208 per attendee, and $54,392 over FY 2002.

The QALY cost savings are calculated based on the baseline and completion QALY scores from surveys of the 25 study participants, valued at $5 per productive hour saved. The annual QALY savings is estimated by multiplying the per-attendee savings estimated in the study of 25 participants by the total 261 participants. QALY cost savings are estimated at $413 per class, $429 per attendee, and $112,032 over FY 2002.

The table then presents the net benefits and the B/C ratios. Net benefits are calculated by subtracting the total costs from the total benefits. For FY 2002 the total net benefits omitting the QALY savings (focused only on medical cost savings) related to the AAEP total $44,051. The total net benefits including QALY savings amount to $156,083.

The costs and benefits are then converted to B/C ratios by dividing the medical cost savings and total cost savings by the program costs. The medical cost B/C ratio for FY 2002 is estimated at 5.3 ($54,392 ÷ $10,341). In other words, for every dollar of cost, the AAEP generates $5.30 in medical care savings. The total program B/C ratio is 16.1 ($156,083 ÷ $10,341), indicating that for every dollar of cost, the AAEP generates $16.10 in benefits overall. These data support the benefits of the AAEP and its continued funding for FY 2003.

One consideration is the opportunity cost of funding the AAEP rather than other health promotion efforts. A review of the literature indicates that the amount of savings for medical costs and QALY productivity is as great or greater for asthma control as for other health promotion efforts such as reduction of dietary fat, exercise programs, or cancer screening.

Additional Evaluation Issues

Several evaluation issues and concerns should be discussed that could not be entered into the CBA calculations. The AAEP was budgeted to accommodate at least 30 more participants than attended over FY 2002. Recommendations are to explore ways to improve the publicity of AAEP throughout the community, to consider weekend classes (Saturday morning or afternoon) for patients reluctant to attend evening classes, and to provide child care for participants. It is also suggested that the RN coordinator explore ways to improve collaboration with clinic and hospital physicians to refer symptomatic patients and to follow up on referrals to ensure that patients attend an asthma management class.

Another recommendation is to employ an instructor who is bilingual in Spanish, to better serve potential participants who experience language barriers. There is also a need for a home visit nurse to conduct environmental assessments in patients' homes, so that they are better able to identify and control asthma triggers.

A final recommendation is to budget for annual evaluation costs, which was not done for FY 2002. The evaluation costs for FY 2002 were considered to be "overhead," but given the time required for the 6-month chart reviews and 15-D Health-Related Quality of Life Index surveys to provide QALY scores, the Patient Education Committee and Financial Office recommend budgeting for these costs in the AAEP budget. Ongoing evaluation is considered essential in assessing the costs and benefits of AAEP, and budgeting these costs gives a more accurate picture of program costs.

A potential opportunity to explore over FY 2003 is a proposed program for children and adolescents, to be conducted in and with the cooperation of the local public school district. A team consisting of members of the Patient Education Committee and the Financial Office is exploring the possibility of grant funding for this expansion of the asthma education program.

In summary, the AAEP demonstrated benefits exceeding its costs over FY 2002, and has the potential for further improvement and expansion over FY 2003.

APPENDIX B

A Cost-Effectiveness Analysis for Proposed Alternative Interventions to Post-Procedure Surgical Pain Reduction

December 3, 2002 Orthopedic Department, Patient Education Department, Pain Clinic, and Financial Office of Healthy Ways Hospital

This document presents a cost-effectiveness analysis (CEA) of alternative interventions to help Healthy Ways Hospital patients reduce or control pain following selected surgical procedures. The CEA was used to help the Surgical Pain Intervention Committee (SPI Committee), made up of representatives from the Orthopedic Department, Patient Education Department, Pain Clinic, and Financial Office of Healthy Ways Hospital, determine which intervention to recommend for funding and support for FY 2003.

The three interventions compared in this CEA are based on complementary and alternative health care approaches to pain reduction and management. Guided imagery is a mental process involving a sensory quality (not just visual, but aural, tactile, olfactory, and kinesthetic perceptions) that is used therapeutically. Hypnosis is achieved via a qualified hypnotist (certified hypnotherapist) who assists the patient to enter into an altered state of consciousness. Biofeedback is a therapeutic method using monitoring instruments to feed back to patients physiological data that normally would not reach their conscious awareness, such as skin temperature. By watching the biofeedback monitoring instrument, patients learn to adjust their mental processes to control bodily processes.

The objective of all of these interventions is to help patients reduce and control post-surgical pain. An in-depth review of the literature and research on guided imagery, hypnosis, and biofeedback indicates that each of these approaches are effective in pain reduction and pain management, including pain experienced in the recovery from surgical procedures. Each of these alternative interventions is considered safe and of low risk to post-surgical patients.

Intangible benefits (benefits that cannot be easily quantified or put in dollar amounts) that the SPI Committee assumes from the interventions (guided imagery, hypnosis, and biofeedback) include increased patient satisfaction and better patient compliance. The SPI Committee also assumes each of the interventions would provide a number of benefits that could be measured and put into dollar terms, including reduced post-operative length of stay, reduced complications, fewer visits to the physician for problems with pain, reduced re-hospitalizations, reduced use of skilled or home health care, and decreased use of pain medications.

These tangible benefits are not quantified for the purposes of the CEA used for the proposal. The reduction of patient post-procedure pain in using a low-risk alternative intervention is an objective the departments represented by the SPI Committee support. However, once a pain reduction and management intervention is implemented from the alternatives of guided imagery, hypnosis, and biofeedback, a one-year evaluation will be conducted using cost-benefit analysis (CBA) methods requiring the quantification and conversion to dollar amounts of as many costs and benefits as possible. A group of physicians from the Pain Clinic will conduct the evaluation to determine the outcomes of the intervention that is selected.

Intervention Costs

Tables B–1, B–2, and B–3 present per-patient and annual costs for the surgical pain interventions of guided imagery, hypnosis, and biofeedback, respectively. Fixed costs include hourly wages for staff implementing the intervention, staff education, and equipment. Annual fixed costs for staff are estimated by multiplying the estimated hourly wage by the number of hours expected each week, then multiplying by 50 weeks for the year (this excludes holiday schedules for the Surgery Department). Non-personnel fixed costs are provided using the best estimates available. Overhead costs (such as housekeeping and administration) are excluded because they are assumed to be negligible for all of the interventions.

Fixed costs per patient are calculated in Tables B–1, B–2, and B–3 by dividing the annual costs by 197 patients estimated to receive selected surgical procedures for FY 2003. These three procedures—spinal fusion, total hip replacement, and auto hema stem cell transplant—are selected for the application of the pain reduction and control intervention over FY 2003. After evaluating the intervention for FY 2003, a decision will be made about continuing and expanding this project to other surgical patients.

Per-patient variable costs in Tables B–1, B–2, and B–3 are estimated using the best available estimates for educational materials. The guided imagery materials are to be mailed to patients in advance of their procedure, so packaging and mailing costs are included. The other two interventions, hypnosis and biofeedback, are implemented during the patient's hospital recovery. Annual variable costs are calculated by multiplying the per patient variable costs by 215. Although the actual number of patients estimated is 197, this provides a somewhat more conservative cost estimate and allows for replacement of lost materials or mailings.

Table B–1 presents the cost estimates associated with the use of guided imagery. The Surgery PA coordinator will identify patients scheduled for the selected procedures, ensure that the educational items are sent to each patient, and contact each patient by telephone to be sure the educational materials are received, that the patient is able to view and use these materials, and to answer any questions. The Surgery PA coordinator will work in consultation with a staff psychologist. The costs of the guided imagery intervention are estimated as $122.08 per patient, and $24,530 for FY 2003.

TABLE B-1

Patient and Annual Cost Estimates for Guided Imagery, 2003

Item	Cost per Patient	Annual Cost
Fixed Costs:		
Psychology Consultant @ $110/hr for 2 hrs/wk	$55.84	$11,000
Surgery PA Coordinator @ $35/hr for 3 hrs/wk	$26.65	$5,250
Clerical @ $12/hr for 3 hrs/wk	$9.14	$1,800
Trainer training for surgery PA	$3.81	750
Variable Costs (patient "toolkit" package):		
Video cassette tape	$4.00	$860
CD	$5.50	$1,183
Audio cassette tape	$3.00	$645
Workbook	$7.00	$1,505
Packaging and mailing	$7.15	$1,537
Total	**$122.08**	**$24,530**

Table B–2 presents the cost estimates associated with the use of hypnosis. A staff psychologist certified in hypnotherapy will perform the hypnosis one day post-procedure for patients recovering from the selected procedures. Patients will require at least two hypnosis sessions, so staff costs are considerable, although equipment and variable costs are minimal. The costs of the hypnosis intervention are estimated as $351.25 per patient, and $69,215 for FY 2003.

Table B–3 presents the cost estimates associated with the use of biofeedback. As in the case of guided imagery, the Surgical PA coordinator will implement biofeedback in consultation with a staff psychologist. More time is required of the Surgical PA than for guided imagery, as at least one visit must be made to each patient while in the hospital to teach the patient how to use the biofeedback monitoring equipment. Equipment costs are highest for biofeedback, as a special video monitor must be purchased that can provide feedback to patients regarding their skin temperature, and special carts must be purchased so the video monitors may be moved to the patient's bedside. The costs of the biofeedback intervention are estimated as $182.57 per patient, and $36,165 for FY 2003.

◯ TABLE B-2

Patient and Annual Cost Estimates for Hypnosis, 2003

Item	Cost per Patient	Annual Cost
Fixed Costs:		
Psychologist @ $110/hr for 12 hrs/wk	$335.03	$66,000
Clerical @ $12/hr for 5 hrs/wk	$15.23	$3,000
Variable Costs:		
Informational Brochure	$1.00	$215
Total	**$351.25**	**$69,215**

CEA of Pain Reduction and Control Interventions

The comparison of per-patient and annual costs shows that guided imagery is the most cost-effective intervention for post-surgical pain reduction. As shown in Table B–4, on a per-patient basis, guided imagery is $229.17 less than hypnosis and $60.49 less than biofeedback. For FY 2003, guided imagery is $44,685 less than hypnosis and $11,635 less than biofeedback.

◯ TABLE B-3

Patient and Annual Cost Estimates for Biofeedback, 2003

Item	Cost per Patient	Annual Cost
Fixed Costs:		
Psychology Consultant @ $110/hr for 2 hrs/wk	$55.84	$11,000
Surgery PA Coordinator @ $35/hr for 8 hrs/wk	$71.07	$14,000
Clerical @ $12/hr for 3 hrs/wk	$9.14	$1,800
Trainer training for surgery PA	$7.61	$1,500
2 video monitors with VCR, portable cart, and skin sensors	$27.92	$5,500
Variable Costs:		
Video cassette tape	$5.00	$1,075
Written information packet	$6.00	$1,290
Total	**$ 182.57**	**$ 36,165**

◯ TABLE B-4

Cost-Effectiveness of Interventions, 2003

Approaches	Cost per Patient	Annual Cost	Guided Imagery vs. Other Intervention per Patient	Guided Imagery vs. Other Intervention, Annual
Guided Imagery	$122.08	$24,530	—	—
Hypnosis	$351.25	$69,215	$229.17	$44,685
Biofeedback	$182.57	$36,165	$60.49	$11,635

Table B–5 presents the costs of the three surgical procedures selected to test the pain reduction and control intervention over FY 2003. The three procedures are spinal fusion, total hip replacement, and auto hema stem cell transplant. Of the three procedures, spinal fusion is most frequently performed in the Healthy Ways Hospital Surgical Department, with 111 procedures estimated for FY 2003 at an average cost per procedure of $6,705. Total hip replacements are expected to number 83 over FY 2003, at an average cost per auto hema stem cell transplant of $6,492. The least frequent and most expensive procedure, auto hema stem cell transplant, is expected to be performed only three times at an average cost per procedure of $75,308.

The addition of guided imagery to the surgical "package" of costs would increase spinal fusion procedures by only 1.8%, total hip replacement procedures by only 1.9%, and auto hema stem cell transplants by only 0.2%. Note that as hypnosis and biofeedback are more costly, they each would increase the costs of these procedures more than the use of guided imagery. Table B–6 also shows that the annual added costs for each of the selected surgical procedures would be lowest for guided imagery.

Funding and Cost-Sharing

One difficulty in designing this pain reduction and control program based on alternative and complementary interventions is funding. Many insurers and government payers will not cover the costs of guided imagery,

◯ TABLE B-5

Selected Surgical Procedure Costs and Additional Costs per Intervention, 2003

Procedure Types and Data			Percent Increase Cost per Procedure			Annual Added Cost per Procedure Type		
Procedure	No. of Procedures	Procedure Cost	Guided Imagery	Hypnosis	Biofeedback	Guided Imagery	Hypnosis	Biofeedback
Spinal Fusion	111	$6,705	1.8%	5.2%	2.7%	$13,551	$38,989	$20,266
Total Hip Replacement	83	$6,492	1.9%	5.4%	2.8%	$10,133	$29,154	$15,154
Auto Hema Stem Cell Transplant	3	$75,308	0.2%	0.5%	0.2%	$366	$1,054	$548
Total	**197**	—	—	—	—	—	—	—

○ TABLE B-6

Shared Departmental Costs for Interventions, 2003[1]

| Approaches | Intervention Costs | | Shared Departmental Costs | | |
	Cost per Patient	Annual Cost	Pain Clinic	Orthopedic Surgery	Patient Education
Guided Imagery	$122.08	$24,530	$8,177	$8,177	$8,177
Hypnosis	$351.25	$69,215	$23,072	$23,072	$23,072
Biofeedback	$182.57	$36,165	$12,055	$12,055	$12,055

[1] Pain Clinic funds 25%, Orthopedic Surgery funds 50%, Patient Education funds 25%.

hypnosis, or biofeedback except for very limited, selected conditions. As a result, it is proposed that the departments represented by the SPI Committee select the most cost-effective intervention, guided imagery, and implement that intervention for the three selected procedures of spinal fusion, total hip replacement, and auto hema stem cell transplant over FY 2003. Guided imagery will then be evaluated using CBA to determine if the benefits of providing this intervention are greater than the costs to fund the program.

It is further proposed that three departments of Healthy Ways Hospital share the FY 2003 costs for providing guided imagery, as shown in Table B–6. If the Pain Clinic, Orthopedic Surgery Department, and Patient Education Department share costs equally, each department will only need to provide $8,177 over FY 2003.

In conclusion, after comparing three alternative and complementary interventions for post-surgical pain reduction and control, guided imagery was found to be the most cost-effective. The SPI Committee recommends implementation of guided imagery for FY 2003, with funding shared equally between the Pain Clinic, Orthopedic Surgery Department, and Patient Education Department of Healthy Ways Hospital. A program evaluation utilizing CBA is recommended to begin early in FY 2003 to evaluate the costs and benefits of using guided imagery as an intervention over FY 2003.

APPENDIX C

Business Plan for a Cardiac Catheterization Laboratory Cardiac Catheterization Project Committee (CCPC) October 8, 2001 SouthSide Hospital, Central City, USA Executive Summary

This business plan, developed by the CCPC, strongly supports the relocation of cardiac catheterization services at SouthSide Hospital to a newly equipped Cardiac Catheterization Laboratory located adjacent to cardiac surgery. This Cardiac Catheterization Laboratory would replace the existing cardiac catheterization services.

Demographic information shows that the population of persons over age 65 is increasing in the Central City area at a higher rate than in the state and the nation, with concurrent estimated higher rates of cardiac disease. The anticipated higher demand for diagnostic procedures like cardiac catheterizations is offset by estimated reduction in referrals if SouthSide Hospital's cardiac catheterization services are not renovated and improved.

Operating budgets and pro forma P&L projections have been estimated by the CCPC for two alternatives (Table C–1). The first alternative is to relocate cardiac catheterization services to a Cardiac Catheterization Laboratory using space in the cardiac surgery department. Relocation of cardiac catheterization services increases patient safety and physician satisfaction because emergency surgery facilities are more readily available. Under the first alternative, cardiac catheterization equipment will be entirely replaced with newer technologies that will provide better diagnostic capabilities.

The second alternative is to maintain current cardiac catheterization services over the coming 4 years, with estimated losses in referrals to SouthSide Hospital for these procedures. The pro forma P&L projections are attached to the executive summary for review.

The CCPC is convinced that a new Cardiac Catheterization Laboratory is both a feasible and a profitable venture for SouthSide Hospital.

TABLE C-1

SouthSide Hospital, Summary Pro Forma P&L Projections for Cardiac Catheterization Proposal Alternatives, FY 2002–2005

	FY 2002	FY 2003	FY 2004	FY 2005
Maintaining Current Cardiac Catheterization Services:				
Volume	498	485	470	454
Charges per Procedure[1]	$7,000	$7,140	$7,283	$7,428
Net Revenue	$1,220,743	$1,142,047	$1,060,816	$977,429
Total Expenses	$1,153,018	$916,167	$945,015	$975,591
pro forma P&L	**$268,619**	**$225,880**	**$115,801**	**$1,838**
Profit Margin	**18.9%**	**19.8%**	**10.9%**	**0.2%**
Implementing the New Cardiac Catheterization Laboratory:				
Volume[2]	505	559	576	593
Charges per Procedure[3]	$8,050	$8,292	$8,540	$8,796
Net Revenue	$1,421,637	$1,529,065	$1,523,871	$1,512,373
Total Expenses	$1,069,716	$1,167,806	$1,192,572	$1,218,446
pro forma P&L	**$351,920**	**$361,259**	**$331,299**	**$293,927**
Profit Margin	**24.8%**	**23.6%**	**21.7%**	**19.4%**

[1] Assumes 2% increase in charges/year.

[2] Assumes 7% drop in projected volume for FY 2002 due to construction.

[3] Assumes 15% increase in base charge of $7,000 and 3% increase in charges/year.

Business Plan for a Cardiac Catheterization Laboratory Cardiac Catheterization Project Committee (CCPC) October 8, 2001 SouthSide Hospital, Central City, USA

SouthSide Hospital is a non-profit, 24-hour acute care facility, with 110 beds and an operating (expense) budget of approximately $51.3 million in FY 2001. Founded by Dr. Wayne Jones in 1949, it is a center of excellence for cardiac care in the Central City service area. The Strategic Plan for SouthSide Hospital, 2001–2005 includes major goals and initiatives to maintain and expand the cardiac services provided to the Central City community. This proposal for a Cardiac Catheterization Laboratory is an important strategic initiative because it will enhance the cardiac services currently provided and help move SouthSide Hospital into the 21st century.

Problem or Need Identification

An Internet search obtained a considerable amount of information on cardiac disorders and cardiac catheterization issues. The Web site for the American Heart Association (www.americanheart.org) has extensive information and statistics on cardiovascular disease. For example, it is estimated that nearly 20% of the general population in the U.S. has some form of cardiovascular disease, with hypertension the most common disorder, and a significant risk factor for stroke and heart disease. Coronary heart disease, stroke, and other cardiovascular disorders cause the deaths of over 2,600 Americans each day. Statistics from the Central County Public Health Department (which serves the Central City service area) confirm that Central County conforms to national and state patterns in that cardiovascular disease is the leading cause of death.

Cardiac catheterizations have increased substantially since the late 1970s as a diagnostic method for cardiovascular disorders. A number of considerations pertinent to the proposed Cardiac Catheterization Laboratory for SouthSide Hospital are presented in the clinical expert consensus document, "Cardiac Catheterization Laboratory Standards," published by the American College of Cardiology on its Web site www.acc.org. One consideration is that, although a minimum recommended number of diagnostic studies performed in a cardiac catheterization facility has not been scientifically validated, the recommendation is that an interventional facility perform at least 400 procedures annually to ensure proficiency. Moreover, hospitals without cardiac surgery back-up should not perform procedures on patients with certain severe disease categories. The document discusses advantages to digital radiological technology and recommends moving away from cineangeography based on improved resolution and the reduction in requirements for film storage space. Credentialing and quality monitoring procedures should be in place in any cardiac catheterization facility.

A search of books and journals produced an abundance of current information on planning, equipping, and licensing a cardiac catheterization facility. However, if this business plan is approved, a consultant with experience in cardiac catheterization facility design and management will be hired to implement this project.

Local cardiology physician groups were targeted for interviews about the need for a Cardiac Catheterization Laboratory. Those interviewed included three cardiologists, each from a different cardiology group practicing in the Central City service area. One of the three cardiologists performs cardiac catheterizations at a competing facility, but expressed concern because the facility does not have a comparable level of cardiac surgery back-up for many of the more serious cases. These more serious cases must be referred 50 miles away to a medical center with cardiac surgery back-up available, or to SouthSide Hospital's current cardiac catheterization services.

All three cardiologists emphasized that SouthSide Hospital's cardiac catheterization services need major upgrading to newer, better technologies, and the current area lacks the space needed. Moreover, although cardiac surgery back-up is available at SouthSide Hospital, the current location of the cardiac catheterization service is not really convenient to the surgical center. Locating the cardiac catheterization procedures within or adjacent to the Surgery Department would allow for a far more timely and effective response should an emergency occur.

All three cardiologists stated that they and the other cardiologists in their groups would increase referrals to SouthSide Hospital for cardiac catheterizations and related interventional procedures if a newer, better-located cardiac catheterization facility were available, but they plan to refer more patients to the out-of-service-area competitor (Rose Woods Medical Center) over the next 5 years if SouthSide Hospital's cardiac catheterization facilities are not upgraded.

Product Definition

The proposed Cardiac Catheterization Laboratory would be located in one of the Cardiac Surgery Center's operating rooms, currently an under-utilized space which is lead lined (for radiology procedures) and meets the state's requirements for size and other related features. An adjoining supply room would be remodeled to create an equipment control room. This new location would remove the cardiac catheterization services from the Radiology Department and much more conveniently locate them within the Cardiac Surgery Center in case of the need for emergency intervention. The Cardiac Catheterization Laboratory would also be much closer to the Recovery Room and Outpatient Observation Room for routine follow-up care and observation of more seriously ill clients.

The proposal includes plans for upgrading or replacing the current cardiac catheterization equipment to utilize the latest technologies available. A consultant with expertise in the design and management of cardiac catheterization laboratories will plan and oversee the purchase of equipment and the creation of the new services. The Cardiac Catheterization Laboratory budget (Table C–2) indicates the remodeling costs and the types and costs of replacement equipment. Budget projections are also included for the alternative scenario, maintaining the current cardiac catheterization services (Table C–3).

Market Analysis or Environmental Scan

SouthSide Hospital's service area is defined as the southern half of Central County and consists of approximately 20 zip codes. The current (FY 2001) service area population is approximately 215,000. The service area has a higher proportion of persons over age 65 (14.3% compared to the state's 11.9%) and a much higher annual growth rate for this age group (12.5% compared to the state's 6.2%), which reinforces not only the need but potential success of a state-of-the-art Cardiac Catheterization Laboratory.

The major competitor for cardiac patients in the market area is Goodman General Hospital, a for-profit facility located in the northern part of Central City. However, Goodman General does not have the cardiac surgery backup required for more serious cases. Rose Woods Medical Center, located in Anywhere, is 50 miles away, but, in addition to cardiac surgery back-up, offers the latest technologies for cardiac catheterization, improving diagnostic accuracy and patient outcomes. Relocating and upgrading the cardiac catheterization services would divert many of these referrals from Rose Woods Medical Center to SouthSide Hospital.

Based on the above demographic data and opportunity for referrals, Table C–4 projects the estimated service population and number of cardiac catheterization procedures for FY 2002–2005. Projections are also provided for actual referrals for cardiac catheterization

TABLE C-2

SouthSide Hospital Capital Budget for Cardiac Catheterization Laboratory, FY 2002

Item	Cost Estimate
Construction (Remodeling)	$1,050,000
New Philips HC5000C Catheterization Laboratory	1,104,128
Extended Warrantee	74,458
Hemodynamic monitoring system	118,779
Extended Warranty	7,794
Intra-Aortic Balloon Pump	43,000
Extended Warrantee	1,050
Emergency Crash Cart & Defibrillator	11,500
Start-up Medical Supplies	12,000
Sub-Total	**2,422,708**
Sales Tax (7% on purchases)	89,418
Total	**$2,512,127**

TABLE C-3

SouthSide Hospital Current Cardiac Catheterization Services Operating Expense Budget, FY 2002–2005

Item	FY 2002	FY 2003	FY 2004	FY 2005
Salaries[1,2]	$180,960	$186,389	$191,980	$197,740
Benefits (25% of salaries)	$45,240	$46,597	$47,995	$49,435
Total Personnel	**$226,200**	**$232,986**	**$239,976**	**$247,175**
Medical Supplies[3]	259,375	278,828	299,740	322,221
Non-Medical Supplies	3,000	3,225	3,467	3,727
Housekeeping	8,000	8,240	8,487	8,742
Linen	3,000	3,090	3,183	3,278
Education & Training	10,000	10,000	10,000	10,000
Service Contracts[4]	77,000	96,250	96,250	96,250
Total Non-Personnel	**360,375**	**399,633**	**421,127**	**444,218**
Total Operating Budget	**$586,575**	**$632,619**	**$661,103**	**$691,392**

[1] Includes 3 FTE clinical staff ($25/hr), 1 FTE unit clerk ($12/hr).
[2] Assumes 3% increase in salaries per year.
[3] Assumes 7.5% increase in medical & non-medical supplies per year.
[4] Service contracts increase by 25% beginning FY 2003.

TABLE C-4

SouthSide Hospital Projected Service Population and Cardiac Catheterization Procedures for Alternative Scenarios, FY 2002–2005

Year	Service Population[1]	Total Procedures[2]	Current Cardiac Cath Services[3]	Cardiac Cath Laboratory[4]
2002	221,450	554	498	543
2003	228,094	570	485	559
2004	234,936	587	470	576
2005	241,984	605	454	593

[1] Assumes 215,000 service population FY 2001 and 3% growth rate FY 2002–2005.

[2] Assumes 2.5 procedures/1,000 FY 2002–2005.

[3] Assumes 10% base and 5% growth in referrals to out-of-service-area competitor each year, based on cardiologist interviews & current referral data.

[4] Assumes 2% average referral to out-of-service-area competitor FY 2002–2005.

to SouthSide Hospital, based on interviews with local cardiologists. Note that under the alternative of maintaining current services, referrals are projected to decrease despite the increased demand estimated for the service area. A renovated Cardiac Catheterization Laboratory is expected to increase referrals significantly.

Budget Estimates

Two sets of budget estimates are prepared. The first includes a capital budget and operating budget projections for a new Cardiac Catheterization Laboratory. The second set of budget estimates are operating budget projections for maintaining current cardiac catheterization services.

Budget Estimates for a New Cardiac Catheterization Laboratory

The capital budget for FY 2002 and the operating budget projections for FY 2002–2005 for the new Cardiac Catheterization Laboratory are in Tables C–2 and C–5. Assumptions are summarized in the notes to each budget table.

Note that the start-up costs for the project are represented in the capital budget, so for FY 2002, the year the proposal would be implemented, the total operating and capital (start-up) costs are $574,575 plus $2,512,127, or $3,086,702 total. The finance office will prepare estimates of 5- and 10-year loan and depreciation costs of this capital investment before project implementation.

Budget Estimates for Maintaining Current Cardiac Catheterization Services

Table C–3 shows the costs of maintaining current cardiac catheterization services. Note that as referrals are estimated to be substantially lower, there are only three clinical staff rather than four. Also note that although the service contract increases by 25% beginning FY 2003, given the age of the equipment, our vendors have warned that there may be additional repair or maintenance costs.

Additional Financial Analyses

Pro forma P&L projections for fiscal year 2002–2005 are presented for the proposed new Cardiac Catheterization Laboratory for SouthSide Hospital. Note that the more profitable alternative is to relocate cardiac catheterization services and update the equipment.

TABLE C-5

SouthSide Hospital Cardiac Catheterization Laboratory Projected Operating Budget, FY 2002–2005

Item	FY 2002	FY 2003	FY 2004	FY 2005
Salaries[1,2]	$232,960	$239,949	$247,147	$254,562
Benefits (25% of salaries)	$58,240	$59,987	$61,787	$63,640
Total Personnel	**$291,200**	**$299,936**	**$308,934**	**$318,202**
Medical Supplies[3]	259,375	272,344	285,961	300,259
Non-Medical Supplies	3,000	3,150	3,308	3,473
Housekeeping	8,000	8,240	8,487	8,742
Linen	3,000	3,090	3,183	3,278
Education & Training	10,000	10,000	10,000	10,000
Service Contracts[4]	0	85,000	85,000	85,000
Total Non-Personnel	**283,375**	**381,824**	**395,938**	**410,752**
Total Operating Budget	**$574,575**	**$681,760**	**$704,872**	**$728,954**

[1] Includes 4 FTE clinical staff ($25/hr), 1 FTE unit clerk ($12/hr).

[2] Assumes 3% increase in salaries per year.

[3] Assumes 5% increase in medical & non-medical supplies per year.

[4] Service contracts begin FY 2003.

Pro forma P&L Projections for the Current Cardiac Catheterization Laboratory

Table C–6 shows the pro forma P&L projections if current cardiac catheterization services are maintained over the next 4 years. Note that administrative overhead costs are higher (related to higher liability costs projected by risk management because of higher estimated rates of misdiagnosis from using older equipment, and from the less convenient location to cardiac surgery). The average profit margin for fiscal year 2002–2005 is only 14.9%, which is well below the 20% profit margin target.

Pro Forma P&L Projections for a New Cardiac Catheterization Laboratory

Table C–7 presents a pro forma profit and loss statement and estimated profit margins for FY 2002–2005 for the proposed Cardiac Catheterization Laboratory for SouthSide Hospital. Note that the average profit margin for FY 2002–2005 is 20.9%, which meets the target profit margin of 20%.

Timeline

Table C–8 presents the timeline for the proposed Cardiac Catheterization Laboratory. The timeline is prepared from business plan submission on October 8, 2001 through beginning patient care services in the newly renovated facility on April 29, 2002, approximately 7 months total.

Conclusion and Feasibility Statement

The demographic study and analysis of profit and loss indicate that the relocation and renovation of cardiac catheterization services at SouthSide Hospital will be a profitable venture. Potential threats include the

TABLE C-6

SouthSide Hospital Current Cardiac Catheterization Services, Pro Forma P&L Projections 2002–2005

	FY 2002	FY 2003	FY 2004	FY 2005
Volume	498	485	470	454
Charges per Procedure[1]	$7,000	$7,140	$7,283	$7,428
Gross Revenue	3,487,838	3,460,749	3,421,988	3,370,445
Deductions[2]	2,267,094	2,318,702	2,361,172	2,393,016
Net Revenue	$1,220,743	$1,142,047	$1,060,816	$977,429
Operating Expenses	586,575	632,619	661,103	691,392
Depreciation[3]	263,191	263,191	263,191	263,191
Administrative Overhead[4]	19,931	20,357	20,721	21,007
Total Expenses	$869,697	$916,167	$945,015	$975,591
pro forma P&L	$351,047	$225,880	$115,801	$1,838
Profit Margin	28.8%	19.8%	10.9%	0.2%

[1] Assumes 2% increase in charges/year.
[2] Assumes 2% increase in deductions/year.
[3] Assumes 10 year straight line depreciation.
[4] Assumes administrative overhead $40 per procedure with 5% increase/year.

TABLE C-7

SouthSide Hospital Proposed Cardiac Catheterization Laboratory, Pro Forma P&L Projections 2002–2005

	FY 2002	FY 2003	FY 2004	FY 2005
Volume[1]	505	559	576	593
Charges per Procedure[2]	$8,050	$8,292	$8,540	$8,796
Gross Revenue	4,061,819	4,633,531	4,915,713	5,215,080
Deductions[3]	2,640,183	3,104,466	3,391,842	3,702,707
Net Revenue	$1,421,637	$1,529,065	$1,523,871	$1,512,373
Operating Expenses	574,575	681,760	704,872	728,954
Depreciation[4]	465,481	465,481	465,481	465,481
Start-up Costs[5]	95,302	0	0	0
Administrative Overhead[6]	17,660	20,565	22,218	24,011
Total Expenses	$1,153,018	$1,167,806	$1,192,572	$1,218,446
pro forma P&L	$268,619	$361,259	$331,299	$293,927
Profit Margin	18.9%	23.6%	21.7%	19.4%

[1] Assumes 7% drop in projected volume for FY 2002 due to construction.
[2] Assumes 15% increase in base charge of $7,000 and 3% increase in charges/year.
[3] Assumes 2% increase in deductions/year.
[4] Assumes 7 year straight line depreciation on equipment, including crash cart, and construction.
[5] Start-up costs include medical supplies & all extended warrantees.
[6] Assumes reduction in administrative overhead to $35/procedure with 5% growth/year.

◯ TABLE C-8

SouthSide Hospital Timeline for Proposed Cardiac Catheterization Laboratory, FY 2001–2002

Date	Activity	Authority/Responsibility
10/8/01	Submission of proposal for Cardiac Catheterization Laboratory (CCL) to CEO and CFO.	Cardiac Catheterization Project Committee (CCPC)
11/19/01	Pending CEO & CFO approval, proposal revised & send to Board of Directors.	CEO, CFO & CCPC
12/10/01	Approval of proposal by Board of Directors.	Board of Directors
1/7/02	Hire consultant to design & start up CCL.	CEO, CFO & CCPC chair
1/21/02	Contract negotiation for construction & capital equipment.	CFO, consultant, CCPC chair
2/18/02	Begin renovation of Operating Room for CCL.	Consultant, construction company project manager
4/1/02	Begin installation of equipment; order start-up medical supplies.	Consultant, construction company project manager, equipment project manager, medical supplies vendor
4/22/02	Finish renovation, installation, testing & trouble shooting, receive start-up supplies.	Consultant, construction company project manager, cardiac cath equipment project manager, medical supplies vendor
4/29/02	Opening of CCL for patient care.	Consultant, chair of CCL

development of enhanced cardiac surgery and diagnostic services by competitors, unanticipated reductions in reimbursement, unanticipated reduction in volume, and technological change rendering the Cardiac Catheterization Laboratory obsolete.

Interviews with local cardiology group representatives and a market analysis indicate it is highly unlikely that competitors in the local service area are planning to add or enhance their cardiac surgery or diagnostic services over the next 5 years. A growth rate of 2% in deductions to charges is included in the pro forma profit and loss analysis; this is the best forecast available at this time. A reduction in the volume is unlikely; the volume figures are relatively conservative, given the growth in the over-65 population in the service area and the anticipated increase in referrals from local cardiologists due to the improved location and equipment following the renovation. Technological changes are not anticipated to affect new cardiac catheterization facilities for at least 5 years, which is the depreciation time period, again a conservative approach.

We strongly recommend review and serious consideration of this proposal to maintain and enhance SouthSide Hospital's reputation for cardiac services in Central City.

APPENDIX D

Education, Outreach, and Screening for Underserved Latina/Hispanic Women in the Anywhere Metropolitan Area

This proposal, submitted by the Rose Woods Medical Center Breast Cancer Screening Program (BCSP), requests a $50,500 grant to enhance our education, outreach, and screening services and to develop a multicultural model for women from the Latino/Hispanic communities of the Anywhere metropolitan areas. Please contact Ms. Grace Smith, Director, BCSP, Rose Woods Medical Center, 1234 Main Street, Anywhere, 99999 if there are any questions regarding this proposal.

Problem Definition

Even though the incidence rates for breast cancer are lower for Latina/Hispanic women than for white women, Latina/Hispanic women are more likely to die from breast cancer. Latina/Hispanic women are underserved and under-utilize breast cancer screening services for many reasons, all of which contribute to late diagnosis and treatment with higher mortality rates. These reasons include the lack of health insurance, under-representation of Latinos/Hispanics in the health care professions, language and cultural barriers, religious and health care beliefs, fear of immigration penalties, and lack of transportation. In addition, fear and lack of knowledge about breast cancer, breast cancer screening, and breast cancer treatment is a disincentive.

Needs Assessment

BCSP provided breast-screening services to 402 Latina/Hispanic women in 2001. Of these, 314 were monolingual or spoke only limited English. Of this 314, only 111 brought someone to translate. In addition, 226 of the 402 Latina/Hispanic women were uninsured (56.2%), compared to 36.4% of the African-American women and 24.3% of the white women screened.

Currently, the BCSP employs only one Spanish-speaking receptionist and one half-time RN, who must do all the translation for the program as none of the other receptionists, technicians, nurses, radiologists, or other BCSP staff speak Spanish. This disparity presents barriers to education and services for the Latina/Hispanic women in the area. There are no breast cancer screening or womens' health programs in the Anywhere Metropolitan Area that meet the linguistic or cultural needs of Latina/Hispanic women.

BCSP recognizes that breast cancer education, outreach, and screening must not only reduce the language barrier for Latina/Hispanic women, but must address the diversity of this ethnic population and provide culturally sensitive care and support. In addition, BCSP recognizes the importance of meeting the needs of Latina/Hispanic women who lack health insurance.

Program Goals and Objectives

The proposed education program targets Latina/Hispanic women age 20 and above. Latina/Hispanic women age 40 and above, and younger women who are identified as at risk (such as those with a reported family history of breast cancer), are targeted for breast cancer outreach and screening. Emphasis will be placed on providing services to women who are of lower income, uninsured, and monolingual or limited in the English language.

The goals of the program are as follows:

1. Increase awareness and knowledge about breast health issues and services among Latina/Hispanic women age 20 and above by providing education and outreach in local churches in the Anywhere Metropolitan Area with large Latino/Hispanic congregations.
2. Increase the number of Latina/Hispanic women in the Anywhere metropolitan area, insured and uninsured, age 40 and above (and younger women identified at risk), who seek breast cancer screening at BCSP facilities, including clinical breast exams and first time or annual mammograms.
3. Increase the number of Latina/Hispanic women age 20 and above in the Anywhere metropolitan area (insured and uninsured) who have routine clinical breast exams at Rose Woods Medical Center facilities.
4. Identify incentives and disincentives (such as attitudes, beliefs, knowledge, language, income, and transportation) and improve access to appropriate mammography services for Latina/Hispanic women in the Anywhere Metropolitan Area.
5. Serve as a resource for BCSP personnel and local health care agencies and clinics to improve access to health services for Latina/Hispanic women in the Anywhere metropolitan area.
6. Coordinate breast cancer screening services with the Cancer Services Center for Women at Rose Woods Medical Center, building on a collaborative relationship to facilitate psychosocial support and breast care follow-up for newly diagnosed Latina/Hispanic women in the Anywhere metropolitan area who have been seen in Rose Wood Medical Center facilities.

The program objectives are as follows, including activities to achieve the objectives and methods for evaluating the extent to which the objectives are achieved:

1) By the conclusion of the grant period, BCSP will provide breast health education to 1,000 Latina/ Hispanic women age 20 and over in local churches in the Anywhere metropolitan area, including linguistically and culturally sensitive information on the importance of mammography when age appropriate, clinical breast exams, routine breast self-examination, BCSP services, and other assistance programs for underinsured and uninsured populations.
2) By the conclusion of the grant period, 330 Latina/Hispanic women in the Anywhere metropolitan area (including at least 130 new clients) will receive medical translation and access assistance services, as needed, for clinical breast exams, screening, and follow-up care at BCSP and/or Rose Woods Medical Center facilities.
3) By the conclusion of the grant period, program staff will identify the major access problems for Latina/Hispanic women and will generate a report with recommendations to BCSP and the Administration of Rose Woods Medical Center.
4) All Latina/Hispanic women from the Anywhere metropolitan area who are newly diagnosed with breast cancer or other breast health problems at Rose Woods Medical Center will receive appropriate referrals and information, with psychosocial, program navigation, and follow-up support as needed.

Program Description and Activities

This program develops a model for breast cancer education, coordinating the efforts of the BCSP and the Rose Woods Medical Center Health Ministries/Parish Nursing Program to serve Latina/Hispanic women in local churches with large Latino/Hispanic congregations.

1. The bilingual Spanish breast health RN hired by the Rose Woods Medical Center Health Ministries/Parish Nursing Program (RN) will have an orientation including the following requisites:
   - Review of the literature and conference proceedings regarding beliefs, barriers to health care, and other behaviors of Latina/Hispanic women related to breast health and breast cancer.
   - Complete the BCSP Clinical Breast Exam Training Course.
   - Complete the BCSP Breast Self Examination Patient Educator's Course.
   - Identify resource persons in churches with large Latino/Hispanic congregations in the Anywhere metropolitan area, at the Clinica Hispanica (a local free clinic for Latino/Hispanic poor and undocumented persons), at the Central County Public Health Department (which serves the Anywhere metropolitan area), and at the Cancer Services Center for Women at Rose Woods Medical Center.

2. The RN will work with BCSP to develop linguistically and culturally sensitive educational programs beginning the first month of the grant period.
3. The RN meets with pastors, ministers, parish nurses, and health ministry board members of churches with large Latino/Hispanic congregations in the Anywhere metropolitan area to collaborate and schedule breast health presentations beginning the second month of the grant period.
4. The RN develops methods to identify and document barriers to access for Latina/Hispanic women, including a bilingual interview.
   - The RN meets routinely with representatives from the BCSP, the Rose Woods Medical Center Health Ministries/Parish Nursing Program, the Cancer Services Center for Women at Rose Woods Medical Center, and churches with large Latino/Hispanic congregations in the Anywhere metropolitan area to report progress, plan program modifications as needed, identify unmet needs, and develop funding and a strategic plan for services beyond the 12-month grant funded period.

5. The RN assesses client needs and provides translation and transportation assistance for up to 350 Latina/Hispanic women in the Anywhere metropolitan area to BCSP services.
6. With assistance from the Director of BCSP, the RN submits timely quarterly and annual reports as required by The Joyce Ogden Breast Cancer Foundation.

Timetable

The timetable for this project is presented as follows, assuming that funding is approved and begins FY 2002 (July 1, 2002):

- July 1 to 31—RN recruitment and hiring
- August 1 to 15—RN orientation
- August 15, 2002 to June 30, 2003—program implementation
- Quarterly reports submitted October 15, 2002; January 15, 2003; April 15, 2003; and the final annual report June 30, 2003.

Resources

Rose Woods Medical Center, through the Health Ministry/Parish Nursing Program and the BCSP, will provide the following in-kind contributions:

- Office space
- Telephone, computer, and fax
- Postage
- Liability insurance premiums
- AV equipment and supplies (slide projector, video monitor, etc.)
- Other indirect costs
- On-going supervision

Resource Needs and Budget

The primary need is for a Spanish bilingual breast health RN hired at 20 hours a week (0.5 FTE). Other resources needed include taxi vouchers, mileage, some administrative costs, and the printing of bilingual educational brochures. The budget is presented in Table D-1.

Evaluation Plan

Some initial methods for program evaluation are as follows, with refinements to the plan as the program is implemented:

- Data collection, analysis, summary, and report on the number and demographic characteristics of the women served by the program, including the number of women referred for follow-up services.
- Identification and analysis of actual barriers to access that are encountered during the course of program implementation.
- Preparation of an internal report and recommendations to the Rose Woods Medical Center's Administration and to the Directors of the BCSP, the Health Ministries/Parish Nursing Program, and the Cancer Services Center for Women.

Future Funding

If funded by The Joyce Ogden Breast Cancer Foundation, we hope to qualify for a second year of funding. If approved, program expansion in the second year will include volunteer training within the local congregations to provide translation and transportation assistance, and publicizing BCSP services in church newsletters and at congregational activities such as Health Awareness Days and Health Fairs.

TABLE D-1

Latina/Hispanic Women's Program Budget, FY 2002–2003

Item	Amount
Spanish speaking bilingual RN (0.5 FTE)[1]	$32,000
RN benefits	$3,500
Taxi vouchers[2]	$10,250
Administration	$3,500
Mileage[3]	$1,100
Educational brochures[4]	$150
Total	**$50,500**

[1] Contract and part-time benefits total $35,500 annually.

[2] Estimated $18 per round-trip for approximately 510 vouchers.

[3] Estimated at $0.34/mile x 30 miles for approximately 110 days.

[4] Estimated as 1,000 brochures at $150.

We will also prepare a report evaluating the program and present a business plan requesting support for this program as an increase to the BCSP and/or the Health Ministries/Parish Nursing budgets at Rose Woods Medical Center, specifically funding the 0.5 FTE breast health RN position to maintain the program activities.

Capability Statement

As mentioned in the cover letter, Rose Woods Medical Center is the oldest acute care facility, and is the largest provider of breast cancer screening services in the Anywhere metropolitan area. The Rose Woods Breast Cancer Screening Program (BCSP) screened over 12,200 women in 2001, resulting in the largest number (500) of newly diagnosed cases in the county. BCSP was the 2001 recipient of the Anywhere Mayor's Office Annual Outstanding Service Award for its breast cancer screening services to women, particularly those without health insurance or with other social or economic disadvantages.

Over the prior 3 years, BCSP developed and implemented a highly successful and nationally recognized model for engaging underserved African American women in breast cancer screening and follow-up care in collaboration with the Health Ministry/Parish nursing program. Based on the success of this prior program addressing diversity and disparity in health care, we believe we are fully capable of developing a model program for breast health and breast cancer education, outreach, and screening for the underserved Latina/Hispanic women in the Anywhere metropolitan area. We also have letters of support and MOUs from the Mayor's Office, collaborating offices and agencies, and representatives of churches with large African-American and Latino/Hispanic congregations lending their support to this proposed program.

We appreciate your review of this proposal, and are available upon request for further information upon request.

Attachments:

- Cover letter
- Letters of support
- MOUs

Note: These attachments appear on the CD-ROM included in the back of this book.

APPENDIX E: Policy Question Worksheet

Policy Question Worksheet for Tracking Future Trends in Health Care

Policy Question	Future Trends
Cost	
Quality	
Access	
Universality	
Equity	
Efficiency	
Choice	
Prevention	

SOURCE: Adapted from Roberts & Clyde, 1993.

Glossary

A/P (see **accounts payable** or **trade credit**): A current liability representing the amounts due to vendors for supplies

Accelerated depreciation: Methods of reporting depreciation in which the depreciation expense is calculated as progressively smaller over subsequent time periods

Accounts payable (see **A/P** or **trade credit**): A current liability representing the amounts due to vendors for supplies

Accounts receivable (AR): A claim for payment for goods or services provided

Accrual basis of accounting: An accounting method in which revenues are recorded when earned—representing an obligation for payment—and expenses are recorded when inputs are employed, used, or consumed

Accrued expenses: A current liability representing expenses generated daily, with periodic payment, such as wages and interest due on loans

Accumulated depreciation: Total depreciation expensed over time (typically year to year) against the original cost of fixed assets

Activity (asset management or turnover) ratios: Help managers determine how effectively the enterprise is using its assets

Activity-based costing (ABC): A cost allocation method that focuses on the indirect and direct costs of specific activities performed within cost centers, with the cost of specific activities used as cost drivers

Acuity: Estimated severity of various disorders, frequently measured by the hours of direct care required per patient day

Adjusted FTE: A full-time equivalent that accounts for non-productive as well as productive time, typically fewer hours than an unadjusted FTE

Adjusted percent variance: A calculation in monitoring flexible budgets to correct the percent variance for the effects of volume, using the formula: Adjusted Percent Variance = Percent Budget Variance − Percent Volume Variance

Adjusted variance: A calculation in monitoring flexible budgets to correct the variance for the effects of volume, using the formula: Adjusted Variance = Budgeted Value × Adjusted Percent Variance

Adjustment authority: Budget control approval to revise the budget during the budget year to correct for uncontrollable, predictable changes in price or quantity variance

Adverse selection: Over-selection of a health plan based on its coverage of populations likely to have high health care costs

Advertising: Mass media communication purchased by a sponsor to persuade a target audience

Agent: The party entrusted with decision-making authority, such as a physician entrusted with decision-making authority on behalf of the patient

Align incentives: Design strategies to reinforce the simultaneous goals of improving health care quality and access while reducing costs

Allocative efficiency: Represents minimizing the amount or cost of inputs while maximizing the value or benefit of outputs, or producing outputs of maximum value or benefit for a given amount or cost of inputs

Allowable costs: Costs directly related to providing an acceptable standard of health services, reimbursed under cost-based reimbursement systems

Amortization: Expensing the value of an intangible asset over its life

Annual report: A financial statement that provides an overall summary of an organization's financial performance, prepared largely for the review of persons outside the organization

AR (accounts receivable): A claim for payment for goods or services provided

Asset management (activity or **turnover) ratios:** Help managers determine how effectively the enterprise is using its assets

Assets: Any of a business organization's tangible or intangible resources that possess or create economic benefit, recorded in the balance sheet as Assets = Liabilities + Equity

Assumption: Expectation or belief about the internal or external environment that influences decision-making

Asymmetric information: Situation in which one party possesses knowledge needed to enable rational decision making that the other party lacks

Average (mean): The sum of a set of values divided by the number of the set of values

Average cost (AC): The total cost of producing a product divided by the quantity produced, calculated as AC = TC ÷ Q

Average daily census (ADC): The sum of the daily count of patients over a month (or specified time period) divided by the number of days in the month (or the same specified time period)

Bad debt: A reduction to charges representing uncollectible reimbursement from patients or third-party payors who are assumed to be able to pay but do not pay

Balance sheet (see **statement of financial position**): A financial statement that reports information about the organization's assets and acquisition of those assets

Balance the budget: Apply budget control or adjustment for variance to equalize budgeted values with actual values, or to allow revenues to equal or exceed expenses

Benchmark: A target indicator that measures the achievement of an industry standard

Benefit: Output or contribution produced by the objective function—in many cases, cost savings achieved by the intervention

Benefit-cost ratio (B/C ratio): Calculation in cost-benefit analysis in which benefits are divided by costs, which allows for comparison across similar interventions

Benefits management: Continual monitoring of a member's benefit status for patients with high-cost conditions in order to conserve the benefit to the greatest possible extent

Board-restricted accounts: Unrestricted accounts established by internal decision-making entities (boards) that can change their funding restrictions relatively flexibly

Book value: The balance sheet value of owner's equity for asset

Break-even analysis: Calculating the amount of revenue-generating volume or revenue required that covers the costs of a program, service, or department, with or without profit, calculated as Total Revenue = Total Costs or Total Revenue = Total Costs + Profit

Budget balancer: Management strategy for generating revenues or reducing expenses to achieve desired profits

Budget control: Use of information from budget monitoring and administrative theory to manage performance to meet budget targets or to resolve undesired variances from targets

Budget cycle: The time frame for budget preparation and approval, budget implementation, and budget monitoring and control

Budget monitoring: Includes management activities, such as reviewing and tracking the budget against actual performance, to identify undesired variances from targets and identify the sources of undesired variances

Budget variance: The difference between the target (budget) value and the actual value of volume, revenue, or expense

Budget year: 12 month time period for budgets that may or may not represent a calendar year, also referred to as the **fiscal year**

Business grant proposal: Application for funding that describes the budget, pricing, and all other financial information related to the proposed program or service, usually as one of two sections of the same grant proposal, with the **technical grant proposal** as the other section

CA (current assets): Cash or other resources of an organization expected to be converted into cash or exchanged within a fiscal year, such as marketable securities, **receivables** or **collectibles**, inventory, and current prepayments

Cap: A limit placed on insurance coverage, usually on an annual or lifetime basis

Capability statement: Grant proposal documentation that presents a convincing description of the qualifications of the applicant agency or agencies and participating staff in implementing the proposed program or service

Capital: In accounting, refers to owner's equity in a for-profit enterprise—in a production function, refers to inputs other than labor

Capital budget: A budget of expenses for high-cost and long-term items such as equipment, major maintenance and repair, renovation, and construction

Capital improvement grant: Provides funding to build or renovate buildings and to acquire capital equipment

Capital in excess of par: An entry under contributed capital in the stockholders' equity section of a for-profit organization's balance sheet that represents capital greater than the face value of the stock

Capital structure (debt management or **leverage) ratios:** Show the capability of an enterprise to manage and pay its debts

Capitalization ratios: Debt management ratios using balance sheet data that indicate the extent to which assets are financed by debt

Capitation: A form of pre-payment in which a fixed payment is established per health plan enrollee and is paid to the provider (or provider system) for a specified set of services over a specified time period

Carve-in: A specialty managed care organization operating within the larger HMO or other medically oriented MCO

Carve-out: A specialty managed care organization operating separately and independently from the HMO or other medically-oriented MCO

Case mix: Combination of clients with various disorders and acuity levels for a given provider or setting, which represents the various levels or amounts of care required; often measured in units such as average hours of direct care per patient day or the average number of patient visits, used in managed care reporting and acute care staffing and budgeting

Cash basis of accounting: An accounting method in which revenue represents and is recorded at the time of payment, and expenses represent and are recorded at the time of expenditures or monetary disbursements

Cash flow budget (cash budget): Shows estimates of the flow of money in and out of the institution, to help anticipate substantial cash shortfalls or surpluses

Cash flow coverage ratio (CFC ratio): A debt coverage management ratio that shows how well the cash flow covers fixed financial needs, calculated as Cash + Marketable Securities ((Expenses less Depreciation less Provision for Uncollectibles) ÷ 365 expressed in days

Cash flow statement (see **statement of cash flows**): A financial report that provides details about the sources of cash assets and how cash is used in the enterprise

Centenarian: Person age 100 or older

Ceteris paribus: A Latin term used in economics meaning "all else remaining equal," or the assumption that all variables are held constant except the variable of interest

Charge: The full price used in calculating gross revenue before any reductions are applied

Charge-based reimbursement: A health care payment system in which the provider bills the payor for the charges provider set for the good or service

Charity care: A reduction to the charge that represents the provision of services to clients who are assumed to be unable to pay

Churning: Scheduling more office visits or procedures than necessary for the patient

CL (current liabilities): A section in the balance sheet which include debts or other financial obligations that must be paid over the short term, usually within the fiscal year

Coinsurance: A percentage of a health care cost paid by the beneficiary, such as 20% of a hospital bed rate per inpatient day

Collateral: An asset pledged to the lender if the borrower defaults on the loan

Collectibles (receivables): A current asset representing cash currently collected or due as payment due for goods or services provided, representing a major item for cash management

Common size analysis: Calculating each line of the income statement as a percent of total revenues, or each line of the balance sheet as a percent of total assets, to compare and assess the organization's financial performance

Common stock: An entry under contributed capital in the stockholders' equity section of a for-profit organization's balance sheet that represents shares of stock at its **par** value

Community rating: A method in which premiums are based on the population characteristic of an entire group, in many cases adjusted for age and sex

Competitive grants: Provides funding to only one applicant when multiple agencies are applying for the program funding available

Complement: Product associated with a specific good or service—an increase in the price of complements decreases demand and vice versa

Compounded: The interest earned in each time period earns interest in future time periods

Concurrent review (utilization review): Evaluating the medical record and determining whether the hospitalization is medically necessary, and whether each additional day of hospitalization is medically necessary and will be authorized for reimbursement

Conflict of interest: An ethical discord between two or more desired but opposing circumstances, for example, when the physician both an agent and a provider billing for services unity

Contra-asset account: A negative asset on the balance sheet; the higher the contra-asset account, the smaller the organization's total assets

Contributed capital: The equity section of a for-profit organization's balance sheet that has entries for common stock and **capital in excess of par** value, representing the **capital** or owner's equity in the enterprise

Contribution margin (CM): The amount available to first cover fixed costs (including overhead), then contribute to profits, as shown in the formula: Total Revenue − Total Variable Costs = Contribution Margin

Contribution margin per unit (CMU): The contribution margin per client or per unit of goods or services produced, as shown in the formulas: Contribution Margin per Unit = Revenue per Unit − Variable Cost per Unit, or Contribution Margin per Unit = Contribution Margin ÷ Volume

Control variance: The internal efficiency in charging and billing for services

Controllable variance: Sources of budget variance within the scope of the manager's authority

Co-payment: A dollar amount of a health care cost paid by a beneficiary, such as $20 of every primary care physician office visit

Cost: Resource required as input to produce an objective function, in other words, to produce goods or services, often referred to as operating expense

Cost allocation: Determining the total direct and indirect costs of cost centers such as an inpatient department by allocating the expenses of cost centers to each other using direct distribution, reciprocal, step-down or other accepted methods

Cost center: A work unit that generates expenses and reports an operating expense budget; also refers to a non-revenue cost center that generates expenses but not revenues; may also refer to a revenue cost center or profit center

Cost driver: The measure or specification for allocation of costs from a cost pool in cost allocation

Cost pool: The costs that are grouped or selected to be allocated to other cost centers in cost allocation

Cost-based reimbursement: A health care payment system in which the provider is paid allowable costs directly associated with providing acceptable standards of appropriate health care

Cost-benefit analysis (CBA): Method of evaluating the benefits produced by resources used within a given intervention

Cost-effectiveness analysis (CEA): Method of evaluating and comparing the benefits produced and the resources used between two or more alternative interventions

Cost-finding: Determining the total direct and indirect costs of a service unit such as a patient day using cost allocation, activity based costing, resource use classification systems or other accepted methods

Costs: Resources required to provide a service or produce a good, represented in the expense budget section of an operational budget

Coverage ratios: Debt management ratios using income statement data that show how well reported profits cover fixed financial charges

Creaming (skimming): Selection of populations at lower risk and lower cost by health care insurers

Current assets (CA or working capital): Cash or other resources of an organization expected to be converted into cash or exchanged within a fiscal year, such as marketable securities, **receivables** or **collectibles**, inventory, and current prepayments

Current liabilities (CL): A section in the balance sheet which include debts or other financial obligations that must be paid over the short term, usually within the fiscal year

Current maturities of long-term debt: Represents the portion of long-term debt that must be paid in the coming year

Current Procedural Terminology (CPT®): A coding system that identifies specific physician services and procedures, used to classify outpatient services and costs

Current ratio: A liquidity ratio used as an indicator of the extent to which short-term claims are covered by liquid assets, calculated as: Current Ratio = Current Assets ÷ Current Liabilities

Debt management (capital structure or leverage) ratios: Show the capability of an enterprise to manage and pay its debts

Debt ratio (debt-to-assets ratio): A debt capitalization management ratio that indicates the extent to which debt is used to finance assets, calculated as Total Debt ÷ Total Assets

Debt-to-capitalization ratio: A debt capitalization management ratio that shows the proportion of debt utilized for permanent capital, calculated as Long-Term Debt ÷ Long-Term Capital

Debt-to-equity ratio: A debt capitalization management ratio that provides lenders with information on how much capital creditors have provided to the organization per dollar of equity capital, calculated as Total Debt ÷ Total Equity

Deductible: Minimum threshold out-of-pocket payment before a plan begins to cover health care costs

Default: Failure of a borrower to repay a loan (interest or principal) to the lender as it becomes due

Degree of operating leverage (DOL): Measure of operating leverage, calculated as Contribution Margin ÷ EBIT

Demand: The quantity of a product for which a consumer is able and willing to pay measured over a specified time period

Demand curve: Graphic depiction of the quantities demanded in a specific market over a specific time period for each possible price

Depreciation: Expensing the cost of a capital asset over its useful life

Derived demand: Product demand for the sake of the ultimate output, not for the product itself, as the demand for nurses to provide hospital care

Diagnostic related groups (DRGs): Classifications of illnesses by their type and standardized expected length of inpatient care used since 1983 by the Medicare **prospective payment system**

Direct costs: Expenses incurred or resources used as inputs in the provision of health care or production of an objective function, such as nursing services for hospital inpatients

Direct distribution: A cost allocation method that assigns indirect costs to revenue cost centers from designated cost pools using accepted cost drivers or an overhead rate

Disclosure: Reporting on all of the aspects of financial transactions as accurately and completely as possible so information is not omitted that would give an unfair view of financial condition or performance

Discount rate: The rate of interest used in the discounting calculation to find the **present value**

Discounted charge: Differs from a negotiated charge because it is a non-negotiated flat fee reimbursed by the payor that is less than the provider's full charge

Discounting: Converting the future value of a monetary investment to its **present value**

Disequilibrium (see equilibrium, market failure): Situation in which supply and demand are not in balance in an economic market

DOL (degree of operating leverage): Measure of operating leverage, calculated as Contribution Margin ÷ EBIT

DRGs (Diagnostic Related Categories): Categories of medical and surgical conditions specified in Medicare prospective payment systems

Dynamic labor shortage: A situation of market failure in which the demand for labor continues to increase, but even with wage increases the supply cannot keep up with demand because of factors such as barriers to entry

Earnings Before Interest and Taxes (EBIT): An entry in the income statement also referred to as **operating profit** or **excess of revenue over expenses from operations** recorded because interest payments and taxes do not contribute to the operations of an enterprise; in non-profit enterprises EBIT reflects earnings before interest payments

EBITDA: Earnings before interest, taxes, depreciation and amortization

Economy of scale: Situation in which the long-run average costs decline as output increases, enabling the producer to maximize profits

Economy of scope: Situation in which a producer can jointly produce two or more products at a lower cost than producing each of these goods or services separately

Efficiency: Maximizing the production of goods and services while minimizing the resources required for production

Elasticity: A measure of responsiveness in the quantity demanded by consumers given the amount of change in price or income

Ending cash balance: The amount of money left at the end of the cash flow budgeting period after all cash expenses are paid for the specified time period

Enrollment variance: A type of volume variance representing changes in revenues based on changes in the size of the population served by the health care setting, usually encountered in capitated systems serving specified numbers of covered lives

Equilibrium (see disequilibrium): Situation in which supply and demand are balanced in an economic market, so that the quantity produced and demanded are equal at a price equaling the marginal cost of production

Equity (see **owners equity** or **OE**): Ownership claim on assets, recorded in the balance sheet, and estimated as Equity = Total Assets − Total Liabilities; in health policy, represents the burden of cost fairly distributed based on the ability to pay

Excess of revenue over expenses from operations: An entry in the income statement also referred to as **EBIT (Earnings Before Interest and Taxes)** or **operating profit** recorded because interest payments and taxes do not contribute to the operations of an enterprise; in non-profit enterprises EBIT reflects earnings before interest payments

Expense budget: The line items and dollar estimates associated with the operating costs for the budget year

Expenses: Inputs or costs incurred in the process of producing goods and services and generating revenue

Expense variance: Difference between budget and actual expenses

Experience rating: A method in which premiums are based on the utilization or claims history of the group, rather than on the characteristics of the group's population as a whole

Externality: Uncompensated social consequence of producing or consuming selected goods and services, for example, the positive effect for society of an individual's influenza vaccination; event beyond the control of the intervention that increases risk or uncertainty about the outcomes in a cost-benefit analysis

Factor substitute: An input that enhances another input, serving as a demand shifter, such as a dental assistant who performs many of the preventive procedures that dentists would otherwise perform

Fair market value: The price paid to the owners for an asset

Favorable budget variance: The difference between actual and budgeted amounts that is beneficial to the health care setting

Fee-for-service (FFS): A health care payment system in which the provider is paid allowable costs directly associated with providing acceptable standards of appropriate health care

Fiduciary agency: An office or agency located internally or externally to the applicant agency's overall organization, which assumes the responsibility for financial management of the grant for a percentage of the grant award as payment

Financial accounting: Collecting, reporting, and analyzing organizational level data to present in financial statements

Fiscal conservatism: An accounting practice in which probable losses to a business are recorded if they may be reasonably estimated, while gains are not recorded until they are actually realized

Fiscal year (FY): 12-month time period for budgeting and other financial reporting which may or may not represent the calendar year, selected to fit funding cycles or the financial activities of the setting

Fixed asset turnover (utilization) ratio: Shows how well property, plant, and equipment are utilized to generate profits and provide services, calculated as Total Revenue ÷ Net Fixed Assets

Fixed assets (see **non-current assets, NCA** or **real assets**): Relatively permanent, illiquid resources of an organization such as property, plant and capital equipment

Fixed budget (static budget): Itemizes estimates of revenues and costs for an unchanging volume of service units, price of inputs, or amount of inputs required

Fixed cost (FC): Cost assumed not to vary over the budget year, regardless of changes in volume, such as rent, capital equipment, and permanent fixed staff

Fixed staff: Employees who must be available at the setting regardless of patient volume or acuity

Flexible budget: Adjusts for variation in volume or in the price or amount of inputs, which change associated patient care costs

Forecasting: In budgeting, a formal process in which systematic qualitative or quantitative methods are utilized to estimate future volume, revenues, and expenses as accurately and reliably as possible

Formulary: An approved list for prescribing generic or brand name pharmaceuticals that are less costly than other brand name pharmaceuticals, established by a health plan or MCO

Free rider problem: A potential concern in the provision of public goods, in which many individuals or parties benefit from the public good, but few or no individuals or parties pay for its production

FTEs (full-time equivalents): Determine how many full-time employees are required to work direct hours; one FTE = 2,080 work hours over a business year

Functional classification: Entering costs in a financial statement based on the purpose of the expense, such as inpatient services or administration

Fund accounting: An equity category on the balance sheets of many nonprofit organizations which represents self-contained individual accounts set up for specific activities, programs or other purposes designated by a donor or grant funder

Gatekeeping: The requirement that access to specialists must be authorized by a primary care provider

General fund (operating fund, unrestricted fund): Assets of a nonprofit organization or enterprise that are not restricted by external donors or grant funders, and that may be used for any legitimate activity or purpose

Generic: Less costly than the equivalent brand name pharmaceutical

Goal: Broad statement describing what is to be accomplished over the long or short term

Goodwill: An intangible asset which represents the difference between the **fair market value** and the **book value** of an asset, often obtained via merger or acquisition

Gross domestic product (GDP, see GNP): Value of all goods and services produced by a country over a year, counting the earnings in the country in which the assets are located, and nearly equal to the GNP in the U.S. economy

Gross national product (GNP, see GDP): Value of all goods and services produced by a country over a year, counting the earnings in the home country of the owner of an asset, and nearly equal to the GDP in the U.S. economy

Gross revenue: The total amount generated for goods or services purchased by the client or payor before any discounts are applied, calculated as Gross Revenue = Service Units × Charge per Service Unit

Health maintenance organization (HMO): A managed care organization providing health care to persons voluntarily enrolled in a pre-paid plan

Health program grant proposal: Application for funding which focuses on planning or providing a specific program or service to a target population with documented problems or needs

Healthcare Common Procedure Coding System (HCPCS): A coding system that incorporates and expands CPT® codes to classify services and products not included in the CPT® codes and to reduce the use of "miscellaneous or non-classified" codes

HMO (health maintenance organization): A managed care organization providing health care to persons voluntarily enrolled in a pre-paid plan

Human capital: An approach to valuing human life in which the present value of a person's future earnings are estimated

IBNR (Incurred But Not Reported expense): A current liability entry on the balance sheet or line in the expense budget reflecting pre-payment by capitation systems leading to unreported expenses accrued near the end of an accounting period

Illiquid asset: An organization's resource that cannot readily be exchanged for or converted into cash, such as long-term investments and fixed assets

Incentive: Reward or reinforcement (financial, choice, or time) influencing one of the major interests in health care: the provider, the client, or the payor

Income statement: A financial statement that reports an organization's overall profit or loss

Incremental budgeting: The next year's budget is based on the current year's budget, plus revisions based on assumptions, variances, and administrative budgetary guidelines

Indirect costs: Expenses incurred or resources used that are not direct inputs in the provision of health care or production of an objective function, and that may be budgeted as overhead depending on organizational policy, such as costs for security or landscaping

Inferior good: A pro product for which income elasticity is negative—demand for a normal good falls as income rises

Information problem: The inability of patients, providers or payers to possess all of the information they need for completely rational decision-making

In-kind contribution: A resource the grant proposal applicant is able to make available to support the program or service, such as space, staff, or transportation vehicles

Input: An expense budget item that generates direct or indirect costs in providing goods and services; a resource used to produce goods or services

Intangible: An input or output that one cannot measure

Intangible asset: Resource of an organization that one cannot measure, such as reputation

Interest: A percentage rate charged by a lender representing the price for borrowing

International dollar: Global unit of currency that takes the price levels of various countries into account

Interval variance: A source of reimbursement variance representing the length of time for receipt of payment for services

Inventory: Asset reported in the balance sheet, which in most health care organizations represents supplies kept on hand

Inverse: The amount calculated as 1 less a given decimal amount, as the inverse of 0.3 is $1 - 0.3 = 0.7$

IPA (independent practice association): An organization such as a physician group practice that contracts with a managed care plan to provide services for a capitation rate

Job positions: Amount of full-time (one FTE) or part-time (portion of an FTE) employees hired, for example, 2 job positions of 0.5 FTE each equals 1 job position of 1.0 FTE

Just-in-time: A method of inventory management in which suppliers manage and deliver supplies just before they are required

Lagged values: Estimates reflecting prior financial activities for set periods of time

Law of diminishing marginal utility: As consumption increases, marginal utility decreases

Letter of transmittal: A cover letter enclosed when sending the health program grant proposal to the funding agency that sets the tone and introduces the applicant agency and specific contacts

Leverage (capital structure or **debt management) ratios:** Show the capability of an enterprise to manage and pay its debts

Liability: Claim on assets established by contractual agreements, and estimated as Total Liabilities = Total Assets − Equity

Line item: A category of volume, expense or revenue defined and coded by the institution as a way to organize the budget, usually making up the rows of a budget report

Line item flexibility: Budget control approval to transfer funds contained within one line item for another line item, within specified policy limits

Liquid asset: An organization's resource that represents cash or that can readily be exchanged for or converted into cash, such as income from short-term investments or net accounts receivable

Liquidation: Dissolving a business and distributing its assets first to fulfill claims on liabilities, then either paid out to shareholders (in for-profit enterprises) or contributed to charity (in nonprofit enterprises)

Liquidity ratios: Describe an enterprise's capability to turn assets into cash or to cover current debts with cash and other assets available

Long-term capital: Long-term debt plus equity

Managed care organization (MCO): A managed care plan that may be structured as an HMO, PPO, EPO, or POS plan or other entity using managed care rules and incentives

Managerial accounting: Budgeting and planning, often focused at the level of departments or work units

Marginal cost (MC): Amount of increase in total costs given 1 unit of additional output

Marginal product: Represents the amount of change in output associated with a one unit change in labor or capital

Marginal utility: The rate of change in total utility given a 1 unit change in consumption

Market: An economic mechanism that in theory enables the efficient allocation of resources

Market failure: Situation in which a market cannot reach a reasonably competitive (efficient) equilibrium so that the distribution of income or production is not socially optimal

Market share: The estimated percentage of the entire market for a product or service that is managed by a provider or organization

Marketable securities: Current assets entered on the balance sheet representing highly liquid, low interest-bearing investments such as bank savings accounts, U.S. Treasury bills and money market mutual funds

Master budget: A budget report combining the strategic plan, long-range budget, operating budget(s), capital budget(s) cash flow budget(s) and budget proposals into one document that links short-term and long-term financial planning

Matching principle: A feature of accrual accounting, in which revenue is matched to the time revenue is earned, and revenue is matched with the expenses used to generate that revenue

Materiality principle: Details (such as categories or exact monetary figures) are recorded in financial statements only if they are relevant, enable the reviewer to understand the financial statements, or are required for the reviewer to obtain a fairly stated view of the entity's financial condition

MCO (managed care organization): A managed care plan that may be structured as an HMO, PPO, EPO, POS plan or other entity using managed care rules and incentives

Mean (average): Value summarizing a set of values calculated as: Sum of a Set of Values ÷ Number of Values in the Set

Median: The 50th percentile, middle, or midpoint value, above which fall 50% of the measures and below which fall 50% of the measures

Member month: Total of all months of coverage of each health plan enrollee, calculated as: Members per 1st Month + Members per 2nd Month. . . + Members per nth Month

Memoranda of understanding (MOUs): Grant proposal documentation of the contributions collaborating agencies agree to provide to support the proposed program or service

Monopoly: Inefficient market conditions in which are few if any competitors, no close substitutes, information problems, and barriers to enter or leave

Monopoly rent: Excess profit that occurs in some monopoly markets resulting from charging a price exceeding the marginal cost per unit

Monopsony: A form of market failure seen in many health care labor markets, in which a few purchasers exert market power (price or wages) paid to many suppliers (workers)

Moral hazard: A beneficiary's higher utilization of covered services than would be utilized otherwise

National health insurance: A national health care system in which the national government guarantees health coverage, but may or may not own or employ the health care providers, as in Canada, Japan, and many European nations

National health service: A national health care system in which the national government not only guarantees health coverage but also owns and employs many of the health care providers, as in Great Britain

Natural classification: Entering costs in a financial statement based on the nature of the expense, such as salaries, medical supplies, or property lease

Natural monopoly: Economic market in which the average cost per unit of production falls as output increases because the marginal cost of production is low

NCA (see **fixed assets, non-current assets**, or **real assets**): Relatively permanent resources of an organization such as property, plant, and capital equipment

NCL (non-current liability): A liability entry in the balance sheet for debts or other financial obligations that must be paid over the long term, not due within a year, such as long-term debt

Needs assessment: Grant proposal documentation that clearly and convincingly presents the extent and seriousness of need for the program or service in the target community or population

Negotiated charges: A health care payment system in which the payor negotiates a rate that is less than the charge, or an enhanced level of care for the rate charged by the provider

Net assets: Represents the equity reported in the balance sheet for nonprofit enterprises, as the earnings of a nonprofit must be reinvested in the business

Net benefits (net contribution): Calculation in cost-benefit analysis in which costs are subtracted from benefits

Net deficit: The amount of loss or excess of expenses over revenues, reported in the income statement by non-profits

Net income (profit): The amount of surplus of revenues over expenses, reported in the income statement

Net receivables: Represent receivables less any discounts, or the amount the organization expects to collect rather than the amount due

Net revenue: Gross revenue less any reductions to the full charges

Net surplus (see **net income, profit**): The amount of surplus of revenues over expenses, reported in the income statement by non-profits

Net working capital: The difference between **current assets (CA)** and current liabilities **(CL)**

Non-current assets (see **fixed assets, NCA**, or **real assets**): Relatively permanent resources of an organization such as property, plant, and capital equipment

Non-current liability (NCL): A liability entry in the balance sheet for debts or other financial obligations that must be paid over the long term, not due within a year, such as long-term debt

Non-personnel expenses: A component of the expense budget that itemizes non-employee costs such as supplies, non-capital equipment, and contracted services

Non-revenue cost center: A cost center that generates expenses but not revenues, and typically provides indirect services; also referred to as a cost center or support service

Non-service revenue (non-operating revenue): Revenue generated from charges for goods and services that are not directly related to the primary operations of the setting, such as hospital lobby vending machines

Normal good: A product for which income elasticity is positive—demand for a normal good rises as income rises

Objective: Clearly stated, measurable task intended to achieve a goal within a specific time frame

Objective function: Tangible, measurable definition of what is to be achieved by an intervention

Occupancy rate: Percent of occupied beds, calculated as: Occupancy Rate = Average Daily Census ÷ Beds in Service

OE (see **owners equity** or **equity**): Ownership claim on assets, recorded in the balance sheet, and estimated as Equity = Total Assets − Total Liabilities

Ongoing activity grant: Provides continual funding (usually up to 3 to 5 years) for a specific program or service

Operating budget: An itemized summary of expenses and associated revenues over a specified budgeting time period

Operating fund (general fund, unrestricted fund): Assets of a nonprofit organization or enterprise that are not restricted by external donors or grant funders, and that may be used for any legitimate activity or purpose

Operating leverage: Indicates the proportion of fixed costs for an enterprise compared to its total costs, indicating the effect of changes in volume on changes in profits

Operating profit: An entry in the income statement also referred to as **EBIT (Earnings Before Interest and Taxes) excess of revenue over expenses from operations** recorded because interest payments and taxes do not contribute to the operations of an enterprise; in non-profit enterprises EBIT reflects earnings before interest payments

Operational assistance grant: Provides funding for overhead expenses and ongoing support of the organization implementing a program or service

Opportunity cost: Economic value of an alternative benefit that could be derived during the same time period or with the same amount of resources as invested in the current activity, for example, the time spent waiting in a clinic for health care could be spent earning wages

Order of operations: Sequence in which mathematical calculations must take place to derive the correct result: operations contained in parentheses, followed by multiplication and division, followed by addition and subtraction

Outlier: A value considerably above or below the expected range, usually referring to the cost or utilization of a provider or patient

Output: Good or service produced or supplied

Overhead: Estimated indirect costs of operating a program which are estimated in individual program, unit or department budgets, depending on policy; also referred to as indirect costs or administrative costs

Owners equity (see **equity** or **OE**): Ownership claim on assets, recorded in the balance sheet, and estimated as Equity = Total Assets − Total Liabilities

P&L (profit and loss) statement: Difference between actual operating revenues and actual operating expenses

Par: The face value of **common stock**

Pareto efficiency: An economic condition in which the amount or value of outputs cannot be increased for one party without increasing inputs or costs (or decreasing the amount or value of outputs) for another party

Pareto improvement: A condition in which a more efficient use of inputs improves the amount or value of outputs for one or more party without making the other party (or parties) worse off

Parity: Relative equality of resource allocation to various disease entities, populations or interventions

Patient days: A volume measure calculated by multiplying the average daily census by the number of days in the month (or specified time period)

Payment variance: A source of reimbursement variance representing changes in the amount of payment for contracted services, including bad debt and denials of reimbursement

Payor: The source of reimbursement or payment, usually the patient or a third party in health care

Payor mix: Various sources of reimbursement with various rates of reimbursement for the same goods and services, such as Medicare, Medicaid, and private insurance plans

Payout ratio: The proportion of net income paid out to shareholders in a for-profit enterprise

Per member per month (PMPM): Measure based on each health plan enrollee per month, calculated as the revenue, cost, or utilization value for a specified time period divided by the member months for the same time period

Per member per year (PMPY): Measure of revenue, cost, or utilization for each health plan enrollee per year, calculated as PMPM × 12

Per thousand members per year (PTMPY): A managed care utilization measure, calculated as utilization PMPY × 1,000

Percent: Proportion made up of part of a total amount divided by the total amount, converted or calculated as a decimal equivalent and multiplied by 100% or subtotal ÷ total × 100%

Percentage change analysis: Calculating the percent of change for each item on a financial statement (income statement or balance sheet) from year to year to compare and assess the organization's financial performance

Percentile: The value below which a given percentage of measures fall, with the 50th percentile as the middle or median value

Perfect competition: Optimally efficient market conditions in which neither consumers or producers have enough market power to control the price, there are no barriers to entry, producers and have **perfect information:** And can make rational decisions, producers bear all the costs of production, and consumers bear all the costs of consumption

Perfect information: Ideal situation for optimally rational economic decision-making, in which consumers are as knowledgeable as producers with free choice among alternative goods or services

Performance (profitability) ratios: Help managers understand how well the enterprise generates profits, related to its assets and revenues

Performance target: A measurable indicator for evaluating the achievement of a performance standard or an objective

Personnel expenses: The costs of full-time and part-time employees itemized in the operating budget

Planning grant: Provides funding (typically for no more than 1-2 years) for community assessment, program planning, community networking, and inter-agency collaboration to address a community problem

Pluralistic health system: A national health care system which combines government and non-government providers and funders but does not provide universal guarantees of health care coverage for its citizens and foreign residents, as in the U.S.

PMPM (per member per month): Measure based on each health plan enrollee per month, calculated as the revenue, cost, or utilization value for a specified time period divided by the member months for the same time period

PMPY (Per member per year): Measure of revenue, cost, or utilization for each health plan enrollee per year, calculated as PMPM × 12

Point-of-service (POS): A managed care plan in which services received from providers within the plan is covered more generously than if the member goes outside the plan to choose a provider (see **preferred provider organization**)

Political monopoly: Economic market controlled by regulatory requirements that create barriers to competition

Pre-authorization (prospective review): Evaluating a provider's treatment plan prior to the intervention, and authorizing whether or not the insurer will pay the costs for the intervention

Pre-existing condition clause: A health plan requirement for the consumer to disclose prior illnesses or conditions, limit coverage, or increase premiums accordingly

Preferred provider organization (PPO): A managed care health plan option in which the plan contracts with independent providers at a discounted rate for services; the plan member receives more generous coverage by selecting from these "preferred providers," even without gatekeeper authorization, than if they choose providers outside the plan (see **point-of-service**)

Present value: Monetary value of an investment and its discount (interest) rate for a specified number of years into the future

Price variance: Variation in the cost paid for supplies or other non-personnel items

Primary benefit: A contribution or savings resulting directly from the objective function in a CBA

Principal: The party delegating decision-making authority to another party, such as a patient delegating decision-making authority to the physician, or the amount borrowed from a lender

Principal proponent: Person or group preparing a business plan who will benefit directly from the plan's approval, such as a nurse manager preparing a business plan to renovate the nursing unit

Priority: Organizational activity or issue believed to be of the greatest importance for profitability or survival

Private good: A good or service usually produced in private markets, which is exhaustible and exclusive

Pro forma P&L (profit and loss): Forecasted or estimated difference between revenues and costs

Problem definition: Grant proposal documentation that describes the nature, extent, and seriousness of the problem in enough detail to convince the funder of the problem's importance

Product line: A group of patients with a common characteristic that allows for grouping, such as a common diagnosis or procedure

Product line budget: Similar to an operating budget, except that the focus is on a clinical specialty or on selected groups of patients with same or very similar diagnoses

Product mix: Production of various goods and services with various combinations of costs, volume, and prices, for example, a hospital unit for both medical and surgical patients

Production efficiency: Represents minimizing the costs of producing outputs, or maximizing the production of outputs at a given cost

Production function: Relationships between the maximum output that can be produced given any combination of inputs, such as labor and capital

Production possibilities curve: A graphed illustration of the efficiencies (trade-offs) between two categories of goods or services, within a specified set of constraints

Productivity: The efficiency of production-labor productivity improves when the units of goods or services produced increases for each hour worked

Profit (P): The price per unit of a product sold less the production cost per unit, the net income, or the extent to which total revenue exceeds total costs, as shown in the formula: Profit = Total Revenue − Total Costs

Profit center: A cost center that generates both expenses and revenues, and typically provides direct services; also referred to as a revenue cost center or a cost center

Profit margin (total profit margin): A profitability ratio that shows the relationship between revenues and expenses accrued to generate those revenues, calculated as: Profit Margin = Net Income ÷ Total Revenue

Profit target: A specified amount of profit required to be generated by a program or service, such as a profit target of $200 per day

Profit variance: The difference between actual and budgeted profit and the most primary type of budget variance, influenced by differences in revenue and expenses

Profitability (performance) ratios: Help managers understand how well the enterprise generates profits, related to its assets and revenues

Program description: Grant proposal documentation that provides a narrative depiction of the program or service and its activities, methods and operations so the funder understands how the program objectives will be achieved

Program evaluation: Application of analytic methods to determine whether a program is needed, utilizes its resources effectively, operates as planned, and meets its objectives

Program objective (objective): Clearly stated, measurable task intended to achieve a goal within a specific time frame

Prospective forecasting: Method assuming current information predicts future events, so based on information that the forecaster knows will be implemented

Prospective payment system (PPS): Medicare reimbursement system established in 1983 which pays fixed reimbursement rates to hospitals based on **diagnostic related groups**

Prospective review (pre-authorization): Evaluating a provider's treatment plan prior to the intervention, and authorizing whether or not the insurer will pay the costs for the intervention

PTMPY (Per thousand members per year): A managed care utilization measure, calculated as utilization PMPY $\times$ 1,000

Public good: A good or service that is inexhaustible and non-exclusive, and usually produced by government

Quality-adjusted life year (QALY): An assessment of the proportion of health experienced by an individual over a year, to evaluate the benefits of health care and the value of life

Quantity variance: A source of budget variance resulting from the quantity or use of personnel or non-personnel inputs

Rate: Calculated by multiplying a decimal value by a constant (k), usually a multiple of 10, or rate = decimal $\times$ k

Ratio: Proportion made up of a value from one source divided by a value from another source, or Value A ÷ Value B, reported as a decimal, percent, rate, or multiple

Ratio analysis: Values from financial statements are converted into proportions for financial statement analysis and interpretation

Rationing: Mandatory policies limiting health care expenditures established by various countries around the world to control health care costs

Real assets (see **fixed assets**, **non-current assets**, or **NCA**): Relatively permanent resources of an organization such as property, plant, and capital equipment

Receivables (collectibles): A current asset representing cash currently collected or due as payment due for goods or services provided, representing a major item for cash management

Reciprocal distribution: A cost allocation method that assigns indirect costs to all cost centers for support services

Reimbursement: Payment for the good or service

Reimbursement variance: A source of revenue variance representing changes in the amount of revenues received for services

Relative Value Unit (RVU): Measurement used in the RBRVS for Medicare reimbursement of physician services, corresponding to a CPT® or HCPCS code and includes the cost components of the physician's work, practice expense, and malpractice liability insurance

Requests for proposal (RFP) or **requests for application (RFA):** A type of **solicited grant** frequently used by government funders in which the application and funding criteria are specific and detailed, and a proposal must target and address these criteria in order to qualify for funding, and adhere without exception to a specific deadline for proposal submission

Research grant proposal: Application for funding which focuses on the research investigator's topic and methodology for study or evaluation, in contrast to a health program grant proposal focused on planning or services

Resource Based Relative Value Scale (RBRVS): A method to quantify physician services for Medicare reimbursement using RVUs as measures

Restricted assets: Contributions that donors or grant funders make to nonprofit organizations or enterprises that must be used for a designated purpose, requiring the use of **fund accounting**

Retained earnings: An entry under the stockholders' equity section of a for-profit organization's balance sheet that section represents accumulated earnings reinvested in the business rather than paid in dividends

Retention ratio: The proportion of net income reinvested in the business

Retrospective forecasting: Method assuming future events are a result of past events, so based on historical data and trends

Retrospective review: Evaluating documentation including the claim for reimbursement after a health care good or service has been provided to determine whether the intervention was medically necessary and is eligible for reimbursement

Return on equity (ROE): A profitability ratio that measures the utilization of investor-supplied capital among for-profits, or how well community-supplied capital is utilized for non-profits, calculated as: ROE = Net Income ÷ Total Equity (Net Assets)

Return on total assets (ROA): A profitability ratio that measures the ability to control expenses and to use assets to generate revenue, calculated as: ROA = Net Income ÷ Total Assets

Revenue (see revenue per unit): Income derived from the reimbursement provided or the price set for goods or services

Revenue budget: All of the revenues generated by the health care setting for which the budget is prepared over the specified budget year, in other words, the "revenue" side of the operating budget

Revenue cost center: A cost center that generates both expenses and revenues, and typically provides direct services; also referred to as a profit center or a cost center

Revenue per unit: Income derived from the reimbursement provided or the price charged, per client or per unit of goods or services, calculated as Total Revenue ÷ Volume

Revenue rate variance: A source of reimbursement variance representing changes in the amount of reimbursement paid by payor contracts

Revenue variance: Difference between budget and actual revenues

Risk pooling: Spreading the risk of health care costs across an entire population of population of predominantly healthy consumers paying the plan's premiums

ROA (return on total assets): A profitability ratio that measures the ability to control expenses and to use assets to generate revenue, calculated as: ROA = Net Income ÷ Total Assets

ROE (Return on equity): A profitability ratio that measures the utilization of investor-supplied capital among for-profits, or how well community-supplied capital is utilized for non-profits, calculated as: ROE = Net Income ÷ Total Equity (Net Assets)

Rule of Seventy: An investment earning 7.2% compounded annually is estimated to double every 10 years, and conversely, the present value of an investment at a 7.2% discount rate is about half the future value in 10 years

Secondary benefit: A contribution or savings resulting indirectly from the objective function in a CBA

Secured loan: A loan that has collateral that the lender can sell to recover the money lent if the borrower defaults on the loan

Seed money (see special project grant): A colloquial term for funding for special project grants that serves to start up a program or service that the recipient is expected to support over the long run

Service revenue (operating revenue): Revenue generated directly from the key health care services, for example, per diem bed charges for an inpatient facility

Shifter: A factor other than price that influences the quantity demanded or supplied for a good or service, such as consumer income or production costs

Shortage: Market disequilibrium in which there is excess demand or a drop in supply, with the market price less than the marginal cost

Skimming (creaming): Selection of populations at lower risk and lower cost by health care insurers

Socialized health service: A national health care system in which the national government guarantees health, but allows little or no privately owned or employed providers, and requires its citizens to seek services solely through government providers, as in the former U.S.S.R. and Cuba

Soft money: A colloquial term for grant funding, representing income which may or may not be available

Sole source grant: Provides funding to the only organization in the community that demonstrates a unique ability to carry out a program or service, selected for funding without competing with other organizations, but is still required to submit a grant proposal

Solicited grant proposal: A grant application that is formally and periodically requested by the funding agency; see **requests for proposal (RFP)** or **requests for application (RFA)**

Special project grant (seed money): Provides funding to establish a new, special, pilot, or demonstration project

Special purpose budget: A budget prepared for any purpose for which the health care setting requires a plan not included in any of the other budgets, such as a budget prepared for a business plan or a new venture

Staff mix: The various types or skill levels of staff required to provide care

Staffing: Determining the number and mix of staff and staff time

Staffing efficiency variance: The difference between the actual hours worked and the budgeted hours multiplied by the hourly wage rate, and adjusting for changes in volume

Staffing rate variance: The difference between the actual and budgeted hourly wage rate multiplied by the direct hours worked

Staffing variance: The difference between the actual hourly staff expense and the flexible budgeted expense for hourly staff

Starting cash balance: The amount of cash on hand at the beginning of the cash flow budget month

Start-up costs: One-time expenses usually estimated in the capital budget required to implement a new program, product or service

Statement of cash flows (see **cash flow statement**): A financial report that provides details about the sources of cash assets and how cash is used in the enterprise

Statement of financial operations (income statement): A financial statement that reports an organization's overall profit or loss

Statement of financial position (see **balance sheet**): A financial statement that reports information about the organization's assets and acquisition of those assets

Statistics budget: A budget that estimates the volume of service units over the budget year (or specified time period) that provides a basis for the estimates used in the operating and cash budgets

Step-down distribution: A cost allocation method mandated for Medicare cost reports that assigns indirect costs to non-revenue and revenue cost centers from designated cost pools in sequence, removing cost centers from the procedure when all their costs are allocated

Step-fixed staff: Employees remaining constant in number until volume reaches a certain point, then staffing increases by a given step or amount

Stockholders' equity: Represents the equity reported in the balance sheet in for-profit enterprises

Stop-loss insurance: Provides coverage for providers or managed care organizations from unusually costly cases or from overall financial losses that exceed a given percentage of the total capitation contract

Straight-line depreciation: A method of reporting depreciation expense which allocates equal amounts of depreciation expense over the estimated years of useful life of the fixed asset

Strategic plan: A long-term (often 2-5 years) proposal that takes a proactive approach to organizational finances and performance

Subtotal: A total of a subset of selected numbers, which is added to the total with the remaining selected numbers

Supplier-induced demand: The agent uses their knowledge and authority over the principal to influence (usually increase) demand

Supplies variance: The overall variation in non-personnel expenses

Supply: The quantity of a product that the producer is willing to sell measured over a specified time period

Supply curve: Graphic depiction of a the quantities supplied in a specific market over a specific time period for each possible price

Support service: Non-revenue cost center or cost pool that contributes costs to revenue cost centers or cost pools

Surcharge: Adding a percent of the inventory value to items such as supplies or pharmaceuticals to cover costs such as storage and processing

Surplus: Market disequilibrium in which there is excess supply or a drop in demand, with the market price greater than the marginal cost

Tangible: An input or output that one can measured, such as monetary amounts

Tangible assets: Resources of an organization that can be measured, such as monetary amounts

Technical assistance grant: Provides funding to assist in developing, implementing, and managing the activities of a community organization

Technical efficiency: Represents the production of the maximum amount of **outputs** given the minimum amount of **inputs,** or maximizing outputs for a given set of inputs

Technical grant proposal: Application for funding that focuses on the objectives, activities, methods, organization and staffing, usually as one of two sections of the same grant proposal, with the **business grant proposal** as the other section

TEFRA (Tax Equity and Fiscal Responsibility Act of 1982): Legislation that provided for prospective payment systems in Medicare reimbursement to hospitals

Third party transaction: An exchange in which the provider supplies goods or services to the consumer but bills a third party for the costs

Third-party payor: The source of reimbursement or payment does not directly receiving the goods or services provided, as a government or privately sponsored health insurance plan

Total cost (TC): cost of all inputs needed to produce a given level of output, calculated as Total Fixed Cost + Total Variable Cost

Total fixed cost (TFC) (see fixed cost): All budgeted fixed costs, plus a required or estimated amount of overhead costs, depending on organizational policy, as shown in the formula: Total Fixed Costs = Fixed Costs (budgeted) + Overhead (if required)

Total fixed cost per unit: Total fixed cost per client or per unit of goods or services produced, as shown in the formula: Total fixed costs ÷ Volume = Total Fixed Costs per Unit

Total profit margin (profit margin): A profitability ratio that shows the relationship between revenues and expenses accrued to generate those revenues, calculated as: Profit Margin = Net Income ÷ Total Revenue

Total revenue (TR): The revenue per unit multiplied by the volume of clients, visits, or other transactions, as shown in the formula: Total Revenue = Revenue per Unit × Volume; also may be calculated in some settings as: Total Operating Revenue + Total Non-Operating Revenue

Total variable costs (TVC): The Variable Costs per Unit multiplied by the volume of clients, visits or other transactions, as shown in the formula: Total Variable Costs = Variable Costs Per Unit × Volume

Trade credit (accounts payable): A current liability representing the amounts due to vendors for supplies

Trade-off: Situation in which acquiring or increasing a benefit or value requires giving up all or part of another benefit or value

Training grant: Provides funding for training and education to address a problem or need

Transaction costs: Administrative, overhead and other costs related to processing a financial matter

Turnover (activity or asset management) ratios: Help managers determine how effectively the enterprise is using its assets

Uncontrollable variance: Sources of budget variance beyond the scope of the manager's authority

Unfavorable budget variance: Represents undesired variability from budget targets, as when expenses are higher than expected

Universality: Relatively equal access for all persons in a population

Unrestricted fund (general fund, operating fund): Assets of a nonprofit organization or enterprise that are not restricted by external donors or grant funders, and that may be used for any legitimate activity or purpose

Unsecured loan: A loan that does not have collateral, therefore not protecting the lender from default

Unsolicited grant proposal: A grant application in which the funder, frequently a private foundation, adheres to some funding policies but does not establish many formal criteria and will allowing submission at any time rather than enforcing specific deadlines

Utility: The amount of satisfaction resulting from consumption of a product sold in the economic market—consumers try to maximize utility

Utilization review (concurrent review): Evaluating the medical record and determining whether the hospitalization is medically necessary, and whether each additional day of hospitalization is medically necessary and will be authorized for reimbursement

Utilization variance: A type of volume variance representing changes in revenues based on changes in the amount of services provided

Variable costs per unit (VCU): The variable costs, or costs that change, associated with each individual client, client visit, or other relevant transaction, for example, wound dressings

Variable staff: Personnel that change in staffing numbers given changes in the workload or volume

Variance analysis: The systematic comparison of actual to budgeted financial performance to identify the extent and source of variance

Volume (Q): Numbers of clients or units of a good or service representing outputs, such as number of patient visits

Volume variance: Variation in the number of clients or units of a good or service generating operating expenses or operating revenues

Wage stickiness: A situation of persistent labor shortage in which wages do not rise to reach equilibrium and end the shortage as would occur in a competitive market

Welfare loss: Measure of loss to society from the misallocation of resources caused by a monopoly (or other inefficient) market

What-if calculation: Budget estimate based on various assumptions, forecasts, scenarios, approaches, or other management strategies to report, compare, and select among alternative budget decisions

Willingness to pay: An approach to valuing human life in which the amount consumers are willing to be reimbursed for risk or pay for safety devices is estimated

Working capital (current assets or CA): Cash or other resources of an organization expected to be converted into cash or exchanged within a fiscal year, such as marketable securities, **receivables** or **collectibles**, inventory, and current prepayments

Write off: Expense the entire depreciated value of a fixed asset so it no longer appears as an asset on the balance sheet

YTD (year to date): Totals of financial performance for the entire budget year up through the current budget month

Zero base budgeting: Treating a continued budget as if it were a new program or service to improve accuracy and control

INDEX

Page numbers followed by the letter "*t*" indicate tables; Page numbers followed by the letter "*f*" indicate figures; Page numbers followed by the letter "*b*" indicate information in boxes.

A

ABC (activity-based costing), 143–145
Accelerated depreciation, 193
Access to care
  expectations of, 2, 259–260
  future trends of, 263
  policy questions on, 259*t*, 260
  specialty care, 255–256
Accounting
  accrual basis of, 182–183, 185*b*
  basic formula of, 190, 201
  basics of, 182–183
  cash basis of, 182, 185*b*
  financial, 182
  fund, 198–199
  managerial, 182
Accounts, board-restricted, 199
Accounts payable (A/P), 194–195, 201*t*
Accounts receivable (AR), 191, 219, 221
Accrual basis of accounting, 182–183, 185*b*
Accrued expenses, 195
Accumulated depreciation, 193
Activity ratios, 213, 219, 221
Activity-based costing (ABC), 143–145
Acuity, 121
ADC (average daily census), 69, 70*t*, 221
Adjusted FTEs, 123, 124*b*
Adjusted percent variance, 96–97, 98*t*–99*t*
Adjusted variance, 97, 98*t*–99*t*
Adjustment authority, 104, 106
Administrative costs. *See* Indirect costs
Admissions, inpatient
  financial reports of, 54–55, 57–59
  in statistics budget, 69–70

Adverse selection, 37
Advertising, 38
Agents, 35
Aging population, 255, 261–262
Aligning incentives, 31
Allocative efficiency, 10
ALOS. *See* Average length of stay
Amortization, 194, 202
Annual depreciation, 192
Annual reports, 184, 185–186
Annualizing, 93–95
A/P (accounts payable), 194–195, 201*t*
AR (accounts receivable), 191, 219, 221
Asset management ratios
  days in patient accounts receivable, 219, 221
  defined, 213
  examples of, 216*t*
  fixed asset turnover ratio, 219
  summary of, 221*b*
Assets
  in balance sheet, 190–194
  current, 190–191, 216
  fixed (real), 191, 192–194, 203
  illiquid, 191
  intangible, 190
  liquid, 190
  net, 196–197
  non-current, 191–194
  other, 194
  restricted, 199
  tangible, 190
  total, 194
  writing off, 193

Assumptions
  in budget preparation, 110, 130–131
  of markets, 5
Asymmetric information, 35
Audits, 184
Average age of plant, 222–223
Average charge per visit
  per PCP, 50, 51*t*, 52
  by specialists, 53–54, 55*t*
Average cost (AC)
  defined, 17
  of inpatient admissions, 56–58, 57*t*
  of PCP visits, 50, 51*t*, 52*t*
  of referral visits, 53–54, 54*t*
Average daily census (ADC), 69, 70*t*, 221
Average length of stay (ALOS)
  calculating, 69–70, 221*t*
  in operating analysis, 221*t*, 222, 223*b*
Averages
  and annualizing, 93–95
  budget, 93–95
  fiscal year, 93
  per-unit, 93

B

Bad debt, 82
Balance sheets, 189–200
  accounting equation in, 190, 201
  and cash flow statement, 201–202
  cash in, 190–191
  components of, 190, 199*f*
  current assets in, 190–191
  defined, 184, 189
  equity in, 195–199